Minimally Invasive Oral and Maxillofacial Surgery

Oded Nahlieli
Editor

Minimally Invasive Oral and Maxillofacial Surgery

Springer

Editor
Oded Nahlieli
Department of Oral and Maxillofacial Surgery
The Barzilai Medical Center
Ashkelon
Israel

Faculty of Medicine
Ben Gurion University of the Negev
Beer Sheva
Israel

Department of Oral and Maxillofacial Surgery
Eastman Institute for Oral Health University of Rochester
Rochester
NY
USA

Department of Oral and Maxillofacial Surgery
University of Michigan Health System
Ann Arbor
MI
USA

ISBN 978-3-662-54590-4 ISBN 978-3-662-54592-8 (eBook)
http://doi.org/10.1007/978-3-662-54592-8

Library of Congress Control Number: 2017960449

Printed on acid-free paper

This Springer imprint is published by Springer Nature
The registered company is Springer-Verlag GmbH Germany
The registered company address is: Heidelberger Platz 3, 14197 Berlin, Germany

Preface

Minimally invasive techniques have an increasing role in all surgical fields because they result in improved morbidity rates and better aesthetic outcomes. Specifically for the oral and maxillofacial area, these better aesthetic outcomes are of greater importance. Thus, the decision for surgical treatment of facial and oral/dental disorders is not as clear-cut as in many other organ diseases since the decision to operate or not is based not only on functional considerations; the aesthetic considerations are sometimes no less important. The Editor has designed this book focusing on maxillofacial problems relevant for minimally invasive interventions. The Editor intends this book to become an important reference presenting the latest information regarding the management of both common and rare disorders of the maxillofacial area. Internationally renowned physicians and surgeons have provided detailed outlines and discussions on operative techniques and treatments accompanied by rationales for particular approaches advocated by the authors. The topics cover the temporo-mandibular joint arthroscopy, fractures, and lavage; salivary gland endoscopy and minimally invasive techniques for benign parotid tumors; minimally invasive orthognathic surgery and implant surgery; minimally invasive approach to orbital trauma; and general overview of tissue engineering. The description of pathologies includes the preoperative surgical evaluation, decision making, and operative strategies including high quality step-by-step illustrations of the current minimally invasive techniques. Moreover, evolving modern minimally invasive operative techniques like the endoscopic approach to the salivary glands and dental implantation are discussed in this book.

The current edition has been designed primarily to meet the requirements of young surgeons specializing in the oral and maxillofacial areas, who wish to acquire profound knowledge of basic clinical concepts as well as surgical techniques regarding the salivary glands, the diseases and traumas of the temporo-mandibular joint, implant surgery, and various other problems of the maxillofacial area, thus complementing the surgeons' or dental training. These principles are presented together with advancements in technologic, molecular, cellular, and biologic sciences, thus meeting the criteria of the twenty-first century definition of each subspecialty involving care of patients with various diseases of the oral and maxillofacial areas. The preparation of the text material represents an honest attempt to provide information that we believe is of clinical importance not only to surgeons and dentists but also to oncologists, radiologists, and pathologists dealing with patients with salivary gland diseases, facial and mandibular traumas, distraction osteogenesis, and other disorders.

It is hoped that the reader will find the material in our book as helpful and exciting as we do.

Ashkelon, Israel Oded Nahlieli

Acknowledgements

The Editor is deeply indebted to all authors and coauthors who have contributed to *Minimally Invasive Oral and Maxillofacial Surgery*. The Editor believes that this textbook is among the most comprehensive international references on surgical diseases of the maxillofacial area that can be treated by minimally invasive means. The diligent efforts of the contributors, who have provided insightful state-of-the-art presentations, are gratefully acknowledged.

The Editor also wishes to pay tribute to the diligent work of the Springer-Verlag staff members, who enabled the realization of this edition. Particularly appreciated were the efforts of Elise M. Paxson, Developmental Editor, who provided strong encouragement and ongoing support during the creation of this textbook. Furthermore, the Editor is most appreciative of the artist, Mr. Efim Egorov, who provided us with excellent drawings for the chapters on salivary gland endoscopy, dental implantology, and orbital trauma. Finally, my profound gratitude goes to all who were involved in the development of this text, including Dr. Michael Shterenshis, who provided editorial assistance and encouragement in the completion of this textbook.

Contents

Contributors

Michael Abba, DMD Department of Oral and Maxillofacial Surgery, Barzilai Medical Center, Ashkelon, Israel

Awfa Abu-Nimer, DMD Department of Oral and Maxillofacial Surgery, Barzilai Medical Center, Ashkelon, Israel

Nardi Casap, MD, DMD Department of Oral and Maxillofacial Surgery, Hadassah Medical Center, Jerusalem, Israel

Stephen E. Feinberg, DDS, MS, PhD Department of Oral and Maxillofacial Surgery, University of Michigan Health System, Ann Arbor, MI, USA

Sara Hinds, MS, DDS Department of Oral and Maxillofacial Surgery, University of Michigan Health System, Ann Arbor, MI, USA

Joseph McCain, DMD Miami Oral and Maxillofacial Surgery, Baptist Hospital, Miami, FL, USA

Mark McGurk, MD, DMD Department of Oral and Maxillofacial Surgery, Guy's Hospital, London, Great Britain

Hadas Lehman Naaman, DMD, MASc Oral and Maxillofacial Surgery Department, The Hebrew University–Hadassah School of Dental Medicine, Jerusalem, Israel

Oded Nahlieli, DMD Department of Oral and Maxillofacial Surgery, The Barzilai Medical Center, Ashkelon, Israel

Faculty of Medicine, Ben Gurion University of the Negev, Beer Sheva, Israel

Department of Oral and Maxillofacial Surgery, Eastman Institute for Oral Health University of Rochester, Rochester, NY, USA

Department of Oral and Maxillofacial Surgery, University of Michigan Health System, Ann Arbor, Michigan, USA

Dorrit W. Nitzan, DMD Oral and Maxillofacial Surgery Department, The Hebrew University–Hadassah School of Dental Medicine, Jerusalem, Israel

Adi Rachmiel, DMD, PhD Department of Oral and Maxillofacial Surgery, Rambam Medical Center, Haifa, Israel

Faculty of Medicine, Technion-Israel Technion of Technology, Haifa, Israel

Heli Rushinek, DMD Department of Oral and Maxillofacial Surgery, School of Dental Medicine Hebrew University-Hadassah Medical Center, Jerusalem, Israel

Dekel Shilo, DMD, PhD Department of Oral and Maxillofacial Surgery, Rambam Medical Center, Haifa, Israel

Michael Shterenshis, MD Department of Sciences, Alexander Muss Institute for Israel Education (AMIIE-AMHSI), Hod HaSharon, Israel

Samer Srouji, DMD, PhD Department of Oral and Maxillofacial Surgery, Galilee Medical Center, Naharia, Israel

Michael D. Turner, DDS, MD, FACS Oral and Maxillofacial Surgery, The Jacobi Medical Center, Bronx, NY, USA

Leandros-Vassilios Vassiliou, DDS, MD, MSc, FRCS Department of Oral and Maxillofacial Surgery, Guy's Hospital, London, Great Britain

1 The History of Minimally Invasive Approach in Oral and Maxillofacial Surgery

Michael Shterenshis

Before we condemn or applaud an operator, before we adopt him as an example, we should carefully examine his reasons for any given mode of operation.
(M. Jourdain. A Treatise on the Diseases and Surgical Operations of the Mouth, 1851)

Abstract

The history of the modern minimally invasive (MI) approach to oral and maxillofacial surgery (OMS) is short, but it has a very rich background. The development of minimally invasive surgery includes progress in endoscopy, development of intraoperative navigation, tissue engineering (TE), and, specifically for maxillofacial surgery, development of mandibular distraction. In endoscopic surgery, the minimally invasive approach started when illumination and observation were combined with irrigation/suction and intervention with microsurgical instruments. Frame-based stereotaxy of neurosurgery did not contribute to maxillofacial surgery. The selective intraoperative localization of anatomical structures of the facial part of the skull became possible with further computed tomography (CT) and magnetic resonance imaging (MRI) progress that stimulated the development of frameless stereotaxy. The method of distraction osteogenesis is based on the tension-stress principle developed by G.A. Ilizarov in the 1950s and 1960s. Osteogenetic treatment of the jaws has its own history which started in 1799, well before Ilizarov was born. The engineering of cartilage and bone tissue brought benefits to the treatment of disorders of the temporomandibular joint (TMJ). Regenerative dentistry became another main field in the application of tissue engineering in OMS.

1.1 Introduction

The history of minimally invasive (MI) surgery began with Hippocrates or even with the Ancient Egyptian *Edwin Smith Papyrus* [1]. It was Hippocrates who described the use of some sort of pre-endoscopic device, the rectal speculum, in his book *On Hemorrhoids* which was included in his larger collection of works, *The Art of Medicine*

M. Shterenshis, MD
Department of Sciences, Alexander Muss Institute for Israel Education (AMIIE-AMHSI), Hod HaSharon, Israel
e-mail: shteren20@yahoo.com

O. Nahlieli (ed.), *Minimally Invasive Oral and Maxillofacial Surgery*,
http://doi.org/10.1007/978-3-662-54592-8_1

[2]. The specula were used for centuries for dilating openings of cavities of the body for better visibility and observation. Their constant improvement and their combination with mirrors enabled them to be used as laryngoscopes in the middle of the nineteenth century (Fig. 1.1) [3].

While this was the beginning of endoscopy, it was not the beginning of minimally invasive surgery because such devices were used only for observational purposes. In endoscopic surgery the minimally invasive approach started when illumination and observation were combined with irrigation/suction and intervention with microsurgical instruments. Yet it was the development of the endoscopy that brought minimally invasive surgery to life.

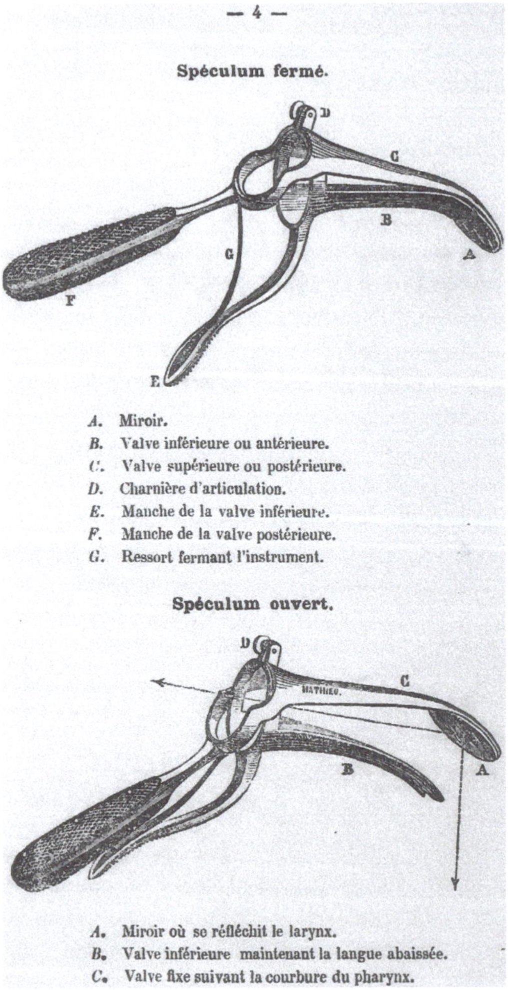

Fig. 1.1 Laryngoscopes in the middle of the nineteenth century. From De Labordette, 1866 [3]

The development of minimally invasive surgery included progress in endoscopy, development of the intraoperative navigation, tissue engineering (TE), and, specifically for maxillofacial surgery, development of the mandibular distraction.

1.2 The Development of Endoscopy

The historical development of the endoscope can be traced through several steps to minimally invasive surgery:

- Observation—mirrors, specula
- Natural illumination + observation—improved specula
- Artificial illumination + magnification + observation—early endoscopes
- Illumination + observation + magnification + delivery of medications—improved endoscopes
- Illumination + observation + magnification + delivery of medications + irrigation/suction + microsurgical interventions—modern endoscopes

In simple terms, the modern endoscope must combine visibility with accessibility. And that is how minimally invasive endoscopically assisted surgery was born. In 1805 the German physician of Italian descend, Philip Bozzini from Frankfurt, combined the light of a candle, mirrors, and lenses inside a light-transmitting device called "the lichleiter" [4]. It was a convex vase-shaped stand, and its tin lamp holder was covered with leather, its upper third being uncovered brass. A candle inside one half of the lamp holder gave light, and the other half had an opening in its posterior wall for the observer's eye. The light was reflected into the examining tube. Later, a concave mirror was fixed inside the lamp holder. The device was designed to view the urethra and the rectum. The Medical Faculty of Vienna, being asked by the Austrian government to report on this, dismissed it as a toy. This somewhat clumsy device (Fig. 1.2) did not, at the time, attract much attention, but with further improvements made by two French physicians, Jean Pierre Bonnafont and Antonin Jean Desormeaux, it became a valuable instrument in the mid-1800s. Desormeaux replaced the candle of Bozzini with a spirit lamp (burning alcohol) as a source of illumination, but his main improvement was in changing the angle of the lens. He understood the importance of a proper light source:

> "The means of lighting are of great importance. The luminous points near the focus of the lens arc useful, the others are useless, if not injurious. Hence, it follows that we must have an intense light of small volume. Large flames will not do; candles, oil-lamps, and petroleum are useless; gazogene (a mixture of alcohol and turpentine) seems to me the best, its flame is intense but small, and the lamp well adapted to the instrument. Before I settled upon this lamp, I thought of the electric light, but it is too cumbersome to be carried around, and requires an assistant. It would, moreover, double the price of the instrument. Sunlight, so convenient for the laryngoscope, would not answer for the endoscope, because its rays cannot be controlled, and we must control light to make it useful in the employment of the endoscope" [5].

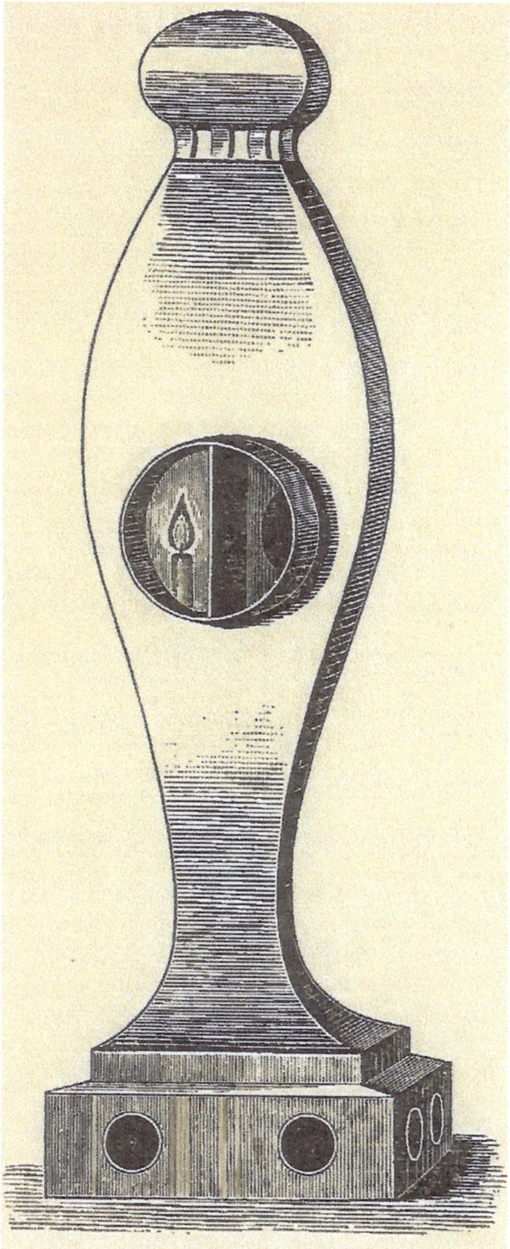

Fig. 1.2 "The lichleiter" of Philip Bozzini from Frankfurt (1805) was the first endoscope. A candle inside one half of the lamp holder gave light, and the other half had an opening in its posterior wall for the observer's eye. From Bozzini P., 1807 [4]

Desormeaux designed his device in 1843 but it came into practice worldwide when he published his main book on the subject in 1865 [6] (Fig. 1.3). It was Desormeaux who invented the word "l'endoscopie." By coincidence, that same year of 1865 Francis Richard Cruise of Dublin published his book "The Endoscope" [7]. He noticed that illumination produced in the endoscope of Desormeaux was not sufficient for distinguishing between certain colors that might be important for the diagnosis of different pathological conditions. He therefore tried to improve visibility by adding a flat silver reflector within the device. The endoscope of Desormeaux, however, was conveniently constructed and portable (Figs. 1.4 and 1.5). The practitioners were able to sketch the observed parts and pathological changes (Fig. 1.6) and these early endoscopic pictures have survived in the books of the time. Both Desormeaux and Cruise indicated that the endoscope could be used, not only for observation, but also for treatment.

This approach was developed further by Robert Newman of New York. While using the Desormeaux-type endoscope, he designed vari-

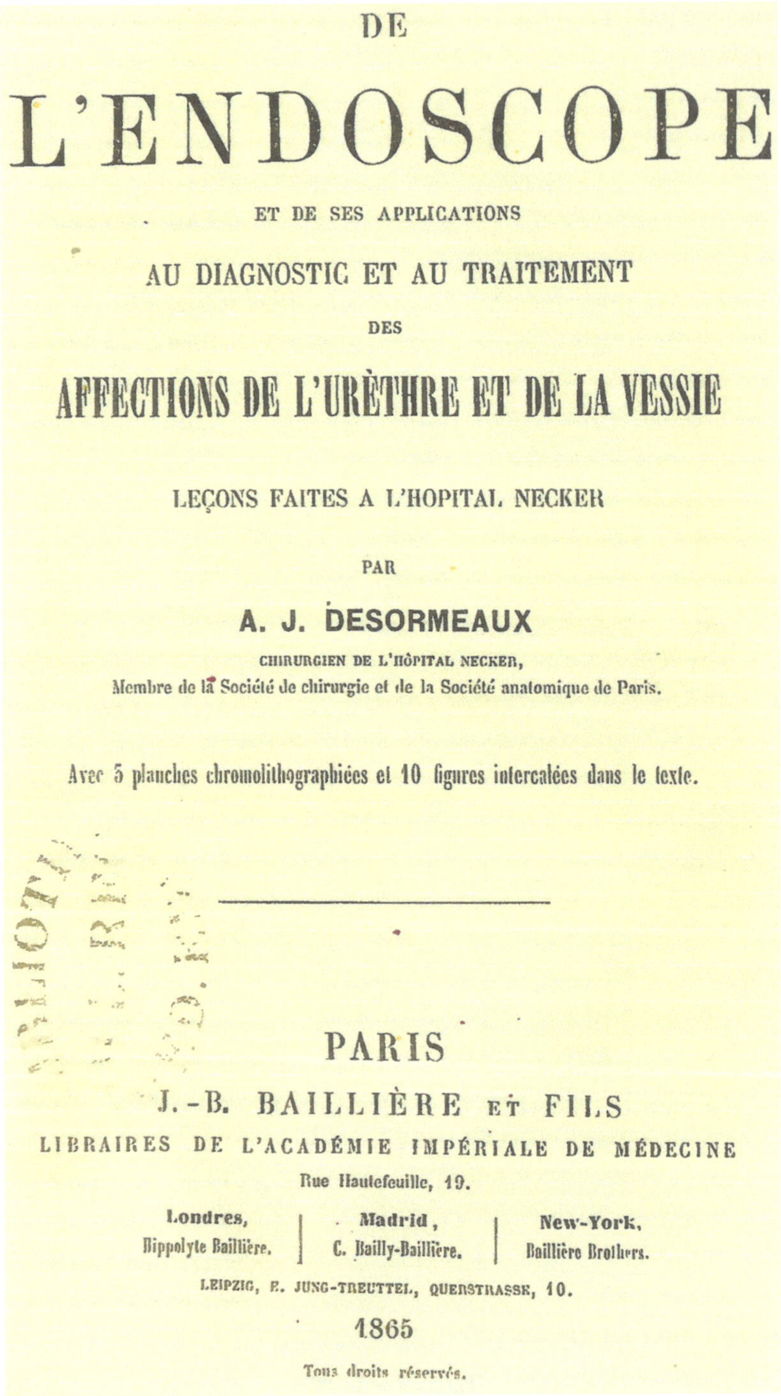
DE

L'ENDOSCOPE

ET DE SES APPLICATIONS

AU DIAGNOSTIC ET AU TRAITEMENT

DES

AFFECTIONS DE L'URÈTHRE ET DE LA VESSIE

LEÇONS FAITES A L'HOPITAL NECKER

PAR

A. J. DESORMEAUX

CHIRURGIEN DE L'HÔPITAL NECKER,

Membre de la Société de chirurgie et de la Société anatomique de Paris.

Avec 5 planches chromolithographiées et 10 figures intercalées dans le texte.

PARIS

J.-B. BAILLIÈRE ET FILS

LIBRAIRES DE L'ACADÉMIE IMPÉRIALE DE MÉDECINE

Rue Hautefeuille, 19.

Londres, Hippolyte Baillière.	Madrid, C. Bailly-Baillière.	New-York, Baillière Brothers.

LEIPZIG, E. JUNG-TREUTTEL, QUERSTRASSE, 10.

1865

Tous droits réservés.

Fig. 1.3 The endoscope of Antonin Jean Desormeaux (1843). Desormeaux replaced the candle of Bozzini with a spirit lamp (burning alcohol) as a source of illumination and changed the angle of the lens. From Desormeaux A.J., 1865 [6]

ous instruments for therapeutic manipulations (Figs. 1.7 and 1.8). Some of the instruments he used were as follows:

> "Holders with sponges at their ends to absorb fluids and cleanse the parts through the tubes. Small cylindrical pieces of silver fitting into a caustic holder. These pieces are dipped into melted crystals of nitrate of silver, and are applied to the diseased parts through the tube as a solid stick. Small glass brushes as a better carrier of solutions through the tubes" [8].

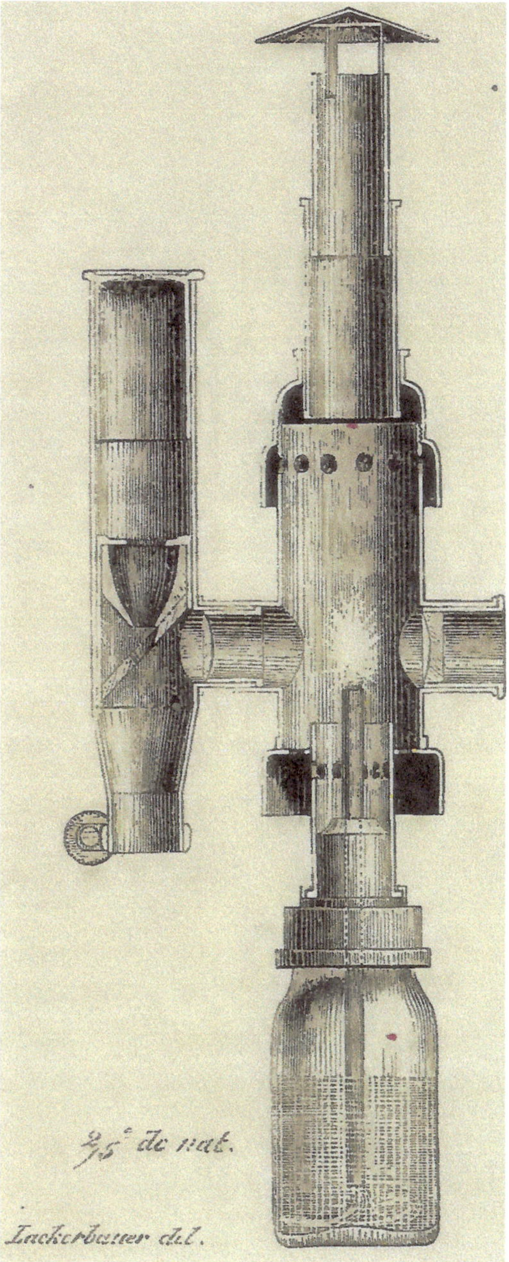

Fig. 1.4 The endoscope of Desormeaux was conveniently constructed and portable. From Desormeaux A.J., 1865 [6]

Yet this was not the beginning of minimally invasive endoscopy-assisted surgery, because the micro-forceps and the basket had not yet been introduced. While the problem of illumination was more or less settled, the problem of magnification remained. By the end of the nineteenth century the practitioners were able to achieve a magnification of only 2.5×. The German urologist Maximilian Carl-Friedrich Nitze (Fig. 1.9) tried to improve visibility by upgrading both illumination and magnification. In 1877, Nitze introduced microscope technology to the endoscope and expanded its field of vision. The combination of lenses he used actually turned an endoscope into a mini-microscope that included a wide-angle lens which was fully immersible in the urine of the bladder. The lenses produced the combined objective, which then magnified the image. Improving magnification and widening the field of vision were major advancements in the ability to visualize the interior of the body. Nitze also improved the light bulb when Tungsten lamps became available; and from this moment on the endoscopes became electrical instruments.

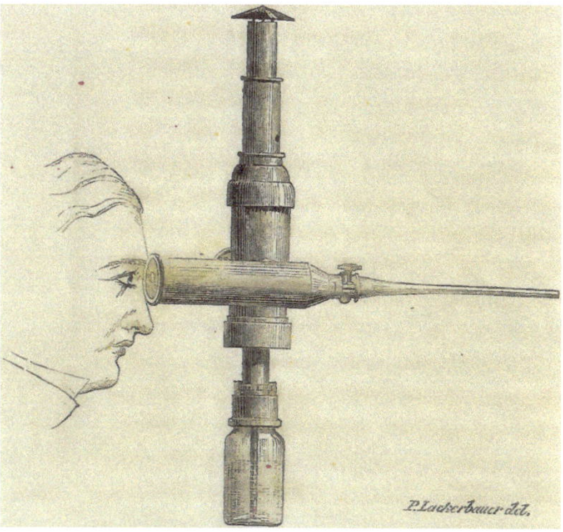

Fig. 1.5 The Desormeaux endoscope in use. From Desormeaux A.J., 1865 [6]

Nitze was irritated by the fact that the image directed back to the eye was upside down and tried, by manipulating the lenses, to improve this situation, but in vain. He became the most distinguished endoscopist of his time, a position that permitted him to publish "The Textbook of Endoscopy," *Lehrbuch der Kystoskopie*, in 1889 [9]. It was already possible, at that time, to take photographic pictures of the endoscopic images and Nitze published his *Atlas* of such images in

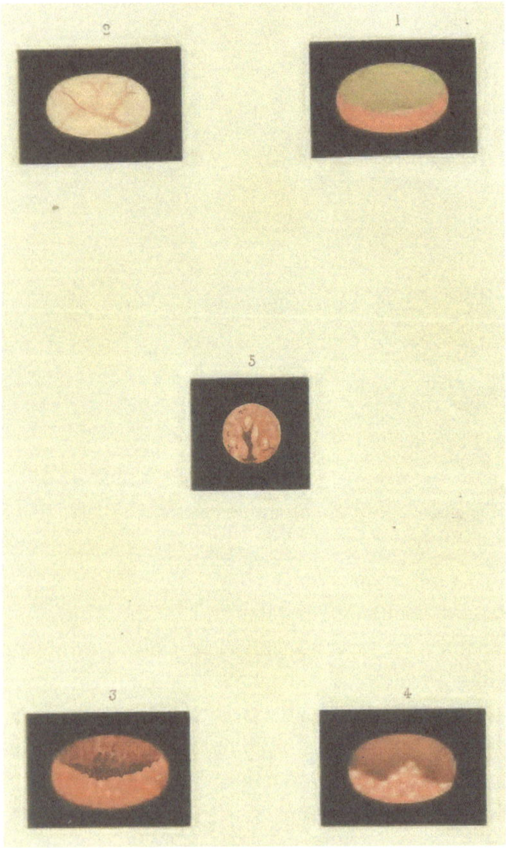

Fig. 1.6 The early endoscopic images as sketched in the 1860s. From Desormeaux A.J., 1865 [6]

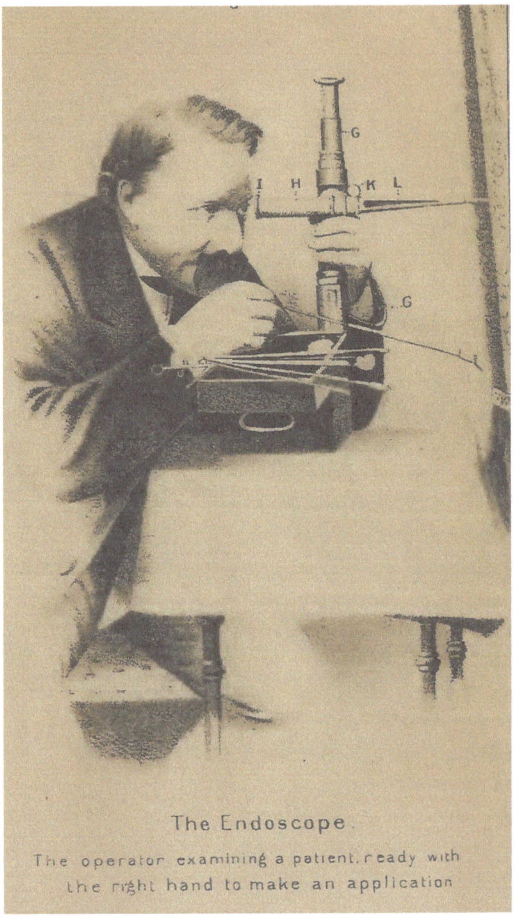

Fig. 1.7 The endoscope designed by Robert Newman of New York. From Newman R., 1872 [8]

1894 [10]. The images taken from the endoscope became more precise but were in black-and-white (Fig. 1.10). Nitze's *Lehrbuch der Kystoskopie* became a classical textbook. In its second edition, which appeared in 1907, he was able to demonstrate a "retrograde-view" scope that had the capability to look at the bladder from all directions (Fig. 1.11). He accomplished this feat by turning the prism system of the endoscope into a small 3-in-1 telescope for endoscopy [11]. By this means the resolution and magnification were both improved. Yet the problem of the upside-down image remained, until it was resolved by the addition of another set of optical lenses that reversed the image. In the beginning of the twentieth century the endoscopic tube had 4.1 mm in diameter.

After these innovations the principal design of the endoscope remained almost unchanged until the 1960s. The endoscopes of the 1930s offered only 20× magnification. Further improvements of the technique were introduced in the following stages: the rigid endoscopes → the semirigid endoscopes → the flexible endoscopes. It was also desirable to design a smaller diameter device.

The situation changed in the 1960s. Quartz rod-shaped lenses were invented in Britain by

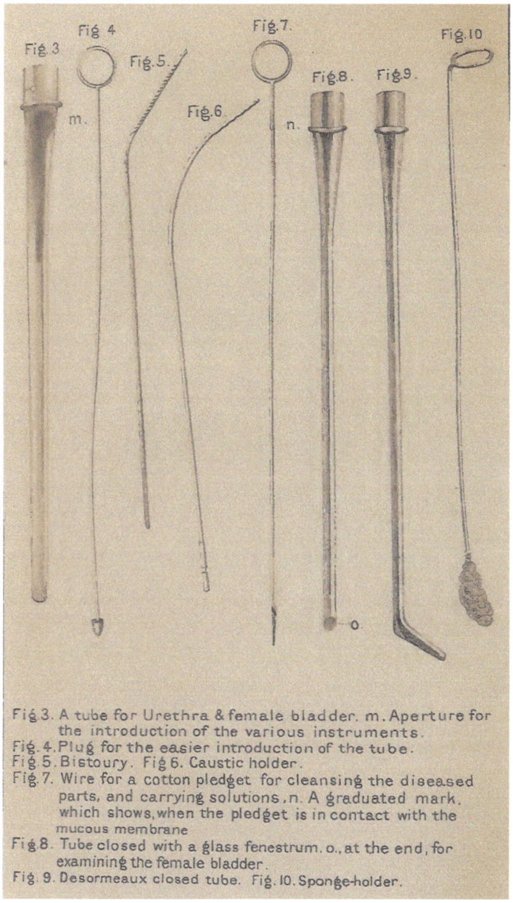

Fig. 1.8 Robert Newman designed various instruments for therapeutic manipulations that can be performed via the endoscope. From Newman R., 1872 [8]

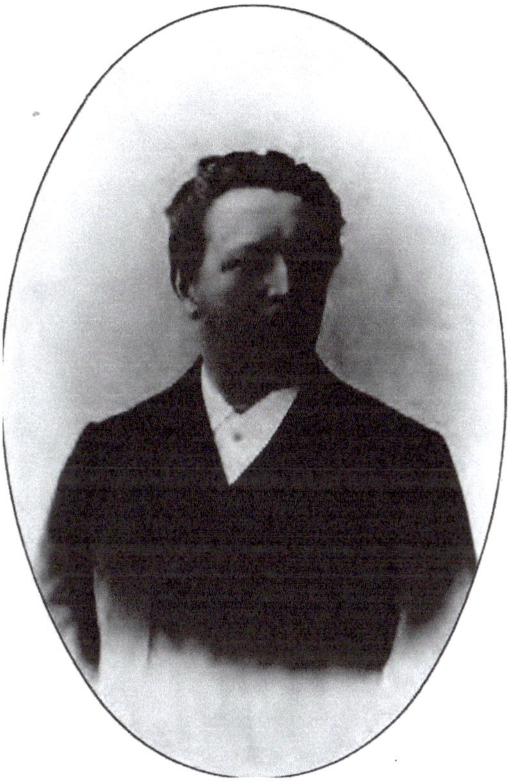

Fig. 1.9 Maximilian Carl-Friedrich Nitze (1848–1906), Germany. Nitze introduced microscope technology to the endoscope and expanded its field of vision

Harold Hopkins. The length of these rod lenses was considerably greater than their width. A light was attached to the lenses. The usefulness of this new generation of endoscopes was quickly recognized by urologists and gastroenterologists [12–14]. The possibility for semirigidity was achieved but the glass contained in these endoscopes made them fragile. Finally, when such prominent medical equipment producers as Karl Storz, Olympus, and Philips turned their attention to this problem in the 1970s, the flexible fiber optic was invented and the problem was solved. These optic fibers were narrower than a human hair, having a diameter between 5 and 25 μm and being able to flex without breaking. Flexible endoscopes were introduced, and these innovations enabled the diameter of the tube to be reduced, leaving more space inside it for an irrigation channel and for microsurgical instruments. Further technical improvements in the 1980s and 1990s gave minimally invasive surgery a very reliable tool.

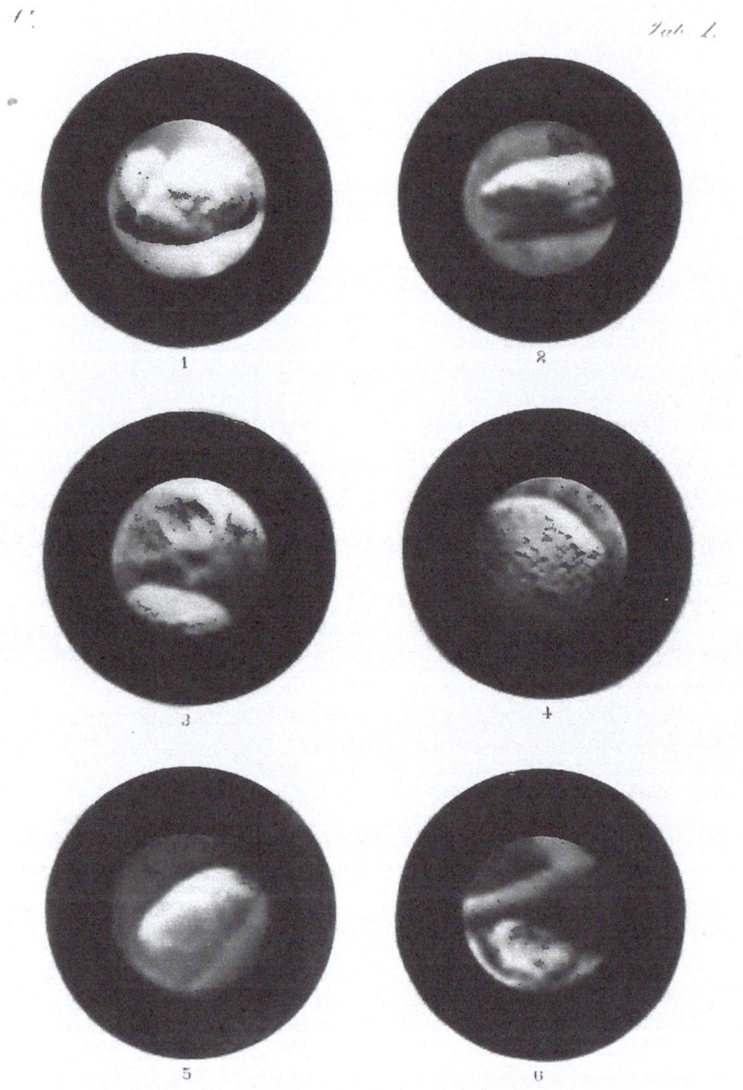

Fig. 1.10 In the 1890s photographic pictures of the endoscopic images replaced early drawings. The images taken from the endoscope became more precise but were in black-and-white. From Nitze M., 1889 [10]

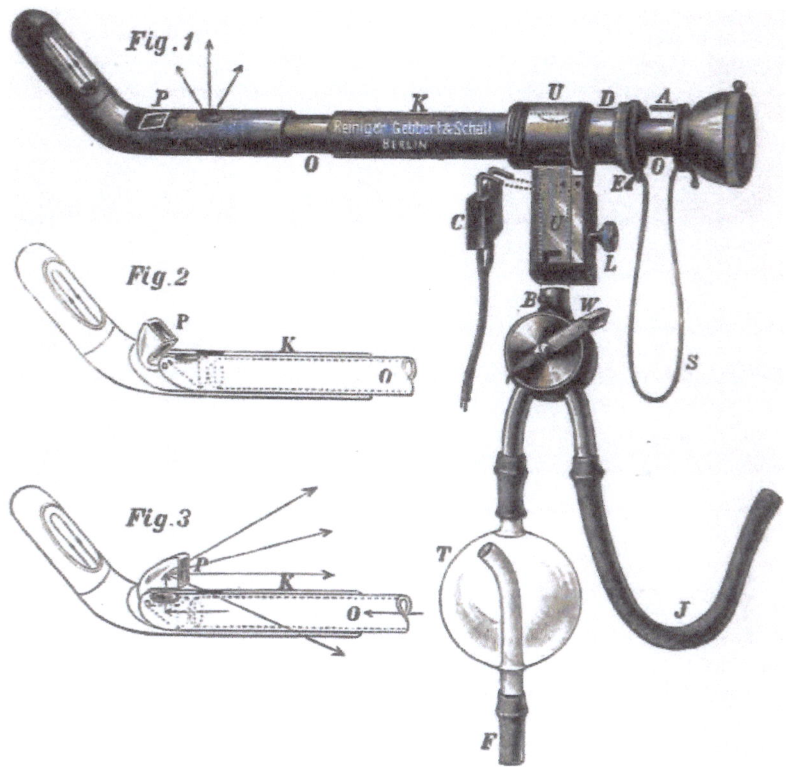

Fig. 1.11 In 1907 Nitze designed a "retrograde-view" endoscope that had the capability to observe the investigated part from all directions. From Nitze M., 1907 [11]

1.3 What About the Maxillofacial Area?

The first endoscopes were designed as rectoscopes, uteroscopes, and urethroscopes. They were quickly followed by endoscopes modified for laryngoscopy, bronchoscopy, and esophagoscopy. By the 1910s these devices had become generally accepted in the medical field [15]. What is important for the current volume is that endoscopy-assisted manipulations performed via the endoscope's channel were readily accepted. Their main application was the removal of foreign bodies from the upper respiratory tract and the bronchi [16]. "Broncho-electroscopes" of that time were now equipped with forceps (Fig. 1.12).

All these devices inevitably used the oral cavity as a passage, but no attention was paid to the cavity itself. For centuries practitioners were satisfied with the direct observation of the oral cavity and the application of simple mirrors. Yet, there was a desire for self-examination of the oral cavity that could be performed with the help of an artificial light source and mirrors. The first attempts for such self-examination were very clumsy (Figs. 1.13 and 1.14). The oral cavity is much more accessible for direct investigation, compared to the uterus or the urine bladder. The mirror and the light reflector were enough for such examination (Fig. 1.15). Therefore the development of the investigation of the organs of the oral cavity came through the combined efforts of endoscopy and direct laryngoscopy [17–19]. The endoscopic approach introduced an artificial light source for such examination in 1860s (Figs. 1.16 and 1.17).

Being concentrated on bronchoscopy and removal of foreign bodies, the peroral endoscopy stimulated the design of various specific instruments to be used for endoscopy-assisted manipulations. In the 1910s and 1920s various practitioners developed "universal non-slipping forceps," "bronchial dilating forceps," ring forceps, single-curette forceps, "curettes of aural type," hooks, aspirator, bellows and bougies, and

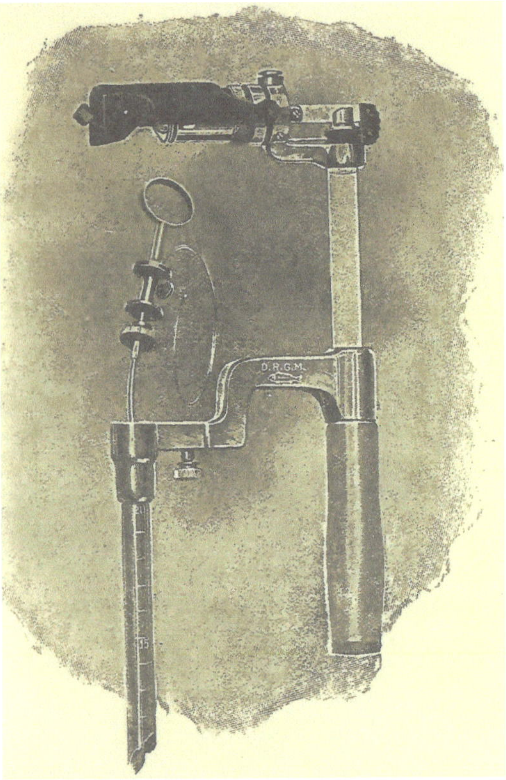

Fig. 1.12 "Broncho-electroscopes" of the 1910s were now equipped with forceps. From Brünings W., 1912 [16]

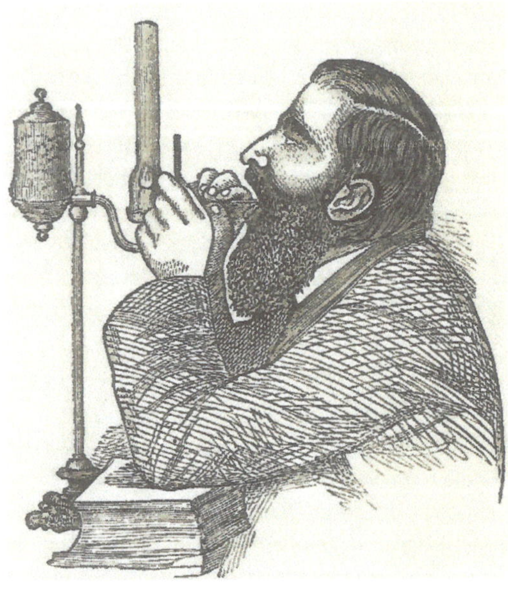

Fig. 1.13 The first attempts for endoscopic self-examination. From Czermak J.N., 1861 [17]

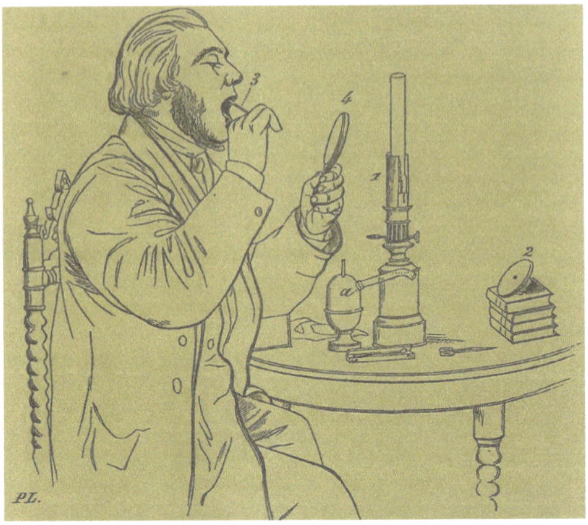

Fig. 1.14 The first attempts for endoscopic self-examination. From Fournié E., 1863 [18]

various other endoscope-applicable instruments were enthusiastically designed [20–22]. The instruments that were most widely used in the 1930s were forceps, suction tubes, and dilators [23]. Some of these instruments were then introduced, after numerous modifications, into minimally invasive endoscopically guided surgery.

While otorhinolaryngologists have, for decades, used endoscopes to observe the nasal cavity, nasopharynx, and larynx, the introduction of endoscopy into maxillofacial surgery was for a while delayed. It was theoretically possible to enter the ducts of the salivary glands with endoscopes, but the device needed some improvements to achieve this. The diameter of the endoscopic tube should be as small as possible. While it is true that more fibers translate to more "pixels," when the fibers are much smaller than 5 µm their physical strength and structural integrity are lost and fracturing can occur. That is why the range of 5–25 µm has become standard. Other possible applications of the endoscope within the oral cavity were endoscopically assisted root canal treatment and dental implantation procedures.

The need for minimally invasive approach to the diseases of the salivary glands was well understood. The morbidity following traditional surgery for parotid and submandibular sialadenectomy included a number of complications

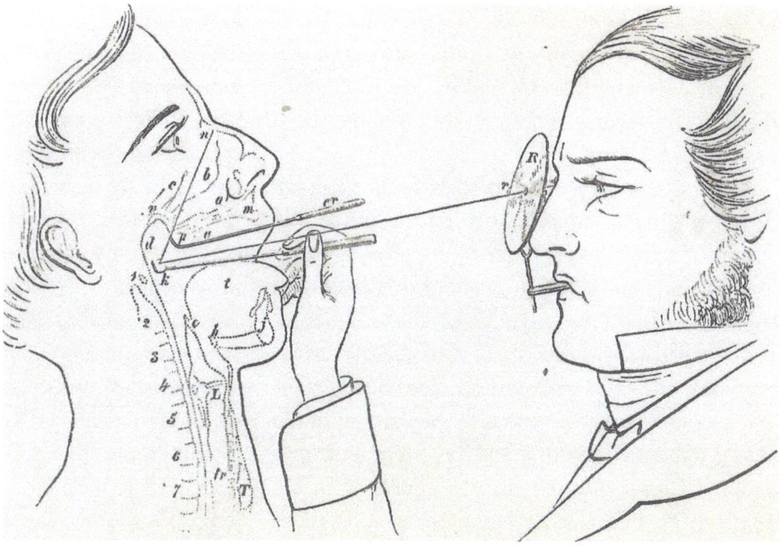

Fig. 1.15 The oral cavity is much more accessible for direct investigation, compared to the other cavities of the human body. The mirror and the light reflector were enough for such examination for a long time. From Czermak J.N., 1861 [17]

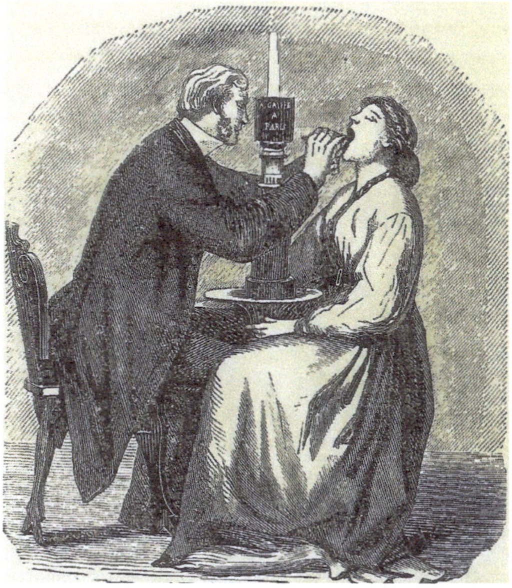

Fig. 1.16 The endoscopic approach introduced an artificial light source for the oral cavity examination in 1860s. From Mackenzie M., 1867 [19]

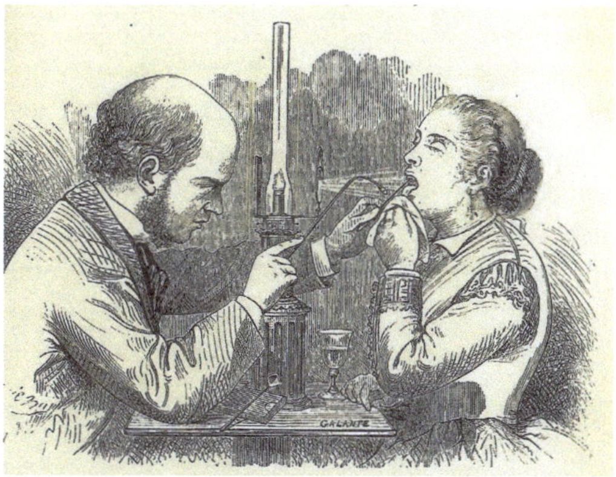

Fig. 1.17 The first attempts for endoscopic examination of the oral cavity. From Walker T.J. The Laryngoscope and its clinical application. London, Richards, 1863

such as the Frey's syndrome, facial scarring, marginal mandibular nerve damage, greater auricular nerve (GAN) numbness, sialocoeles, and salivary fistula. The calculi inside the salivary glands could be the primary target of minimally invasive interventions. The first approach to removing them without major surgery, however, was not connected with endoscopy. In the 1980s, a method for salivary gland calculus disintegration by shock waves was proposed [24, 25]. Shock waves produced by a Dornier lithotripter were able to disintegrate large sialoliths, but no practitioner could be sure that all their fragments are washed out from the gland with the saliva flow.

Therefore, the endoscopic approach was tried. In the beginning of the 1990s the endoscopes could already be about 1 mm in diameter and obtain illumination from the cold light technology designed in 1960 by Karl Storz (Germany). In the 1990s, diagnostic and surgical endoscopy of the salivary glands was developed in France [26–29], Germany [30], Israel [31, 32], Japan

[33], and Britain [34]. The shock-wave lithotripsy of salivary stones was impressively developed in Germany [25, 35] and by the 2000s [36] there were further attempts to combine both methods.

During the same period there was growing desire for increased visualization in endodontic surgery. Surgical microscopes were already being applied for the visualization of root apices, but the microscope takes up a lot of space, whereas endoscopes were quite small and readily transportable, allowing a magnified view of the root-end preparation before and after placement of the filling material. The first articles on endoscopy-assisted endodontic diagnostics appeared in the 1970s [37], but real development of this technique began in the 1990s [38, 39]. Since then, any fractures of the root or extraneous material can easily be identified. This technique was sometimes called "orascopy" and at the very end of the twentieth century it was postulated that "orascopic endodontics" is "a vision for the new millennium" [40, 41]. The development of implantation surgery further stimulated the use of the endoscopes in prosthetic dentistry and minimally invasive implant surgery was born. But this is a story of the 2000s and is well dealt with in the following chapters of this book.

In addition to salivary gland diseases and endodontics, the endoscope was used for some other interventions within maxillofacial surgery. Endoscopic section of the sensory trigeminal root, the glossopharyngeal nerve, and the cranial part of the vagus was already performed in 1981, and that was followed by successful endoscopically assisted suspension in facial palsy [42, 43].

1.4 Intraoperative Navigation in Oral and Maxillofacial Surgery

Compared with the development of endoscopy, the history of intraoperative navigation is much shorter, and is a subject to which Hippocrates did not contribute. We might think that navigational surgery is either image guided or computer assisted. Indeed, its development started when X-ray images became available at the very end of the nineteenth century and was further stimulated with the development of computer science. Its immediate predecessor, however, the stereotaxic approach, appeared somewhat earlier. C. Dittmar from Leipzig designed a guiding device for localization of intracranial structures in 1873 [44]. He performed his experiments by making incisions in the medulla oblongata in rabbits, but this device was never tested on humans. In 1889, professor of anatomy D.N. Zernov from Moscow designed an "encephalometer" for stereotactic navigation (Fig. 1.18). While Dittmar's device looked more like a supportive arm, Zernov's invention looked like a real stereotaxic instrument (Fig. 1.19) [45]. This apparatus was the first stereotaxic device to be used for neurosurgical operations on human patients. It was successfully used in cases of traumatic brain injury, Jacksonian epilepsy, and for the evacuation of pus from the cranial cavity. All these cases were summarized

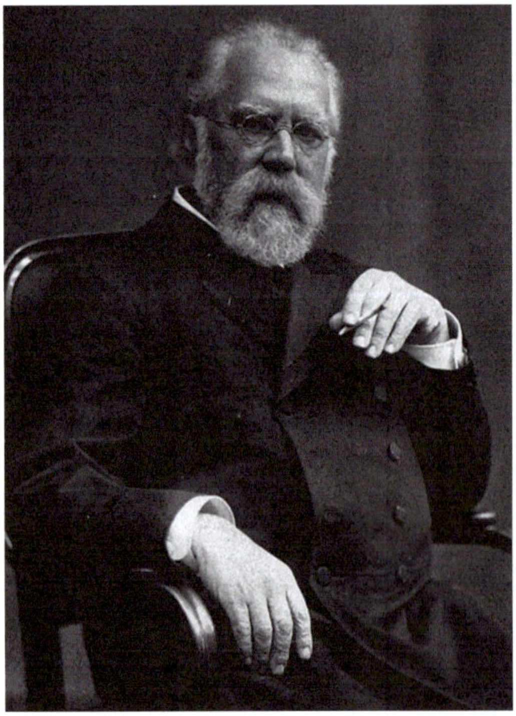

Fig. 1.18 Professor of anatomy Dmitry N. Zernov (1843–1917) from Russia invented an "encephalometer" as a device for localization of intracranial structures in 1889

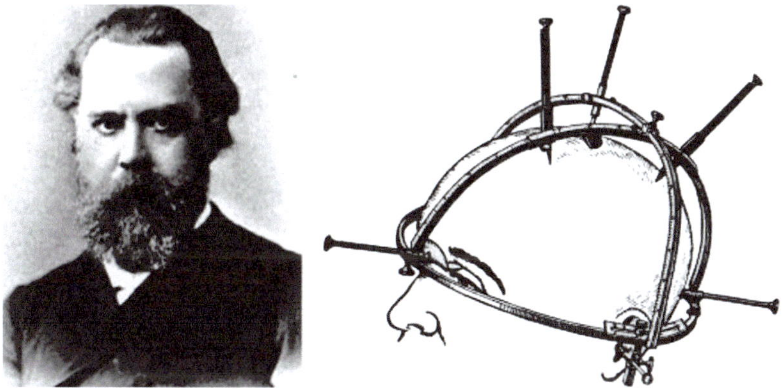

Fig. 1.19 Zernov's invention was the first stereotaxic instrument to be used for neurosurgical operations on human patients. From Altukhov NV., 1891 [46]

and described in a larger work on anatomy written by Zernov's pupil N. Altukhov in 1891 [46]. The stereotactic considerations were also described in the *Textbook of Anatomy* by Zernov that went into many editions in the 1890s and 1900s (Fig. 1.20). All these reports were published in Russian and did not attract the attention of practitioners outside Russia.

The discovery of X-rays did not immediately give any new stimulus to stereotaxic investigations. V. Horsley and R. Clarke applied a tricoordinate system to design their device for brain investigation in animals in 1908 [47]. This was followed in 1918 with a modification for the human skull (Fig. 1.21). No immediate human application followed, however, despite the fact that the device was successfully used on animals during the 1920s and 1930s [48]. Finally, E.A. Spiegel used a head frame for orientation and instrument guidance for human neurosurgery only in 1947 [49]. The use of the Horsley-Clarke apparatus was now combined with X-ray images [50]. During the 1950s R. Hassler and T. Riechert designed a variant of the device in Germany that became known as the Riechert-Mundinger stereotactic instrument [51, 52]. In the 1960s the practitioners already had several devices for stereotaxic X-ray image-guided neurosurgery (Figs. 1.22, 1.23, and 1.24).

Unfortunately, the frame-based stereotaxy of neurosurgery did not contribute to maxillofacial surgery. There was just one isolated case report published in 1971 on stereotactic localization of a facial foreign body [53]. The selective intraoperative localization of anatomical structures of the facial part of the skull became possible with further computed tomography (CT) and magnetic resonance imaging (MRI) progress that stimulated the development of frameless stereotaxy. Ultrasound-based navigation was also suggested. This change of the paradigm happened in the 1990s [54]. Since 1994 S. Hassfeld and other surgeons started to use the intraoperative navigation in oral and maxillofacial surgery (OMS) [55–57]. It proved to be very effective in paranasal sinus surgery, foreign body removal, optic nerve decompression, and surgical removal of tumors of the maxillofacial area. The Springer book of 2007 *Navigational Surgery of the Facial Skeleton* [58] already described navigations useful for biopsies, traumatic optic nerve injury, resections, and reconstruction of the lateral and anterior skull base and the temporomandibular joint (TMJ) and the midface. It also proved to be effective in secondary reconstructions after tumor resections, traumatological procedures, and implant insertions.

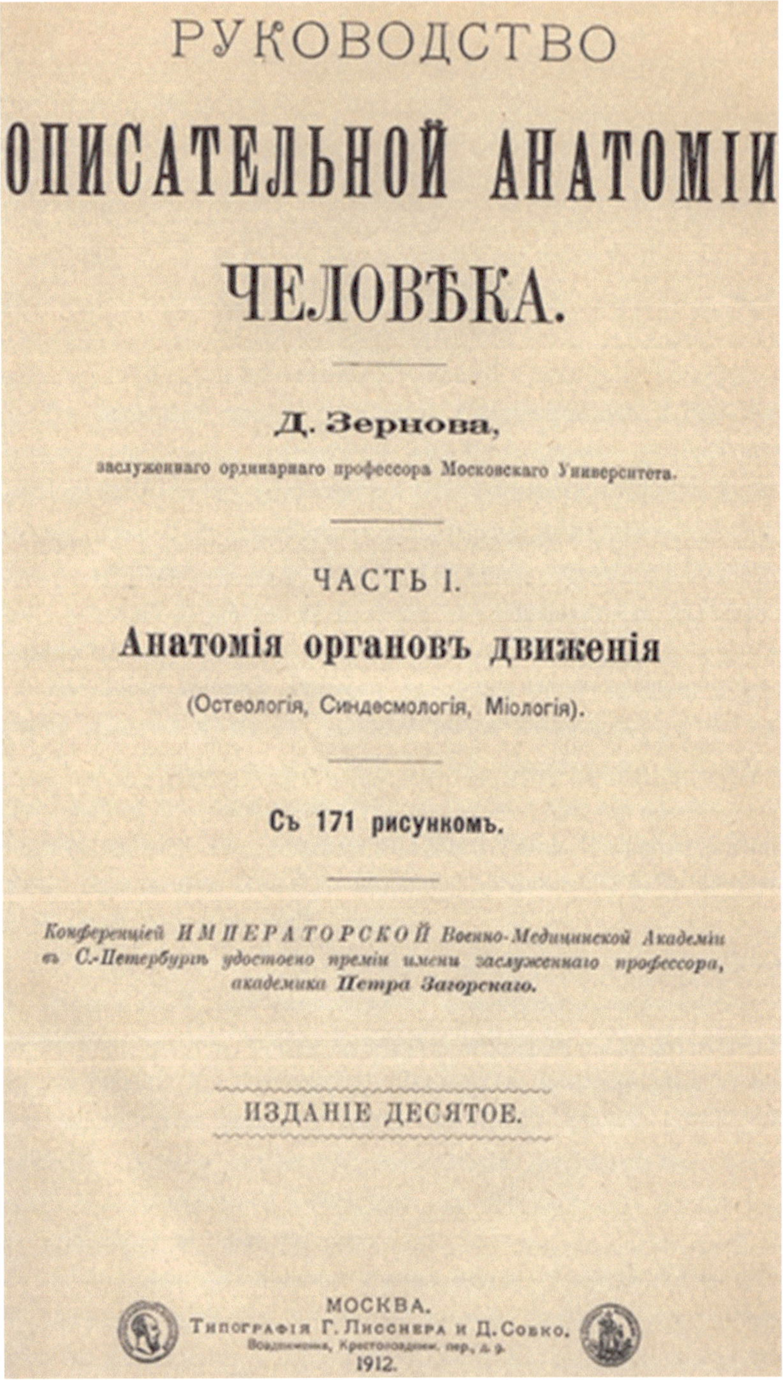

РУКОВОДСТВО

ОПИСАТЕЛЬНОЙ АНАТОМІИ

ЧЕЛОВѢКА.

Д. Зернова,

заслуженнаго ординарнаго профессора Московскаго Университета.

ЧАСТЬ I.

Анатомія органовъ движенія

(Остеологія, Синдесмологія, Міологія).

Съ 171 рисункомъ.

*Конференціей ИМПЕРАТОРСКОЙ Военно-Медицинской Академіи въ С.-Петербургѣ удостоено преміи имени заслуженнаго профессора, академика **Петра Загорскаго.***

ИЗДАНІЕ ДЕСЯТОЕ.

МОСКВА.
Типографія Г. Лисснера и Д. Совко.
Воздвиженка, Крестовоздвиж. пер., д. 9.
1912.

Fig. 1.20 The stereotactic considerations were described in the *Textbook of Anatomy* by D. Zernov that went into many editions in the 1890s and 1900s. This is the title page of the 10th edition of 1912

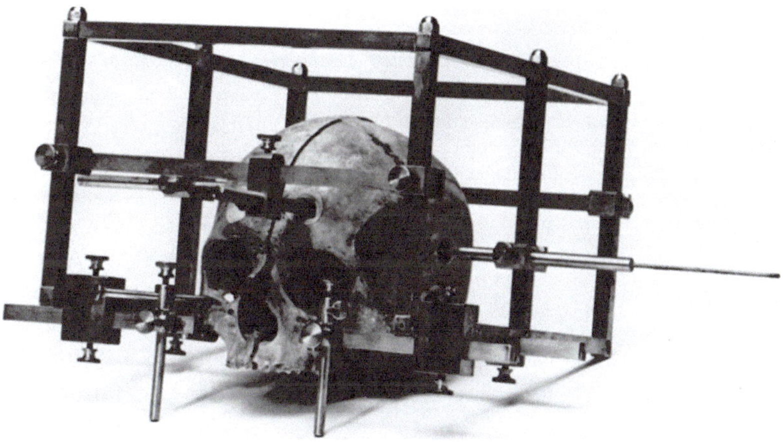

Fig. 1.21 V. Horsley and R. Clarke applied a tricoordinate system to design their device for brain investigation in animals in 1908. This was followed in 1918 with a modification for the human skull. From Clark G., 1939 [48]

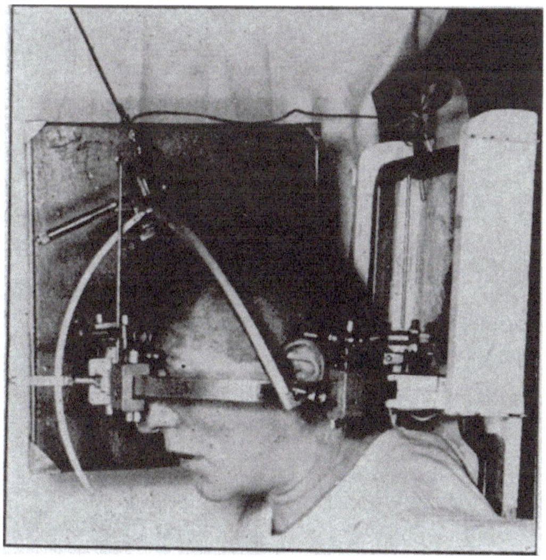

Fig. 1.22 During the 1950s R. Hassler and T. Riechert designed a device in Germany that became known as the Riechert-Mundinger stereotactic instrument. A head frame was used for orientation and instrument guidance during human neurosurgery. From Hassler R, Riechert T., 1955 [51]

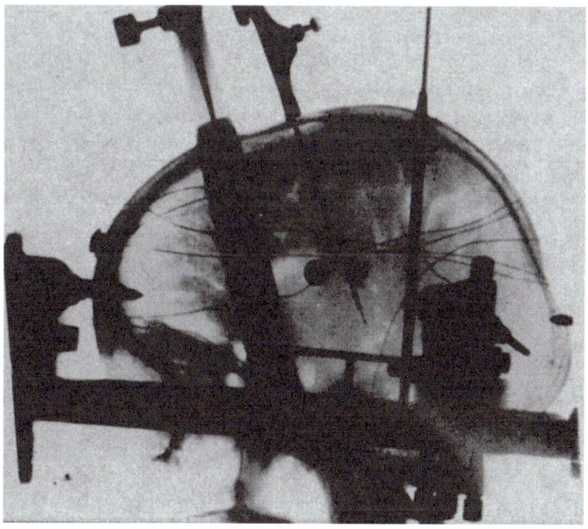

Fig. 1.23 The use of the Riechert-Mundinger device as well as the Horsley-Clarke apparatus was combined with X-ray images for better navigation during human neurosurgery. From Hassler R, Riechert T., 1955 [51]

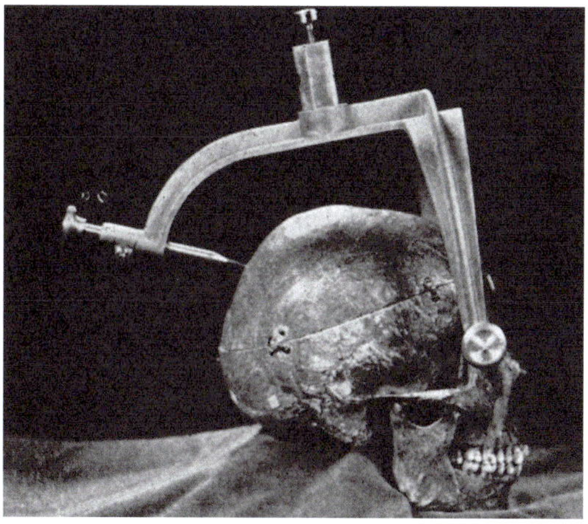

Fig. 1.24 A simplified "stereotactic machine" of the 1960s. The device was applied to the skull within without the use of incisions. Sharply pointed skull supports were tapped into the bone at the lined temporalis just above the superolateral corner of each orbit anteriorly and in the midsagittal plane posteriorly. The apparatus was sturdily fixed to the skull at these three points. From Mark VH, Sweet WH, McPherson PM. Stereotactic surgery: a note on instrumentation. J Neurol Neurosurg Psychiat, 1962, 25:86–89

1.5 Distraction Osteogenesis and Tissue Engineering

> "A miller, imprudently approaching too near the arms of his wind-mill, was caught up by the sleeve, and had his arm dislocated at the shoulder, his clavicle broken, and, in some singular way, *the anterior half of one side of the lower jaw torn completely away*, with the investing flesh and integument. By perfect repose and the use of poultices, we aided nature in the almost unhoped for cure of this horrible accident. A callus was formed, replacing the lost bone, and the soft tissues were renewed, except near the angle of the mouth. By the aid of slight scarification, liniments and an incarnative, this deficiency was filled up, and *all the operations of the mouth restored, except mastication on that side*" [59].

A giant step forward in distraction osteogenesis (DO) of the jaws was made since this case was published in 1718 by Jacob Baier (Baierus). In general, the method of distraction osteogenesis is based on the tension-stress principle developed by G.A. Ilizarov (USSR) (Fig. 1.25) in the 1950s and described by him in the 1960s and the 1970s [60–62]. Ilizarov proposed the method of generating new bone and stressed the influence of blood supply and loading on the shape of bones and joints. This method was adopted in Italy, Germany, and France [63, 64] but the first English article on the method appeared only in 1987 [65]. Almost all Ilizarov's works were dedicated to osteogenesis in the areas of the lower and upper extremities. He tried his approach on the spine (Fig. 1.26) but he never touched the jaws.

The osteogenetic treatment of the jaws has its own history and it started well before Ilizarov was born. A combination of external and internal splints was invented by Rutenick, a German surgeon, in 1799, and improved by Kluge. Bush invented a similar apparatus in 1822, and Houzelot in 1826, since which the apparatus has been variously modified by Jousset, Lonsdale, Malgaigne, and others in the 1860s and the 1870s. These sometimes almost Ilizarov-looking devices (Figs. 1.27, 1.28, 1.29, and 1.30) were primary used to treat the fractures of the mandible but were also employed to restore defects of the lower jaw after abscesses and necrosis [66, 67].

Since the 1950s a non-Ilizarov approach to the osteogenesis of the jaws was tried [68], when the cortical bone and transplants of the sustentacular tissue were tried to stimulate osteogenesis. The Ilizarov approach was implemented in OMS in 1992 [69] and its development is further described in a subsequent chapter of this book.

> "So the Lord God caused the man to fall into a deep sleep; and while he was sleeping, he took one of the man's ribs and closed up the place with flesh. Then the Lord God made a woman from the rib he had taken out of the man, and he brought her to the man."

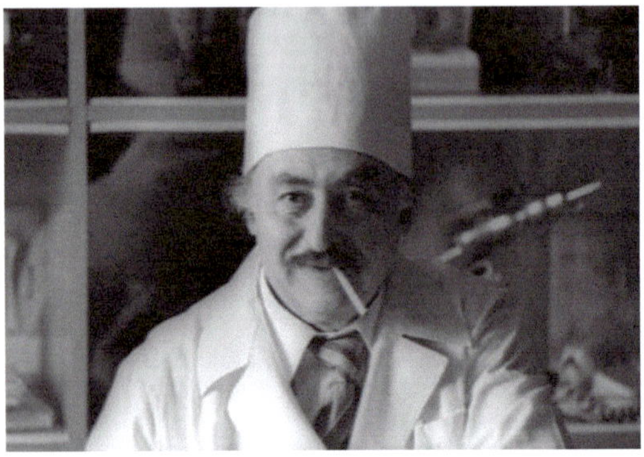

Fig. 1.25 Gabriel Abraham Ilizarov (Gavriil Abramovih Ilizarov, 1921–1992, Russia). Ilizarov proposed the method of generating new bone and stressed the influence of blood supply and loading on the shape of bones and joints. Private picture

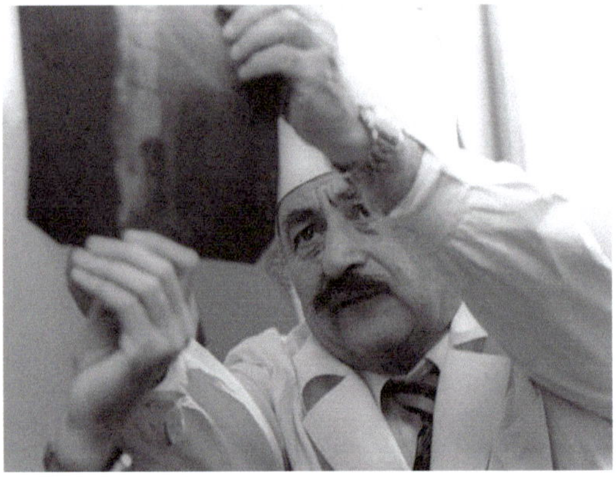

Fig. 1.26 While the Ilizarov's approach is applicable to the area of maxillofacial surgery, almost all his works were dedicated to osteogenesis in the areas of the lower and upper extremities. He tried his approach on the spine but he never touched the jaws. Private picture

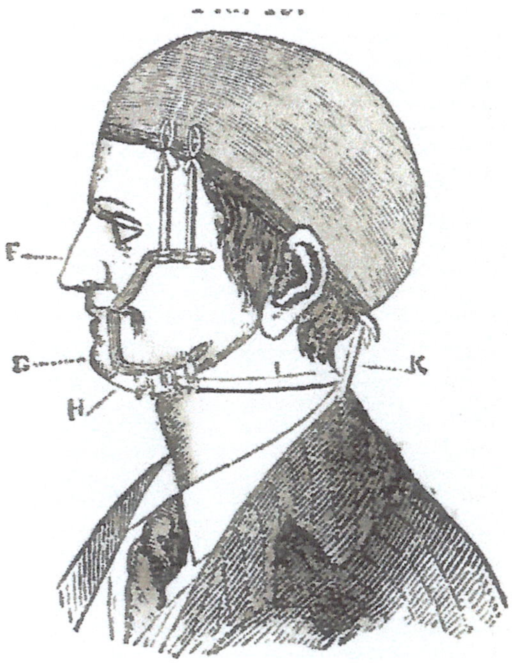

Fig. 1.27 A combination of external and internal splints for osteogenetic treatment of the jaws. The picture shows the wings for cases having no teeth in either jaw—the ends of the wings within the mouth being imbedded in a vulcanite splint. F, upper wing. G, lower wing. H, mental band to hold the jaw up in the splint. I, neck strap to keep the band back. K, balance strap to hold the cap in place. From Heath C., 1872 [67]

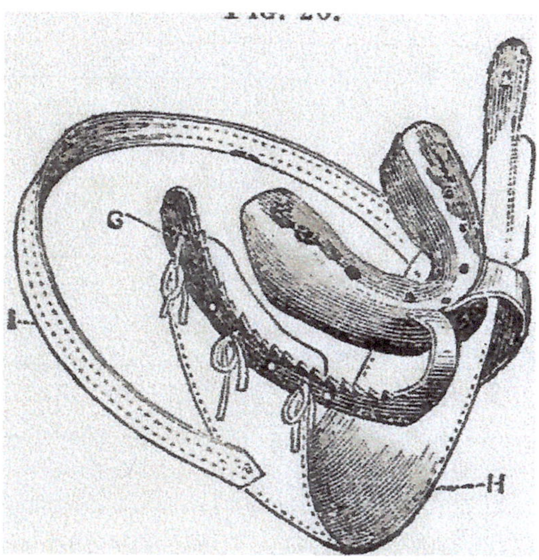

Fig. 1.28 The jaw and splint are supported by the cap in front of its center. This is counterbalanced by the elastic strap which passes from the back of the cap down around a nonelastic, and much heavier, strap, extending across and fastened to the shoulders by elastic ends. The balance strap returns to the cap, and is buckled tight enough to hold the jaw up. At night it may be slackened to do this with the neck flexed. It slides on the shoulder strap as the head inclines to either side. The picture shows a splint made of tin and lined with gutta-percha. From Heath C., 1872 [67]

This quotation from Chapter 2 of the Book of Genesis is sometimes used by the pioneers in tissue engineering to prove that their subject is the first known medical skill [70]. Coming to more recent times, developments in the organ and tissue transplantation, plastic surgery, and reconstructive surgery lavishly contributed to the new medical specialty. The first tissue culture of a frog was performed at Johns Hopkins University in 1907. As happened with endoscopy and with surgical navigation, maxillofacial surgery long remained the Cinderella of medical science. The term "tissue engineering" was formally defined only in 1988 during the Workshop at Lake Tahoe, CA, that was organized by National Science Foundation (USA). It is true that the Italian surgeon Gaspare Tagliacozzi performed many successful autografts to the nose in the sixteenth century and that the transplantation of teeth was common in Britain in the eighteenth century [71]. Yet modern tissue engineering was, in its early days, preoccupied mostly with internal organs, the skin, and the nerve regeneration. Cartilage and bone tissue engineering, however, brought benefits to the treatment of disorders of the TMJ. In 2000 and 2001 Weng reported that a polymer template using a scaffold composed of polyglycolic acid and polylactic acid can be seeded with osteoblasts isolated from a bovine periosteum formed in the shape of the mandible condyle [72, 73]. It was outlined in 2003 that the tissue engineering of the TMJ disc is somewhat specific because the cells of the disc are not chondrocytes, but rather resemble fibrocytes and fibrochondrocytes [74].

Regenerative dentistry is another main field of application of tissue engineering in OMS. The

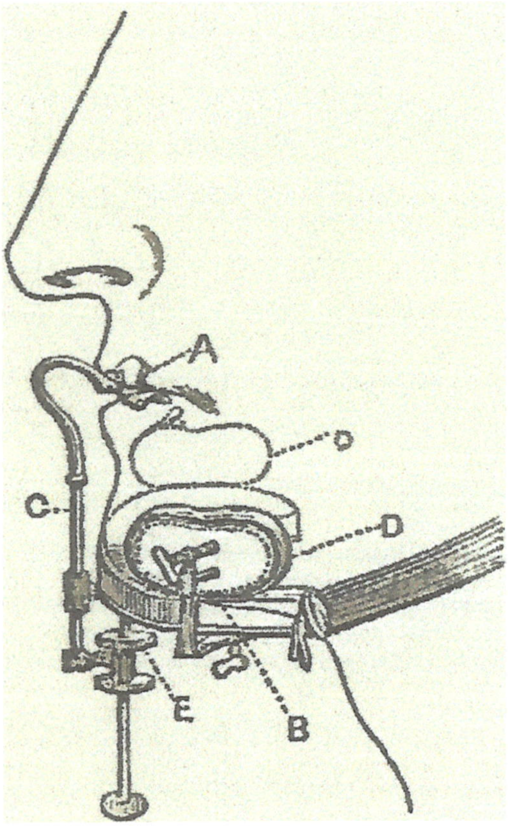

Fig. 1.29 The picture shows the Lonsdale-Hill apparatus (1867–1872) for treatment of the fractures of the lower jaw. The rod carrying the ivory cap (a) for the incisors slides freely up and down a bar projecting downwards from the chin piece (b) and, when in the required position, is fixed by a pin. There is a screw thread cut on the bar, on which a nut (e) travels so as to force down the rod carrying the cap (a) and thereby approximate the cap on the incisors to the chin piece. From Heath C., 1872 [67]

alveolar bone, the periodontal tissues, and the pulp-dentin tissue were successfully regenerated during the 2000s and it is highly probable that the twenty-first-century humans will have the healthiest teeth ever.

The rest of this book is proudly dedicated to the present state of minimally invasive techniques in the field of OMS.

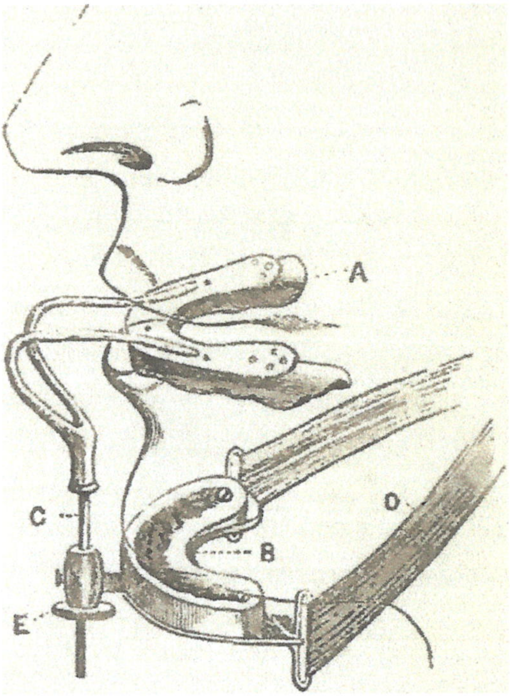

Fig. 1.30 The picture shows the modification of Lonsdale's splint, made by Mr. Berkeley Hill, for the treatment of a complicated case of double fracture in University College Hospital, USA, in 1866. The ivory cap of the incisors was replaced by a metal mold of the alveolar arch, and the lateral pads were removed. From Heath C., 1872 [67]

References

1. Radojcić B, Jokić R, Grebeldinger S, Meljnikov I, Radojić N. History of minimally invasive surgery. Med Pregl. 2009;62(11–12):597–602.
2. Hippocrates. On hemorrhoids. In: Adams F, editor. The Genuine works of Hippocrates. Vol. 2. London: Sydenham Society; 1848. p. 825–30.
3. De Labordette. Note sur le Spéculum Laryngien. Paris: Adrien Delahaye; 1866.
4. Bozzini P. Der Lichtleiter oder Beschreibung einer einfachen Vorrichtung und ihrer Anwendung zur Erleuchtung innerer Höhlen und Zwischenräume des menschlichen Köpers. Weimar; 1807.
5. Desormeaux AJ. The endoscope, and its application to the diagnosis and treatment of affections of the

genito-urinary passages (Engl. transl. by R.P. Hunt). Chicago: Robert Pergus' Suns; 1867. p. 8.
6. Desormeaux AJ. De l'Endoscope et de ses Applications au Diagnostic et au Traitement des Affections de l'Urèthre et de la Vessie. Paris: Baillière et Fils; 1865.
7. Cruise FR. The endoscope as an aid in diagnosis and treatment of disease. Dublin: Fannin and Company; 1865.
8. Newman R. The endoscope. Albany: Weed, Parsons and Company; 1872. p. 6.
9. Nitze M. Lehrbuch der Kystoskopie. Ihre Technik und Klinische Bedeutung. Wiesbaden: Verlag von Bergmann; 1889.
10. Nitze M. Kystophotographischer Atlas. Wiesbaden: Verlag von Bergmann; 1889.
11. Nitze M. Lehrbuch der Kystoskopie. Ihre Technik und Klinische Bedeutung. Zweite Auflage. Wiesbaden: Verlag von Bergmann; 1907.
12. Bush IM, Whitmore WF Jr. A fiberoptic ultraviolet cystoscope. J Urol. 1967;97(1):156–7.
13. Lopresti PA, Hilmi A, Cifarelli P. The foroblique fiberoptic esophagoscope. Am J Gastroenterol. 1967;47(1):11–5.
14. Rider JA, Puletti EJ, Moeller HC. The fiber duodenoscope: a preliminary report. Am J Gastroenterol. 1967;47(1):21–7.
15. Jackson C. Peroral endoscopy and laryngeal surgery. Saint Louis: The Laryngoscope Company; 1915.
16. Brünings W. Direct laryngoscopy, bronchoscopy, and Oesophagoscopy (Transl. and ed. by W.G. Howarth). London: Baillière, Tindal and Cox; 1912.
17. Czermak JN. On the laryngoscope and its employment in physiology and medicine (Transl. G.D. Gibb). In: Selected monographs. London: The New Sydenham Society; 1861.
18. Fournié E. Étude Pratique sur le Laryngoscope et sur l'Application des Remèdes Topiques. Paris: Delahaye; 1863.
19. Mackenzie M. Du laryngoscope. Paris: Baillière et Fils; 1867.
20. Howarth W. A set of modified Jackson's tubes and instruments for peroral endoscopy. Proc R Soc Med. 1925;18(Laryngol Sect):48–9.
21. Moore I. Demonstration of some new instruments recently designed for the removal of foreign bodies from the lungs by per-oral endoscopy. Proc R Soc Med. 1919;12(Laryngol Sect):20.
22. Tilley H. A surgical contretemps, illustrating the value of endoscopy. Proc R Soc Med. 1918;11(Laryngol Sect):73–4.
23. Negus VE. Peroral endoscopy: simplified technique. Br Med J. 1939;2(4120):1223–4.
24. Marmary Y. A novel and non-invasive method for the removal of salivary gland stones. Int J Oral Maxillofac Surg. 1986;15:585–7.
25. Iro H, Benzel W, Zenk J, Fodra C, Heinritz HH. Minimally invasive treatment of sialolithiasis using extracorporeal shock waves. HNO. 1993;41:311–6.
26. Katz P. New method of examination of the salivary glands: the fiberscope. Inf Dent. 1990;72(10):785–6.
27. Katz P. Endoscopy of the salivary glands. Ann Radiol (Paris). 1991;34(1–2):110–3.
28. Trappe M, Marsot-Dupuch K, Le Roux C. Study of the salivary glands in 1990. Ann Radiol (Paris). 1991;34(1–2):98–109.
29. Katz P. New treatment method for salivary lithiasis. Rev Laryngol Otol Rhinol (Bord). 1993;114(5):379–82.
30. Gundlach P, Hopf J, Linnarz M. Introduction of a new diagnostic procedure: salivary duct endoscopy (sialendoscopy) clinical evaluation of sialendoscopy, sialography, and X-ray imaging. Endosc Surg Allied Technol. 1994;2(6):294–6.
31. Nahlieli O, Neder A, Baruchin AM. Salivary gland endoscopy: a new technique for diagnosis and treatment of sialolithiasis. J Oral Maxillofac Surg. 1994;52(12):1240–2.
32. Nahlieli O, Baruchin AM. Sialoendoscopy: three years' experience as a diagnostic and treatment modality. J Oral Maxillofac Surg. 1997;55(9):912–8;discussion 919–20.
33. Yuasa K, Nakhyama E, Ban S, Kawazu T, Chikui T, Shimizu M, Kanda S. Submandibular gland duct endoscopy. Diagnostic value for salivary duct disorders in comparison to conventional radiography, sialography, and ultrasonography. Oral Surg Oral Med Oral Pathol Oral Radiol Endod. 1997;84(5):578–81.
34. McGurk M, Esudier M. Removing salivary gland stones. Br J Hosp Med. 1995;54(5):184–5; discussion 185–6.
35. Iro H, Wessel B, Benzel W, Zenk J, Meier J, Nitsche N, Wirtz PM, Ell C. Tissue reactions with administration of piezoelectric shock waves in lithotripsy of salivary calculi. Laryngorhinootologie. 1990;69(2):102–7.
36. Nahlieli O, Shacham R, Zaguri A. Combined external lithotripsy and endoscopic techniques for advanced sialolithiasis cases. J Oral Maxillofac Surg. 2010;68(2):347–53. https://doi.org/10.1016/j.joms.2009.09.041.
37. Detsch SG, Cunningham WT, Langloss JM. Endoscopy as an aid to endodontic diagnosis. J Endod. 1979;5(2):60–2.
38. Held SA, Kao YH, Wells DW. Endoscope—an endodontic application. J Endod. 1996;22(6):327–9.
39. Bahcall JK, DiFiore PM, Poulakidas TK. An endoscopic technique for endodontic surgery. J Endod. 1999;25(2):132–5.
40. Bahcall JK, Barss JT. Orascopy: a vision for the new millennium, Part 2. Dent Today. 1999;18(9):82–5.
41. Glickman GN, Koch KA. 21st-century endodontics. J Am Dent Assoc. 2000;131(Suppl):39S–46S.
42. Oppel F, Mulch G, Brock M. Endoscopic section of the sensory trigeminal root, the glossopharyngeal nerve, and the cranial part of the vagus for intractable facial pain caused by upper jaw carcinoma. Surg Neurol. 1981;16(2):92–5.

43. Adant JP. Endoscopically assisted suspension in facial palsy. Plast Reconstr Surg. 1998;102(1):178–81.
44. Dittmar C. Über die Lage des sogenannten Gefässzentrums in der Medulla oblongata. Ber Sächs Ges Wiss Leipzig. 1873;25:449–69.
45. Zernov DN. Encephalometer. The device for estimation of the parts of the brain in humans. Proc Soc Physicomed Moscow Univ. 1889;2:70–80. [Russian].
46. Altukhov NV. Encephalometric investigations of the brain relative to the sex, age, and skull indices. Moscow; 1891. [Russian].
47. Horsley V, Clarke RH. The structure and functions of the cerebellum examined by a new method. Brain. 1908;31:45–124.
48. Clark G. The use of the Horsley-Clarke instrument on the rat. Science. 1939;90(2326):92.
49. Spiegel EA, Wycis HT, Marks M, Lee AJ. Stereotaxic apparatus for operations on the human brain. Science. 1947;106(2754):349–50.
50. Hayne RA, Stowell A, Darrough JB. The use of the human Horsley Clarke stereotaxic apparatus; selective section of the thalamo-frontal tracts. Surg Forum. 1951:380–5.
51. Hassler R, Riechert T. A special method of stereotactic brain operation. Proc R Soc Med. 1955;48(6):469–70.
52. Hassler R, Riechert T, Mundinger F, Umbach W, Gangberger JA. Physiological observations in stereotaxic operations in extrapyramidal motor disturbances. Brain. 1960;83:337–50.
53. Horton CE, McFadden JT. Stereotactic localization of a facial foreign body. Case report. Plast Reconstr Surg. 1971;47(6):598–9.
54. Jones D, Christopherson DA, Washington JT, Hafermann MD, Rieke JW, Travaglini JJ, Vermeulen SS. A frameless method for stereotactic radiotherapy. Br J Radiol. 1993;66(792):1142–50.
55. Hassfeld S, Mühling J, Zöller J. Intraoperative navigation in oral and maxillofacial surgery. Int J Oral Maxillofac Surg. 1995;24(1 Pt 2):111–9.
56. Bohner P, Holler C, Hassfeld S. Operation planning in craniomaxillofacial surgery. Comput Aided Surg. 1997;2(3–4):153–61.
57. Hassfeld S, Muehling J, Wirtz CR, Knauth M, Lutze T, Schulz HJ. Intraoperative guidance in maxillofacial and craniofacial surgery. Proc Inst Mech Eng H. 1997;211(4):277–83.
58. Schramm A, Gellrich N-C, Schmelzeisen R. Navigational surgery of the facial skeleton. Berlin, New York: Springer; 2007.
59. Baierus JJ. Adagiorum medicinalium centuria, quam recensuit variisque animadversionibus illustravit. Francofurti et Lipsiae Kohlesius; 1718.
60. Ilizarov GA, Deviatov AA. Surgical lengthening of the shin with simultaneous correction of deformities. Ortop Travmatol Protez. 1969;30(3):32–7.
61. Ilizarov GA, Soĭbel'man LM. Clinical and experimental data on bloodless lengthening of lower extremities. Eksp Khir Anesteziol. 1969;14(4):27–32.
62. Ilizarov GA, editor. The Transosseous Tension-Stress Osteosynthesis in Traumatology and Orthopedics. [Чрескостный компрессионный и дистракционный остеосинтез в травматологии и ортопедии.]. Vol. 1. Kurgan: Sovetskoe Zauralye; 1972.
63. Bignardi A, Boero G, Barale I, Mazzinari S, Marro P. Our experience in the bloodless treatment of fractures with the DOS (dynamic osteosynthesis) external fixation apparatus based on the Ilizarov principle. Chir Organi Mov. 1982;68(1):51–68.
64. Schewior T, Schewior H. Mechanical and technical aspects of an external fixator made of rings and Kirschner wires (using the Wittmoser and Ilizarov methods). Alternatives to plate osteosynthesis. Aktuelle Traumatol. 1984;14(6):263–5.
65. Louis R, Jouve JL, Borrione F. Anatomic factors in the femoral implantation of the Ilizarov external fixator. Surg Radiol Anat. 1987;9(1):5–11.
66. Jourdain M. A treatise on the diseases and surgical operations of the mouth. Philadelphia: Lindsay and Blakiston; 1851.
67. Heath C. Injuries and diseases of the jaws. London: Churchill; 1872.
68. Huebsch RF. The use of cortical bone to stimulate osteogenesis. Oral Surg Oral Med Oral Pathol. 1954;7(12):1273–5.
69. McCarthy J, Schreiber J, Karp N, Thorne C, Grayson B. Lengthening the human mandible by gradual distraction. Plast Reconstr Surg. 1992;89(1):1–10.
70. Patrick CW Jr, Mikos AG, McIntire LV, editors. Frontiers in tissue engineering. Oxford, New York: Elsevier Science; 1998. p. 4.
71. Deaton JG. New parts for old: the age of organ transplants. Palisades: Franklin Publishing Company; 1974.
72. Weng YL. The experimental study of tissue engineered mandible condyle in the shape of human. Shanghai Kou Qiang Yi Xue. 2000;9(2):94–6.
73. Weng Y, Cao Y, Silva CA, Vacanti MP, Vacanti CA. Tissue-engineered composites of bone and cartilage for mandible condylar reconstruction. J Oral Maxillofac Surg. 2001;59(2):185–90.
74. Detamore MS, Athanasiou KA. Motivation, characterization, and strategy for tissue engineering the temporomandibular joint disc. Tissue Eng. 2003;9(6):1065–87.

2 Modern Temporomandibular Joint Arthroscopy: Operative Single-Cannula Arthroscopy

Samer Srouji and Joseph McCain

Abstract

Since the introduction of arthroscopy, the management of temporomandibular joint (TMJ) disorders has improved significantly. The arthroscope facilitates both assessment of the joint and its pathologies as well as visualized surgical interventions. The traditional arthroscopy technique requires the creation of one puncture for diagnosis and two punctures to enable visualization and operation. The alternative operative single-cannula arthroscopy (OSCA) technique presented here is an advanced TMJ arthroscopy technique which requires only a single cannula, through which a single-piece instrument containing a visualization canal, irrigation canal, and a working canal is inserted. OSCA empowers performance of "one-track arthrocentesis" and standard arthrocentesis under diagnostic visualization and supports introduction of hand or mechanical instruments or laser (holmium:YAG) to perform visually guided surgery. The technique has proven as efficient as the traditional technique, with the added benefits of a short learning curve and simplicity of execution. This chapter provides a detailed protocol for the management of TMD using the OSCA technique.

2.1 History and Goals

Masatoshi Ohnishi performed the first temporomandibular joint (TMJ) arthroscopy in 1974 [1]. In 1982, Murakami and Hoshino developed the nomenclature of TMJ arthroscopic anatomy [2]. Modifications and new arthroscopy techniques have since been introduced by McCain [3, 4], Sanders [5], Holmlund and Hellsing [6], Nitzan and colleagues [7], Koslin [8], and others, with the overall goal of establishing a safe and accurate diagnosis, effectively reducing pain and joint

S. Srouji, DMD, PhD (✉)
Department of Oral and Maxillofacial Surgery, Galilee Medical Center, Road 89, Nahariya 22100, Israel
e-mail: Dr.samersrouji@gmail.com

J. McCain, DMD
Miami Oral and Maxillofacial Surgery, Baptist Hospital, Miami, FL, USA
e-mail: jmccain@miamioms.com

O. Nahlieli (ed.), *Minimally Invasive Oral and Maxillofacial Surgery*,
http://doi.org/10.1007/978-3-662-54592-8_2

pathologies, and providing a favorable joint environment for ideal function restoration. Today, two main approaches to TMJ arthroscopy exist, the first being the single-puncture technique, suitable only for diagnostics and basic interventions, while the second, the traditional double-puncture arthroscopy technique, requires insertion of two cannulas; the first cannula is used for the introduction of the endoscope, while the second cannula is for surgical intervention, as described by McCain triangulation technique [9]. In line with the trends in modern surgery, all contemporary arthroscopy techniques aim to allow for minimalized and less invasive surgeries. Yet, the relative complexity of arthroscopy requires a high level of coordination and demands a steep learning curve, presenting major obstacles to heightened embracement of advanced arthroscopy by maxillofacial surgeons. In this chapter, the operative single-cannula arthroscopy (OSCA) technique, which precludes the need for coordination of two instruments inside the joint space, is presented. The proposed technique provides the surgeon with the ability to perform a single-hand operation, and a platform for performing advanced, visually guided arthroscopic surgery [10].

2.2 Anatomy of the Temporomandibular Joint Region

While a detailed anatomical description of the TMJ and surrounding structures extends beyond the scope of this chapter, a brief review of structures associated with possible complications is presented here. The TMJ is a bilateral synovial articulation between the glenoid fossa and articular eminence of the temporal bone, the condylar head of the mandible, and the dense fibrous connective tissue structure known as the articular disc [11] (Fig. 2.1). The biconcave articular disc divides the joint into two compartments. The lower compartment permits hinge motion or rotation (ginglymoid), while the superior compartment allows for sliding (or translatory) movements (arthrodial), hence the term ginglymoarthrodial joint. The superior head of the lateral pterygoid muscle penetrates into the anterior portion of the disc, while posteriorly, the articular disc is connected to the retrodiscal tissue, a highly vascularized and innervated structure. The temporomandibular, stylomandibular, and sphenomandibular ligaments are associated with the TMJ, and define the border movements of the mandible.

The facial nerve has intracranial and extracranial branches distal to the stylomastoid foramen, with the temporal, zygomatic, buccal, marginal mandibular, and cervical branches comprising the five major extracranial facial branches. The temporal and zygomatic branches can be injured when approaching the TMJ, as detailed below. The trigeminal nerve, responsible for sensory function in the face and motor innervation to the mastication muscles, is another important nerve which must be preoperatively identified. The auriculotemporal nerve is a branch of the mandibular nerve (V/1) that

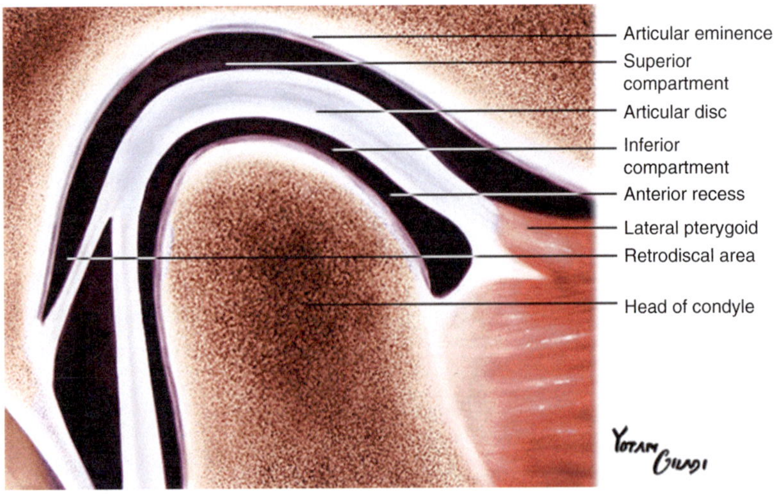

Fig. 2.1 The temporomandibular joint (lateral view)

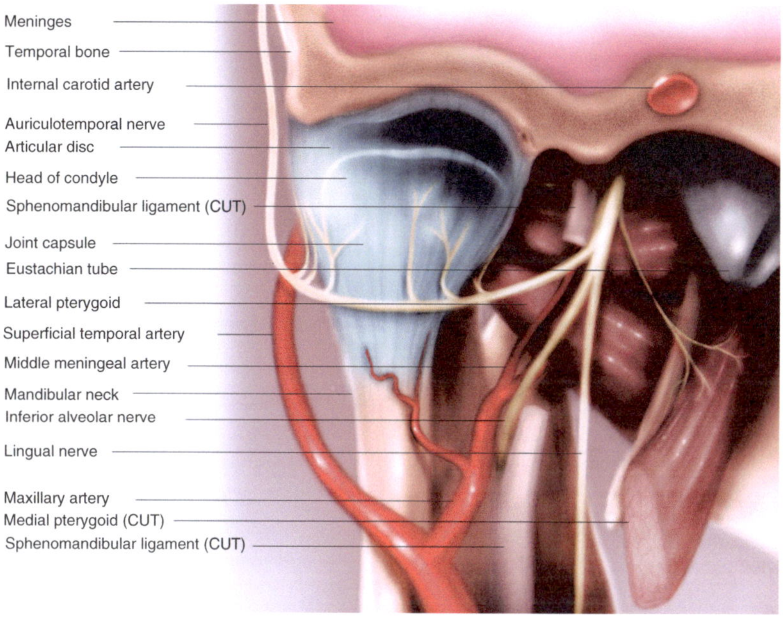

Fig. 2.2 Anatomy of the temporomandibular joint region

runs with the superficial temporal artery and vein. It passes between the neck of the mandible and the sphenomandibular ligament in proximity to the fossa puncture site. The most important blood vessels in this region are the superficial temporal artery and vein. The superficial temporal artery is the smaller of two terminal branches of the external carotid artery and passes behind the neck of the condyle, superficially over the posterior root of the zygomatic process of the temporal bone, before splitting into frontal and parietal branches (Fig. 2.2).

2.3 Temporomandibular Joint Disorders

The term temporomandibular disorders (TMD) is a term that encompasses pathology of the TMJ itself and myofascial pain dysfunction (MPD) syndrome. The prevalence of TMD in the general population is 40–60%, while females are more likely to be affected than males, females are more likely to request treatment, and their symptoms are less likely to resolve. TMD can be caused by injury to the joint, degenerative diseases such as rheumatoid arthritis, and parafunction of the jaw (tooth grinding/clenching), and in some cases there is no known cause. TMD can interfere with speech, eating, and sleeping, resulting in additional psychosocial effects and health risks.

2.3.1 Diagnosis

Patients suffering from TMD should undergo an initial assessment that includes a detailed history, and clinical and general examination. Imaging of the TMJ should be performed. Conventional radiographs and panoramic X-ray are used to evaluate the bony elements of the TMJ only, while computed tomography (CT) is useful in evaluating both the bony elements of the TMJ and the adjacent soft tissues. Magnetic resonance imaging (MRI) has proven to be extremely reliable in assessing the shape, position, mobility, and intrinsic structural integrity of the disc itself and for providing additional information on the status of the soft tissue. Subjective parameters include pain assessment using the ten-point visual analog scale (VAS) (0 = no pain, 10 = severe pain), reported change in diet consistency, and required nonsteroidal anti-inflammatory drugs (NSAIDs). Objective parameters include maximal inter-incisal opening (MIO) measurements (Fig. 2.3a), joint noises,

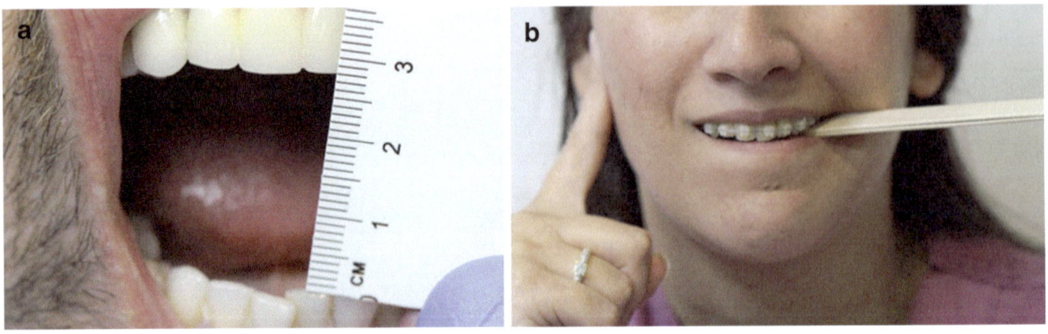

Fig. 2.3 (**a**) Patient with a limited maximal inter-incisal opening. (**b**) Positive direct-pressure loading (Mahan test) to assess contralateral pain upon biting

Table 2.1 Clinical, radiologic, and anatomical/pathological signs for Wilkes classification of TMJ ID

Stage	Clinical	Radiologic	Anatomic/pathologic
I. Early stage	No significant mechanical symptoms other than early opening, reciprocal clicking; no pain or limitation of motion	Slight forward displacement; good anatomic contour of the disc; negative tomograms	Excellent anatomic form; slight anterior displacement; passive incoordination demonstrable
II. Early/ intermediate stage	One or more episodes of pain; beginning major mechanical problems, loud clicking, transient catching, and locking	Slight forward displacement; early signs of disc deformity with slight thickening of posterior edge; negative tomograms	Anterior disc displacement; early anatomic disc deformity; good central articulating area
III. Intermediate stage	Multiple episodes of pain; major mechanical symptoms including locking (intermittent or fully closed), restricted motion, and functional difficulty	Anterior disc displacement with significant disc deformity/prolapse (increased thickening of posterior edge); negative tomograms	Marked anatomic disc deformity with anterior displacement; no hard tissue changes
IV. Intermediate/ late stage	Slight increase in severity as compared to intermediate stage	Positive tomograms showing early-to-moderate degenerative changes—flattening of eminence; deformed condylar head; sclerosis	Hard tissue degenerative remodeling of both bearing surfaces; multiple adhesions in anterior and posterior recesses; no perforation of disc or attachments
V. Late stage	Crepitus; scraping, grating, grinding; episodic or continuous pain; chronic motion restriction; functional difficulty	Disc or attachment perforation; filling defects; gross anatomic deformity of disc and hard tissues; positive tomograms with essentially degenerative arthritic changes	Gross degenerative changes of disc and hard tissues; perforation of posterior attachment; multiple adhesions; flattening of condyle and eminence; subcortical cystic formation

and direct-pressure loading (Mahan test) (Fig. 2.3b), performed using two wooden spatulas placed between the posterior teeth, where contralateral pain suggests some extent of joint inflammation.

2.3.2 Classifications

The Wilkes classification system is the broadly accepted terminology used to define internal derangement (ID) disorders (Table 2.1) [12].

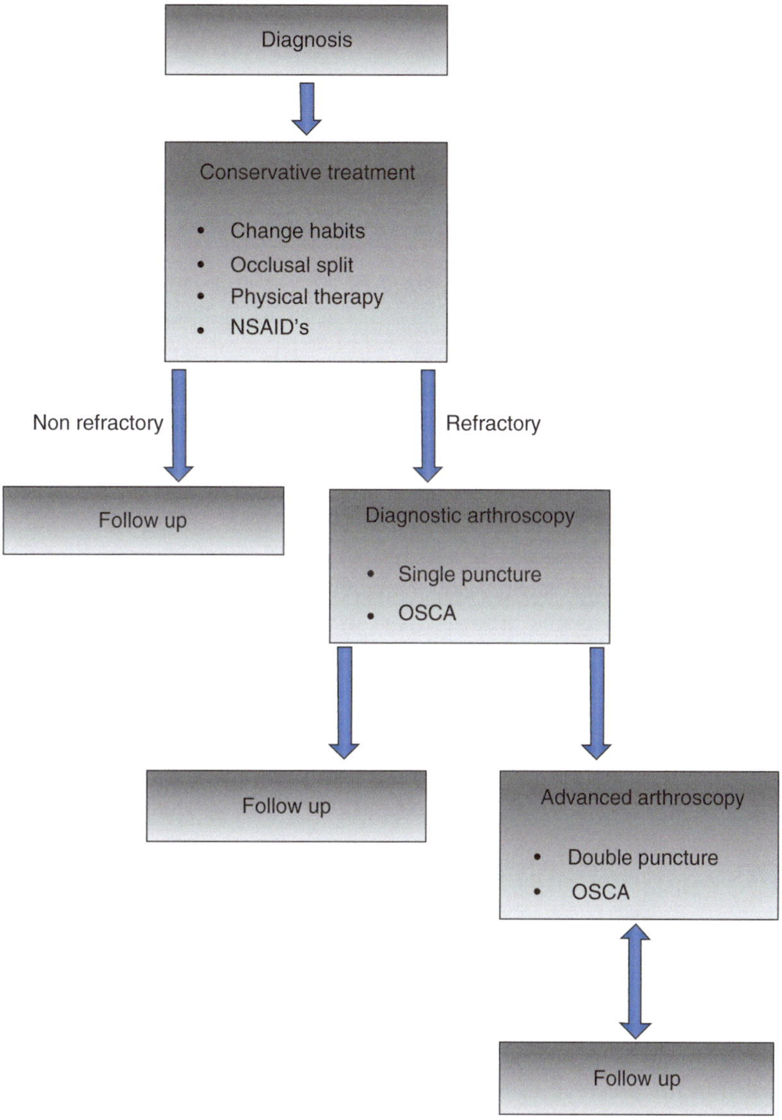

Fig. 2.4 Cascade for the management of patient with TMD

2.3.3 Conservative Treatment

Treatment usually begins with a conservative regimen, which includes advice, reassurance and change of habitual habits, NSAID administration, use of a stabilization (flat-plane) appliance at night for a period of at least 3 months, and physical therapy [3]. Effectiveness of conservative treatment is assessed by improvements in VAS scores and MIO, changes in the consistency of diet from soft/semiliquid to a more solid one, and decreased dependency on NSAIDs for pain management. Patients refractory to conservative treatment, who continue to suffer from pain during physiological function, presenting hypomobility or hypermobility, or with degenerative joint diseases, subluxation, or dislocation, are referred for diagnostic arthroscopy (Fig. 2.4). Diagnostic arthroscopy can be performed using the traditional two-port technique or by OSCA, which enables visualization of various pathological signs of TMJ, such as adhesions, synovitis, internal derangement, and disc perforation. An advanced arthroscopy, employing the double-puncture technique or OSCA, is performed as needed.

2.4 Arthroscopy

2.4.1 Indications for Arthroscopy

The American Association of Oral and Maxillofacial Surgeons (AAOMS) established the following main indications for arthroscopy of the TMJ [11, 13–15]: internal derangement of TMJ, mainly Wilkes stages II, III, and IV; degenerative joint disease (osteoarthritis, OA); synovitis; painful hypermobility; hypomobility caused by intra-articular adherences; inflammatory arthropathies (systemic arthritis); and articular symptoms subsidiary to orthognathic surgery.

2.4.2 Contraindications for Arthroscopy

The OSCA technique, like the traditional arthroscopy technique, is ineffective in cases of severe fibrous or osseous ankylosis. Bony ankylosis usually requires alloplastic or autogenous joint replacement, while fibrous ankylosis responds better to open-joint surgery (debridement or joint replacement). The approach is also contraindicated in the presence of tumor or metastasis in the TMJ. Skin infection over the puncture site contraindicates arthroscopy, since it increases the risk of contamination of the joint space during surgery. Medical conditions that may contraindicate general anesthesia or surgery must be taken under consideration as well.

2.4.3 Armamentarium

2.4.3.1 The Arthroscope

The ideal arthroscopic system should provide an angle of view of at least 30°, and a focal distance, i.e., the distance over which initially collimated rays are brought to a focus, as close to zero as possible. Image resolution is a key parameter, as it sets the limits of visualization details. A color temperature of 5000 °K accurately reproduces natural daylight illumination. Color response and brightness vary across the available systems. Capacity to perform "white balance," to adjust the electronic red, green, and blue signals, is important as well. In the OSCA technique described below, the authors used a Polydiagnost (Hallbergmoos, Germany) interdisciplinary semirigid, 0.9 mm diameter endoscope (PD-DS-1083), which provides high resolution (10,000 pixel), a 120° viewing angle, and a focal distance of 1–15 mm. The device is 181 mm long and uses a standard light connection (ACMI/Storz/Wolf) (Fig. 2.5a).

The optic fiber is passed through the middle connection of a three-way female Luer lock connection handle, while the other two connections are designated for irrigation and instrumentation (Fig. 2.5b). A 26 mm optic shifter is used to adjust the optic fiber length (Fig. 2.5c). The system setup is shown in Fig. 2.6.

The endoscope can be connected to various recording and visualization instruments. In the authors' operation room setup, an AESCULAP endoscopy cart with a 26″ full HD flat-panel display, full HD 3-Chip Camera, AXel 300 xenon light source, and an Eddy Full HD Digital Documentation System is used (Fig. 2.7).

2.4.3.2 Cannulas

A 1.6, 2, or 2.4 mm cannula can be used (Fig. 2.8). When using a 2 mm cannula, instruments or laser fibers of a diameter <1 mm can be introduced into the joint space. The authors have a special set of small-diameter manual and mechanical instruments which will soon become commercially available. The 2.4 mm cannula can accommodate a wider variety of mechanical and manual instruments. A sharp trocar (Fig. 2.9a) is introduced into the superior joint space and removed after penetrating the joint. A blunt obturator (Fig. 2.9b) is then inserted to separate soft tissues within the TMJ. Using a special elastic rubber, the cannula should be marked 25 mm from the working end, to allow the surgeon to monitor the depth of penetration into the joint space during the procedure (Fig. 2.10).

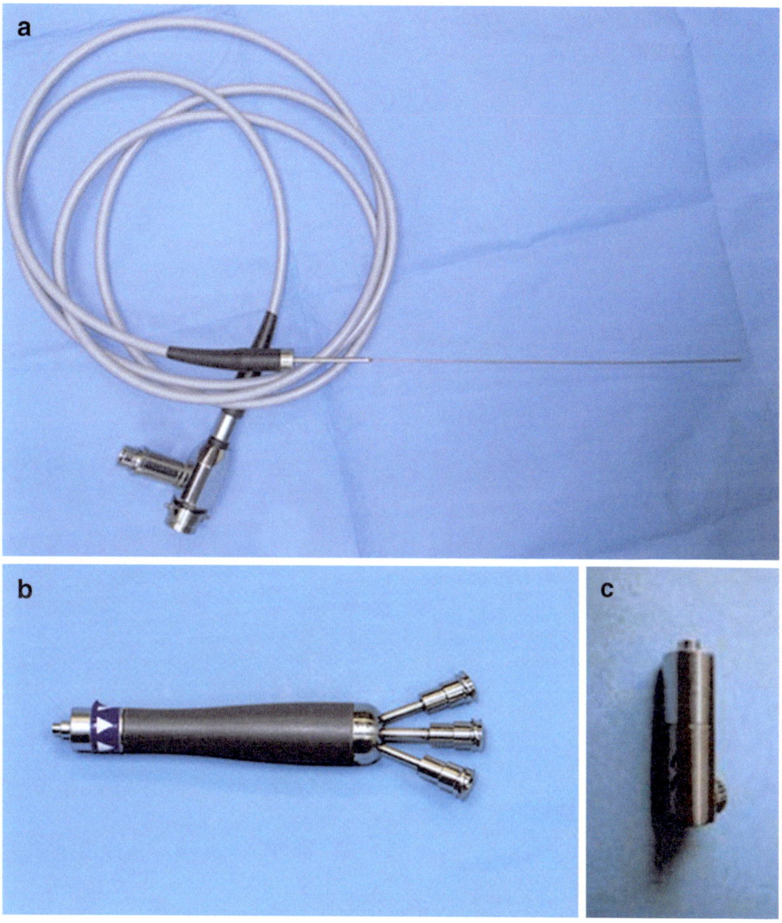

Fig. 2.5 (**a**) Polydiagnost, interdisciplinary semirigid 0.9 mm diameter endoscope. (**b**) Three-way female Luer lock connection handle. (**c**) Optic shifter

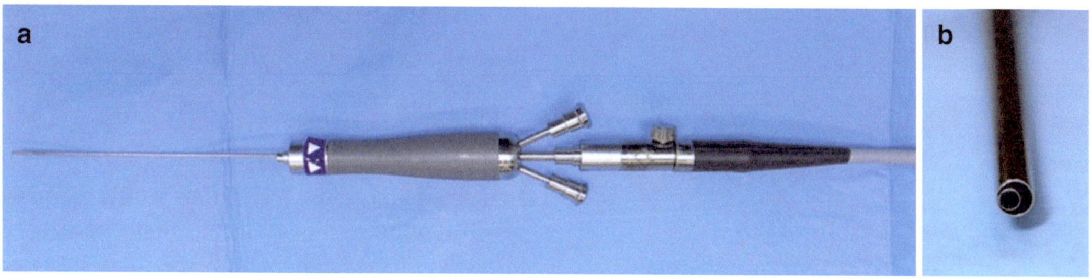

Fig. 2.6 (**a**) Endoscope, handle, and optic shifter attached in tandem. (**b**) Optic fiber emerging from the cannula

2.4.3.3 Probes

Any straight or hooked probe, with a diameter <1 mm, can be used. The probe is the most basic hand instrument used for palpation, severing adhesions, and mobilization/temporary immobilization of tissue. In cases of chondromalacia, the hooked probe is the preferred instrument for palpation and is typically used to elevate the anterior aspect of the disc after anterior releasing procedures and to complete the dissection of the disc from the capsule and the pterygoid muscle.

2.4.3.4 Graspers and Biopsy Forceps

Graspers and biopsy forceps are used when collecting small biopsy samples and for debridement of pathologic or fragmented tissues (Fig. 2.11).

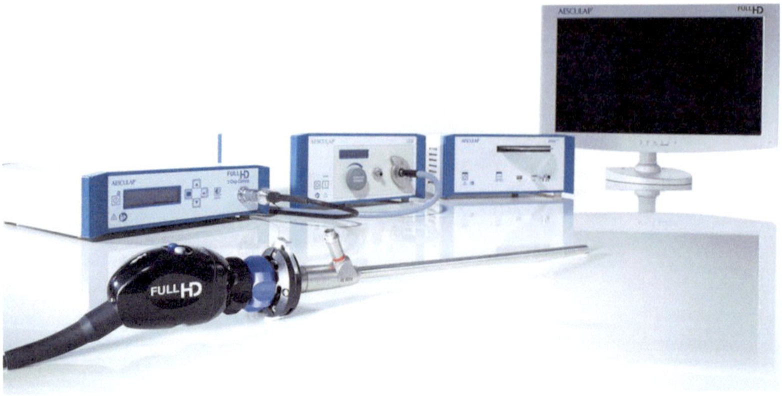

Fig. 2.7 AESCULAP endoscopy system

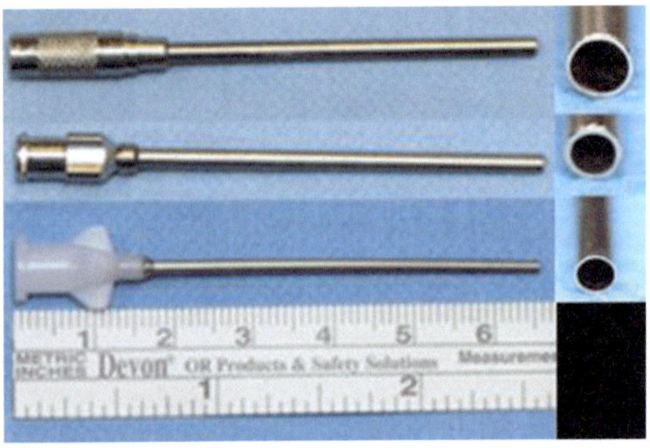

Fig. 2.8 1.6, 2, or 2.4 mm cannulas

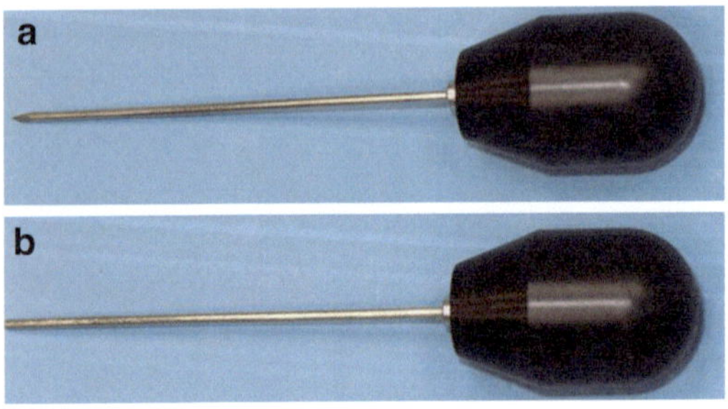

Fig. 2.9 (**a**) Sharp trocar. (**b**) Blunt obturator

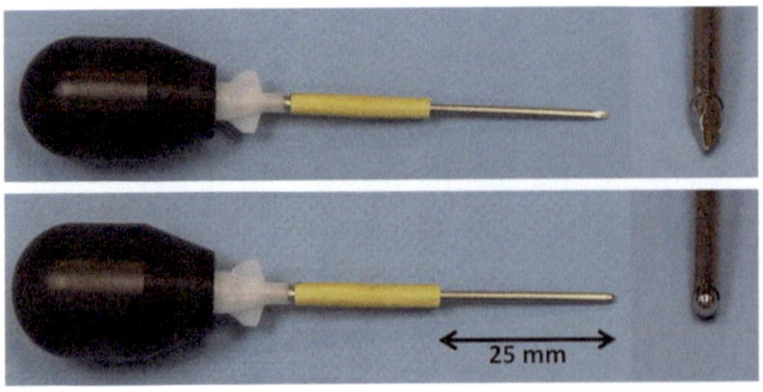

Fig. 2.10 Sharp trocar and blunt obturator inserted into a 1.6 mm cannula marked 25 mm from the working end

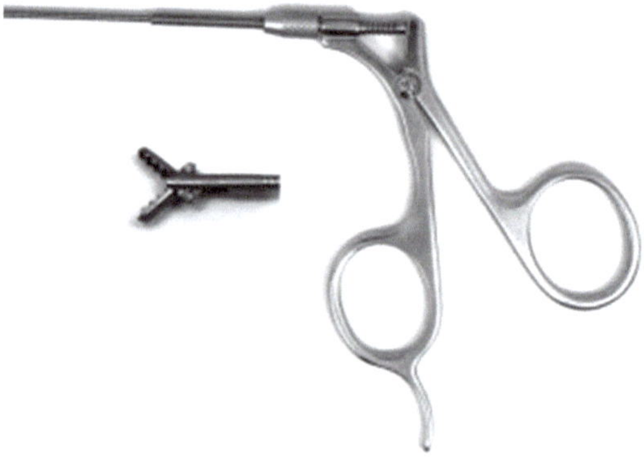

Fig. 2.11 Semiflexible grasper

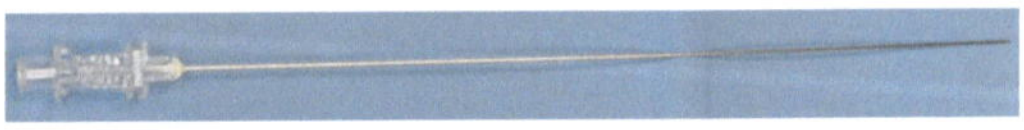

Fig. 2.12 Spinal needle, 150 mm long with diameter of 0.72 mm

2.4.3.5 Spinal Needles

Long spinal needles ($\geq$150 mm) with a diameter of <1 mm are necessary for accurate, visualized injection of medications into the joint space or adjacent structures (lateral pterygoid, connective tissue, or articular disc) (Fig. 2.12).

2.4.3.6 Laser

Lasers emit light based on the stimulated emission of radiation and can operate in either a pulsatile or continuous mode and their physical properties provide for an array of laser setting, each eliciting well-defined and localized effects. Although there are many types of lasers, most have been found ineffective in treating TMJ. The

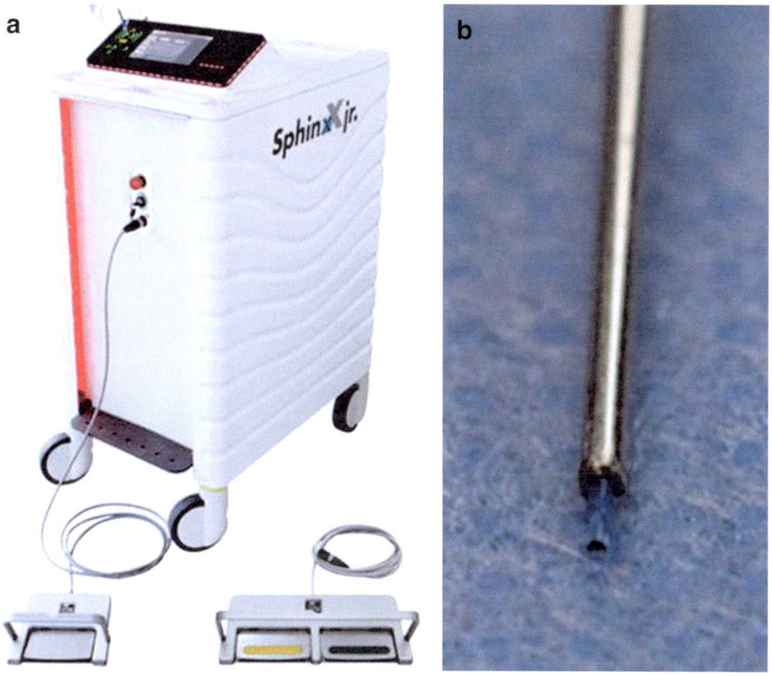

Fig. 2.13 (**a**) LISA LASER PRODUCTS Sphinx jr. Holmium:YAG laser. (**b**) The laser fiber emerging from its metal protection

Table 2.2 Holmium:YAG laser settings for specific purposes

Laser setting for cutting	10 Hz	9 W	0.09 J
Laser setting for ablation	8 Hz	4 W	0.5 J
Laser setting for contracture	5 Hz	2 W	0.4 J

authors recommend use of the air-cooling holmium:YAG laser, and themselves use the relatively compact (H 1000 × W 450 × L 740 mm) and lightweight (approx. 95 kg) LISA LASER PRODUCTS Sphinx jr. Holmium:YAG laser (Fig. 2.13), which operates at a wavelength of 2123 nm. The laser produces 30 W at the fiber tip, 0.3–5 J pulse energy, 100–650 μs pulse duration, and 1–25 Hz frequency. The holmium:YAG laser beam is strongly absorbed by water and therefore can target most biologic tissues. It has a limited depth of penetration (0.3–0.5 mm), rendering it very practical and safe for intra-articular use. In the OSCA technique, a 230 μm fiber laser is used, and is sufficiently small to safely access the small-sized TMJ. The laser can be set for cutting, ablation, or contracture (Table 2.2) and is used for synovectomy, retrodiscal scarification, cutting of tissue, and debridement of fibrocartilage [9] (Table 2.3).

Table 2.3 Comparison of OSCA to the single- and double-puncture arthroscopy techniques

Parameter	Single puncture	Double puncture	OSCA
Main indication	Diagnosis and basic interventions	Advanced arthroscopy	Advanced arthroscopy
Proficiency required	Low	High	Low
Duration of operation	Short	Long	Short
Number of punctures	1	2	1
Number of working cannulas	1	2	1
Risk for facial nerve injury	Low	High	Low
Risk for facial scar	Low	High	Low
Effectiveness is pain relief	Low	High	High
Effectiveness is mouth opening improvement	Low	High	High

2.5 The Operative Single-Cannula Arthroscopy Technique

OSCA is a single-puncture arthroscopy procedure, appropriate for both diagnostics and operative needs; it can be performed under either sedation and local anesthesia or general anesthesia, in a fully equipped operating room. Usually preoperative antibiotics and glucocorticosteroids are intravenously injected to prevent skin contamination and for edema management, respectively. The patient is then placed in a supine position on the operating table and subjected to nasal endotracheal intubation. The skin is prepared and disinfected with chlorhexidine gluconate solution (Unisept), povidone iodine, or any comparable antibacterial solution. The surgical field is then isolated and the anatomical landmarks are identified to avoid possible complications. A tragocanthal line is first established, and the penetration point of the cannula is set at 10 mm anterior to the midtragus and 5 mm caudally to the tragocanthal line (Fig. 2.14a, b).

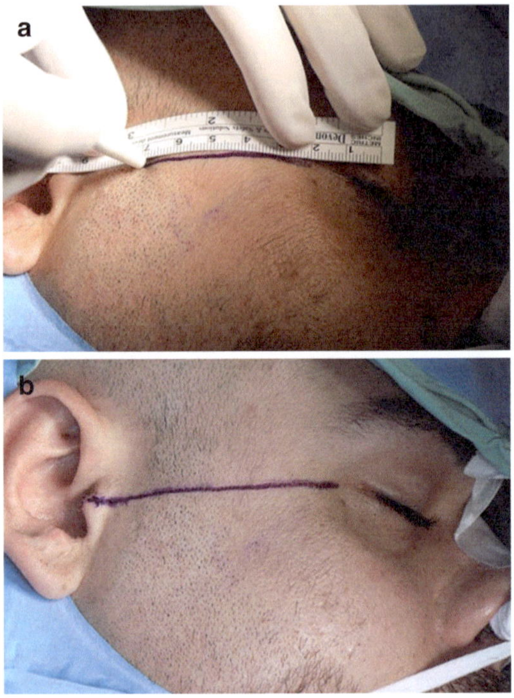

Fig. 2.14 (**a**) Marking of the tragocanthal line. (**b**) The tragocanthal line and penetration point of the cannula 10 mm anterior to the midtragus and 5 mm caudally in relation to tragocanthal line

Before penetrating the TMJ capsule, 2 mL of bupivacaine (Marcaine) is injected into the superior joint capsule, using a 22-gauge needle, in order to expand the structures. A 3 mL syringe is used so that backpressure can be felt when the joint space is entered (Fig. 2.15).

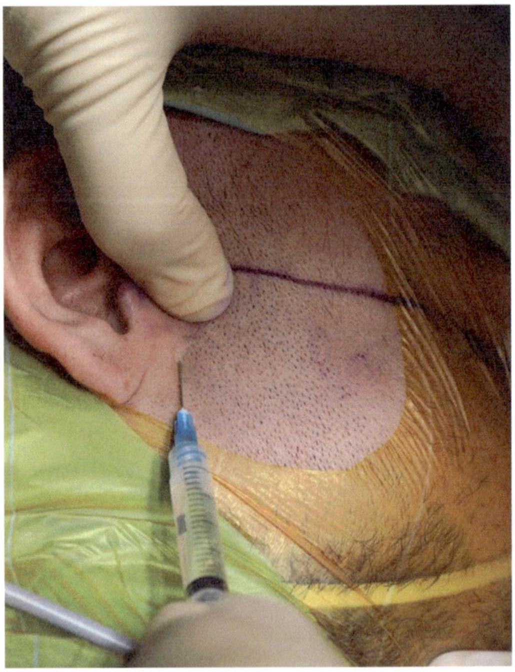

Fig. 2.15 Injection of 2 mL bupivacaine (Marcaine) into the superior joint capsule, using a 22-gauge needle

Injection of epinephrine directly into the joint space remains a topic of debate, since it may affect visualization of the synovial vasculature. The pattern and character of synovial vessels may indicate the level of inflammation present; therefore, any administration of a vasoconstrictor should be after the initial evaluation. Puncture is made using a sharp trocar, which introduces a cannula into the superior joint space, using a standard inferiolateral technique, to a depth of 25 mm [16] (Fig. 2.16).

A cannula is introduced into the superior joint space to a depth of 25 mm. Once penetrating the joint, the sharp trocar is removed and a blunt obturator is inserted to separate the soft tissues within the TMJ (Fig. 2.17). The arthroscope is inserted through the middle connection of the three-way female Luer lock.

2.5.1 One-Track Arthrocentesis

One-track arthrocentesis enables initial location of the TMJ, in addition to its visualization while performing irrigation and arthrocentesis. Two female Luer lock connector pipelines are connected to the other two ports. "One-track arthrocentesis" is performed through the irrigation canal and rinsing is performed through the working canal (Fig. 2.18). Ringer's lactate solution is the preferred irrigation fluid, but standard saline may also be used. A large syringe (50 mL) can be used with a pumping motion, or when there is a need for continuous irrigation (Fig. 2.19), the bag can be placed in a pressure cuff. Caution must be exercised due to possible fluid extravasation.

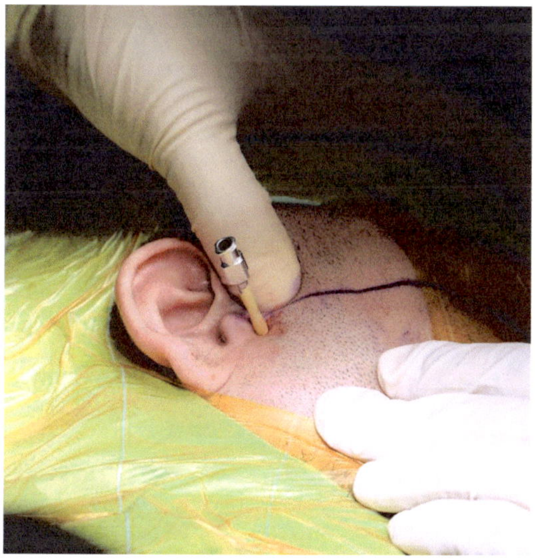

Fig. 2.16 A cannula is introduced into the superior joint space to a depth of 25 mm

2.5.2 Standard Arthrocentesis Under Diagnostic Visualization

An 18-gauge needle is inserted 5 mm anteriorly and 5 mm caudally from the puncture point of the working cannula (Fig. 2.20). This needle serves as an outflow port, while the outflow canal becomes the operating canal of the OSCA system. Depending on the pathological findings within the superior space of the TMJ, the operator can decide to proceed with the full OSCA technique, using hand or mechanical instruments or a laser fiber.

A diagnostic sweep of the TMJ is then performed, during which seven points of interest should be visualized and assessed (Fig. 2.21):

1. The **medial synovial drape** has a gray-white translucent lining and a tense appearance, with distinct superior-to-inferior striae (Fig. 2.22). This articular entity represents one of the most important barometers of TMJ synovitis (Fig. 2.23). In acute inflammatory states, capillary proliferation with hyperemia of the medial synovial drape is increased. In chronic synovitis, the drape has a fibrotic or whitish appearance.
2. The **pterygoid shadow** is located anterior to the medial synovial drape. In pathologic

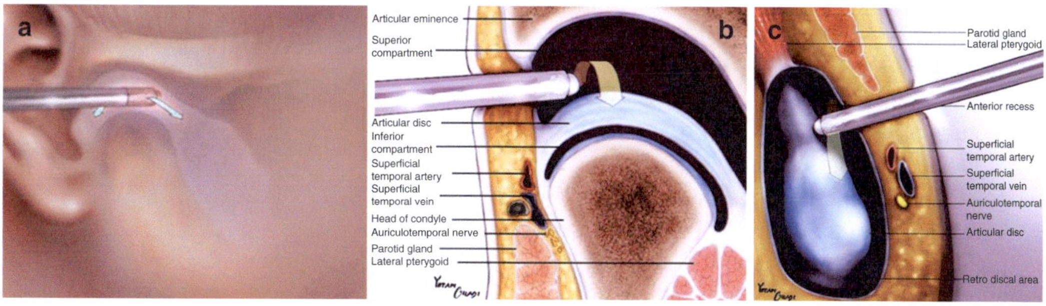

Fig. 2.17 (**a**) Illustration of the sweeping motion of the obturator used for soft-tissue separation. (**b**, **c**) Illustration of the obturator and cannula introduced into the upper compartment of the TMJ (coronary (*left*) and horizontal (*right*) sections)

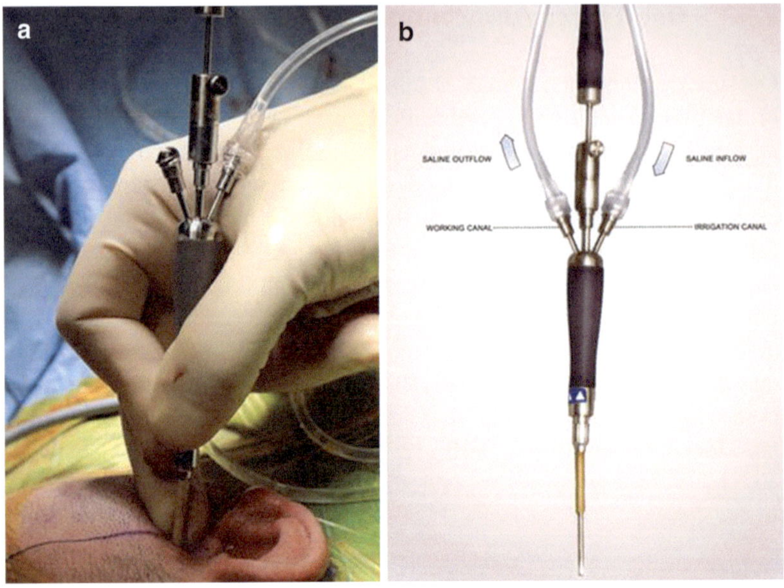

Fig. 2.18 One-track arthrocentesis. (**a**) The arthroscope is introduced into TMJ through the middle connection of the three-way female Luer lock; the irrigation pipeline is also seen. (**b**) Illustration of the arthroscope, showing inflow through the irrigation canal and rinsing through the working canal

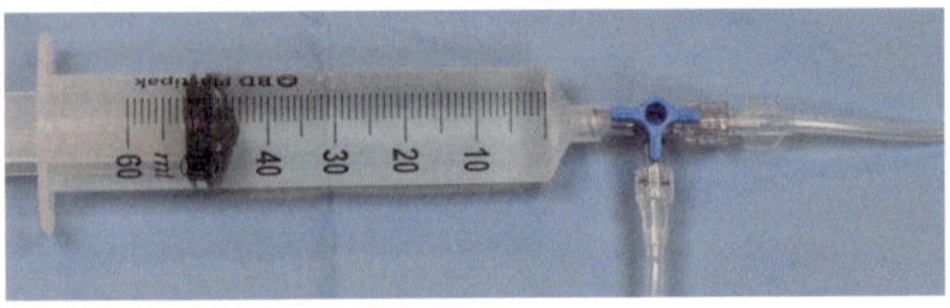

Fig. 2.19 A 50 mL syringe is used for irrigation

states, it exhibits marked erythema and hypervascularization, and can thin to the extent of perforation, coupled with herniation of the pterygoid muscle directly into the anteromedial aspect of the superior joint space (Fig. 2.24).

3. The **retrodiscal synovium**: Here, the synovial membrane covers the posterior insertion of the disc and is reflected superiorly to the temporal fossa. While the mouth is open, the posterior insertion covered by the synovial lining appears as a crest, called the oblique protuberance (zone 1). The retrodiscal tissue is located posterosuperiorly, attached to the posterior glenoid process (zone 2), while the lateral recess of the retrodiscal/synovial tissue (zone 3), which in pathologic states imparts a hyperemic or petechial appearance to the synovium, can be lateral to the oblique protuberance. Chronic synovitis in this area is characterized by synovial hyperplasia, with

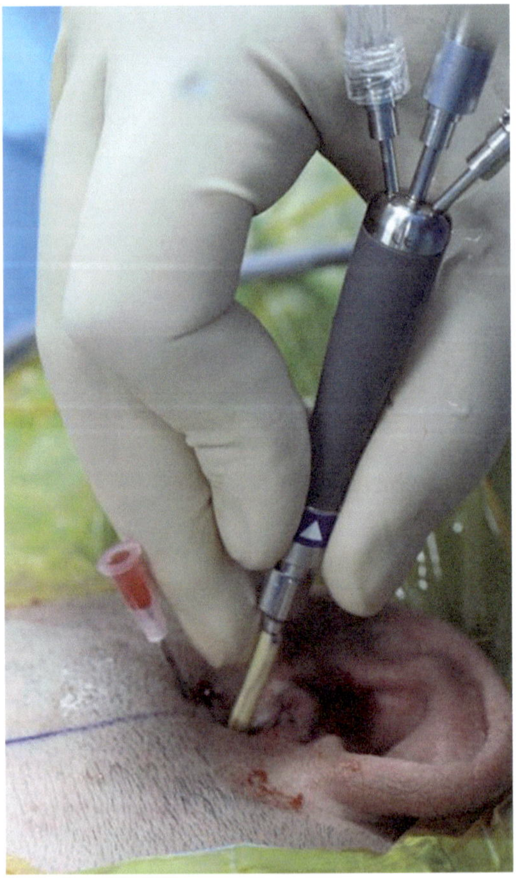

Fig. 2.20 Standard arthrocentesis under diagnostic visualization

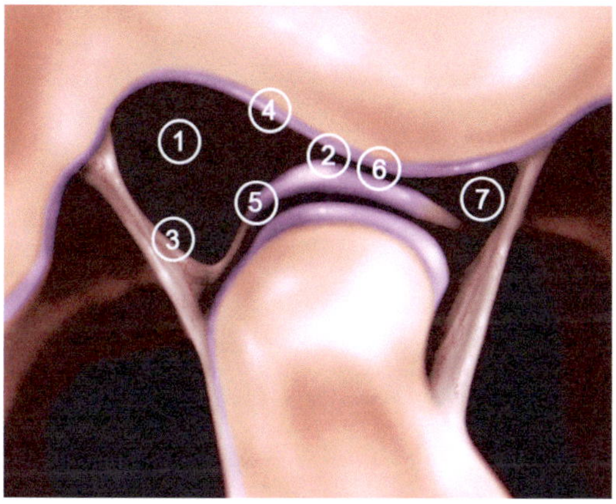

Fig. 2.21 The seven points of interest of the TMJ arthroscopic examination. (*1*) Medial synovial drape. (*2*) Pterygoid shadow. (*3*) Retrodiscal synovium. (*4*) Posterior slope of the articular eminence. (*5*) Articular disc. (*6*) Intermediate zone. (*7*) Anterior recess

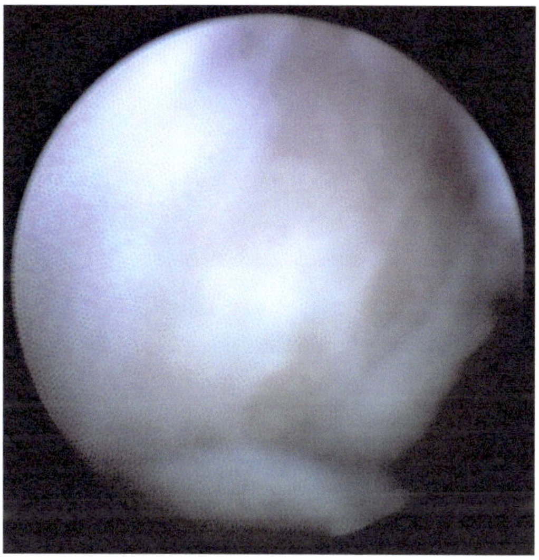

Fig. 2.22 Medial synovial drape

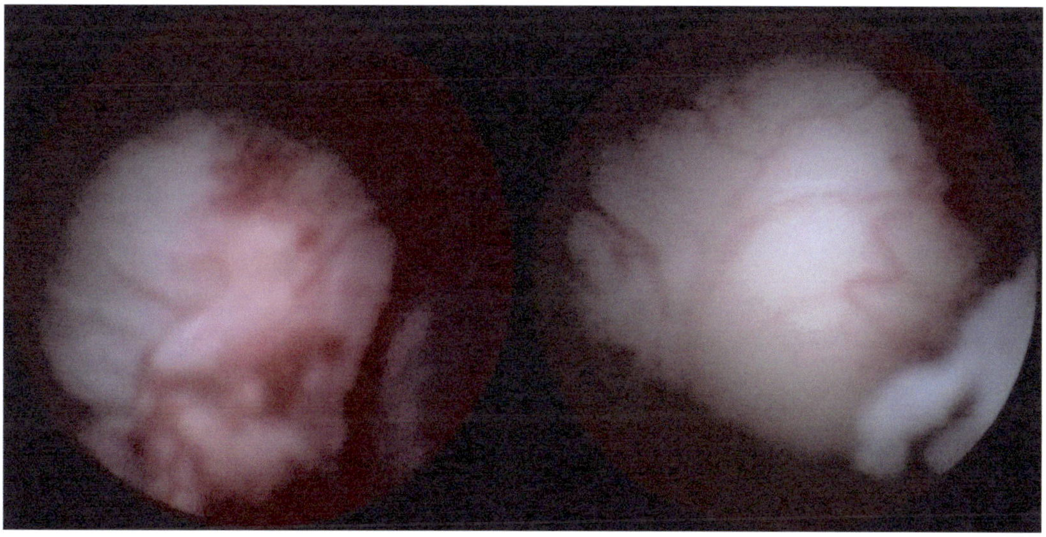

Fig. 2.23 TMJ synovitis with capillary proliferation

increasing proliferation of tissue folds (Fig. 2.25).

4. The **posterior slope of the articular eminence** is characterized by thick, white, and highly reflective fibrocartilage, with anteroposterior striae within. In pathological states, various stages of chondromalacia, i.e., softening of the articular fibrocartilage caused by digestion by proteoglycan collagenases from injured chondrocytes, is often detectable, and can reach a grade of crater formation and subchondral bone exposure. In inflammatory states, creeping of the synovial tissue can be observed in the glenoid fossa and the posterior slope of the eminence (Fig. 2.26).
5. The **articular disc** is milky white, highly reflective, and without striae. In pathologic states, the synovium creeps onto the surface of the disc. Fragmentation of the disc surface is usually an indication of imminent or existing

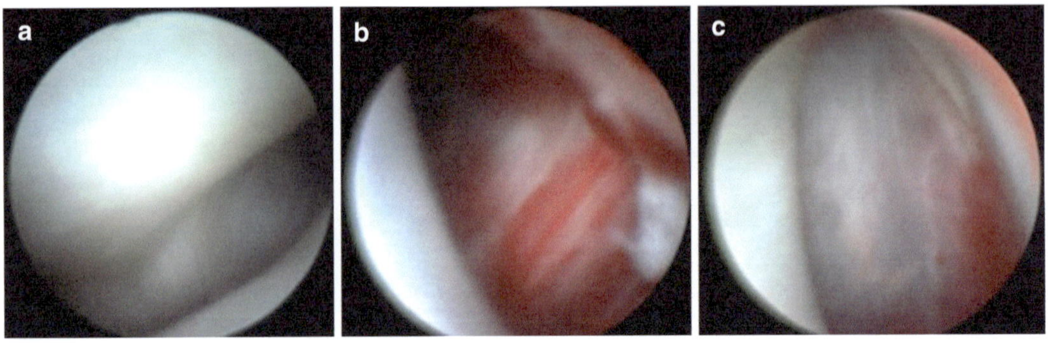

Fig. 2.24 (**a**) The pterygoid shadow (normal arthroscopic appearance). (**b**, **c**) Erythema at the pterygoid shadow

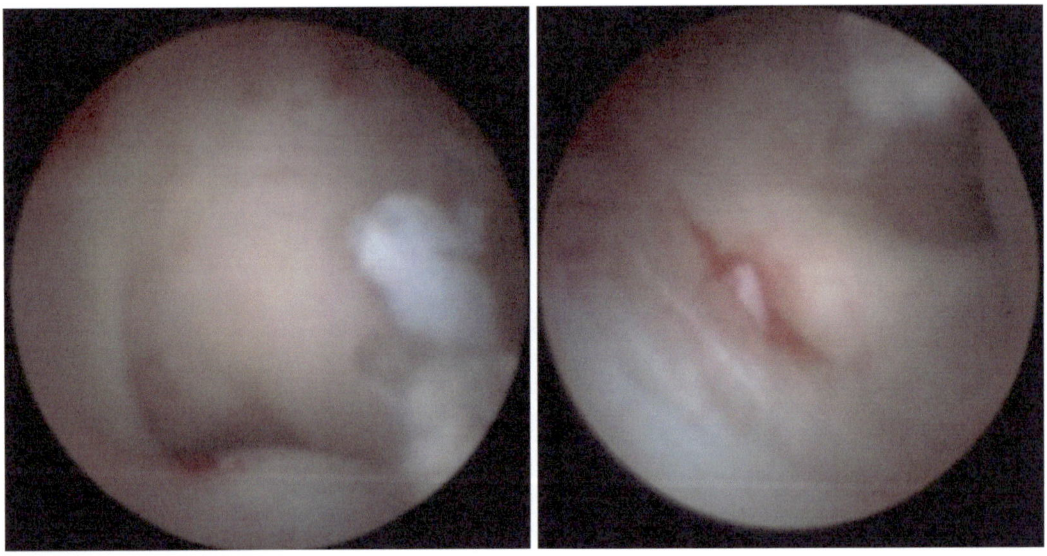

Fig. 2.25 Retrodiscal area

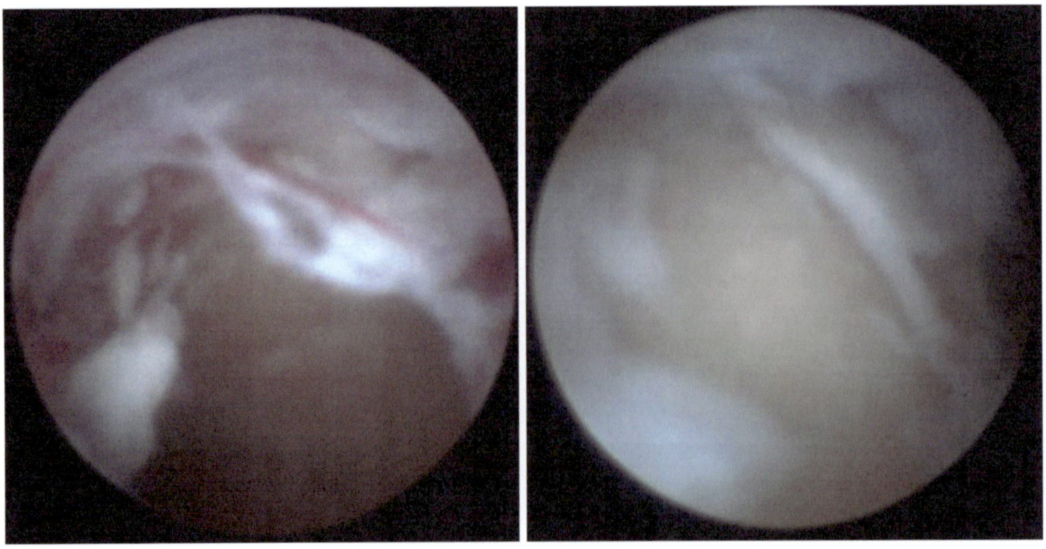

Fig. 2.26 Various stages of chondromalacia

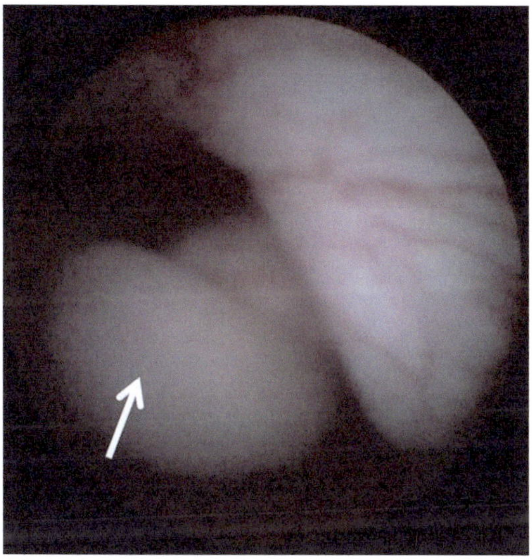

Fig. 2.27 Normal articular disc (*arrow*)

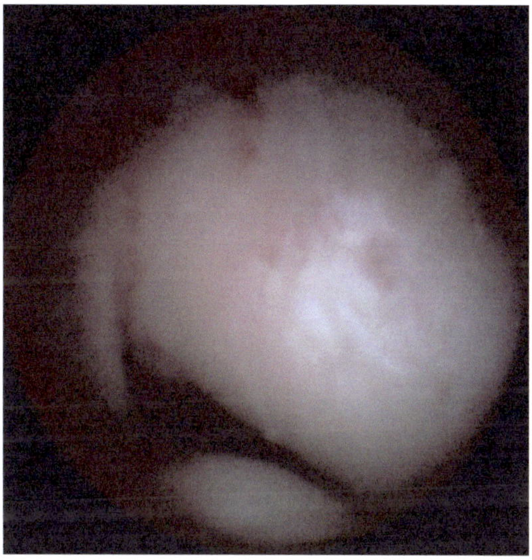

Fig. 2.28 Normal anterior recess

disc perforation. In cases of disc perforation, the inferior joint space can be examined by introducing the scope through the perforation into the inferior joint space (Fig. 2.27).

6. The **intermediate zone** has a white-on-white appearance, and the concavity of the disc can be seen.
7. The **anterior recess** begins with the condyle seated, in which the anterior disc synovial crease is identified. The crease is examined by following it to the terminal medial point, the most extreme medioanterior corner of the crease, and the pterygoid shadow. At the anterolateral site, the union between the lateral synovial capsule and the anterior disc synovial crease can be observed. In pathological states, the vascularity of the anterior synovial pouch increases and all characteristics of synovial inflammation are present. Occasionally, synovial redundancy and synovial plicae are also present (Fig. 2.28).

2.5.3 Visually Guided OSCA

As stated before, many different hand or mechanical instruments can be used during OSCA; the most suitable instrument is selected based on pathological findings or indication (Fig. 2.29). The Ho:YAG laser provides for a wide range of treatment options for internal pathologies and derangements of the joint and also secures precision and safety (Figs. 2.30 and 2.31). Its cutting options can be exploited to sever adhesions and to execute anterior release combined with discopexy. Its ablative capacities are applied on the dilated blood vessels of the synovial and chondromalatic tissue. The contracture mode is used to induce contraction of the retrodiscal synovial tissue for posterior disc repositioning. Of note, the cannula can be inserted through the second port, as in the triangulation technique, to gain better access to the anterior recess, primarily necessary for anterior release during discopexy.

2.5.4 Surgical Interventions Using the OSCA Technique

2.5.4.1 Anterior and Posterior Recess Adhesion Release

Sequential lysis of adhesions in the superior joint space, aimed at restoring the volume and architecture of the joint, should follow an anterior-to-posterior pattern, avoiding repeated motion of instrumentation from the back to the front of the joint, which could increase the risk of unnecessary articular surface scuffing. The probe is first placed

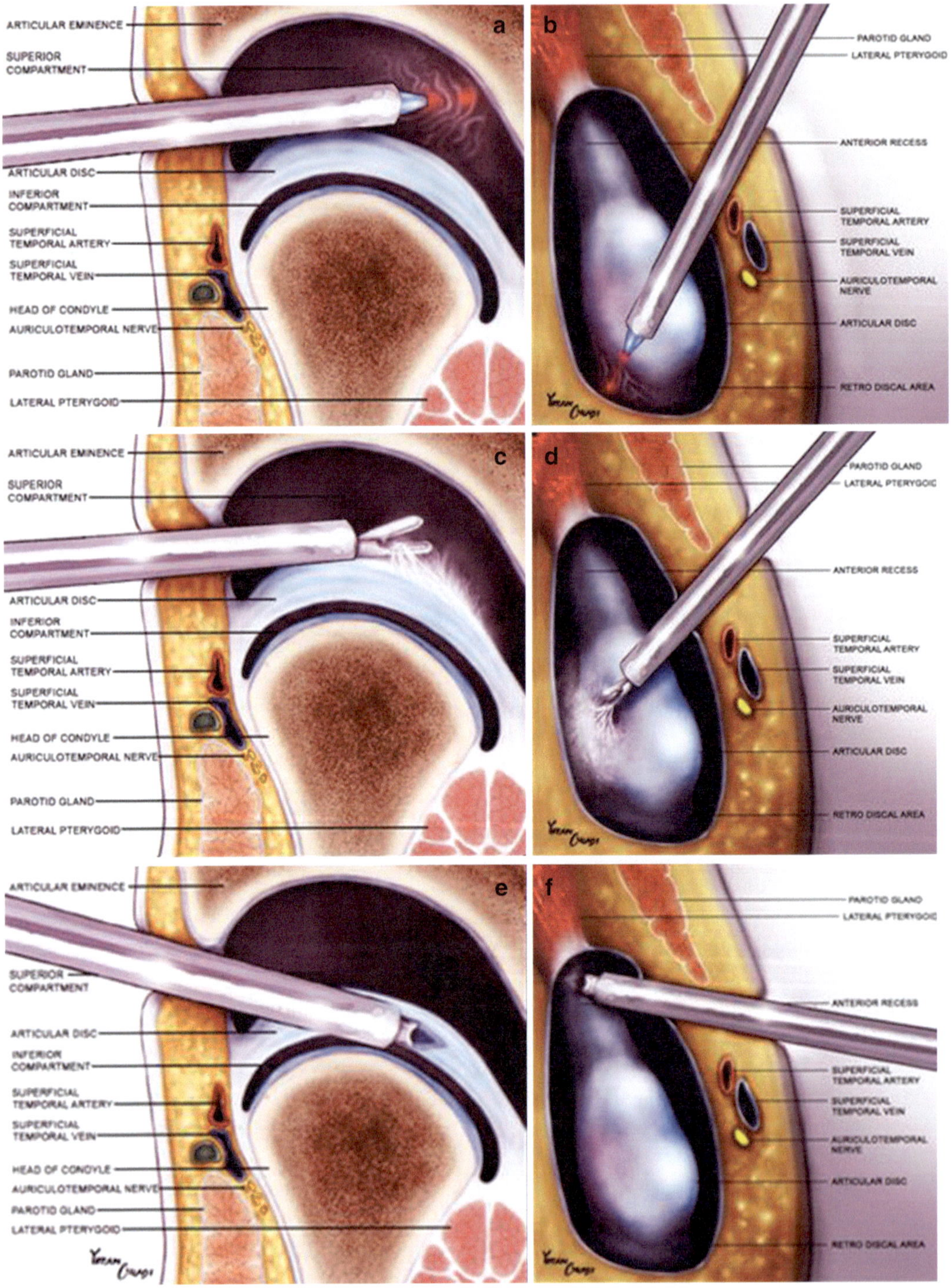

Fig. 2.29 Illustration of visually guided OSCA showing various instruments introduced into the TMJ. (**a**, **b**) Ho:YAG laser used for contraction of the retrodiscal synovial tissue. (**c**, **d**) Grasper used for biopsy or chondromalacia removal. (**e**, **f**) Spinal needle used for injection of intra-articular medication into lateral pterygoid muscle

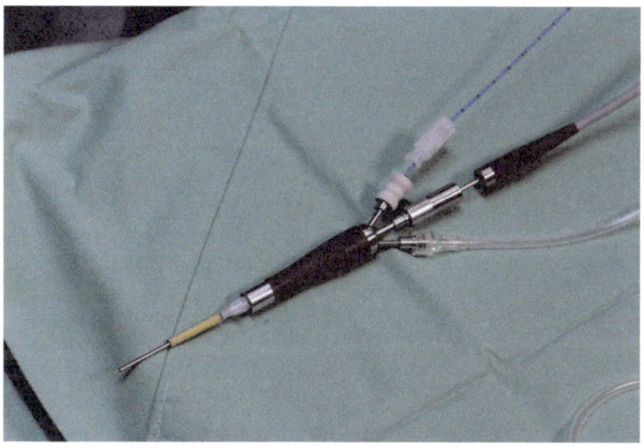

Fig. 2.30 Setup of the Ho:YAG laser fiber with the arthroscope, in tandem

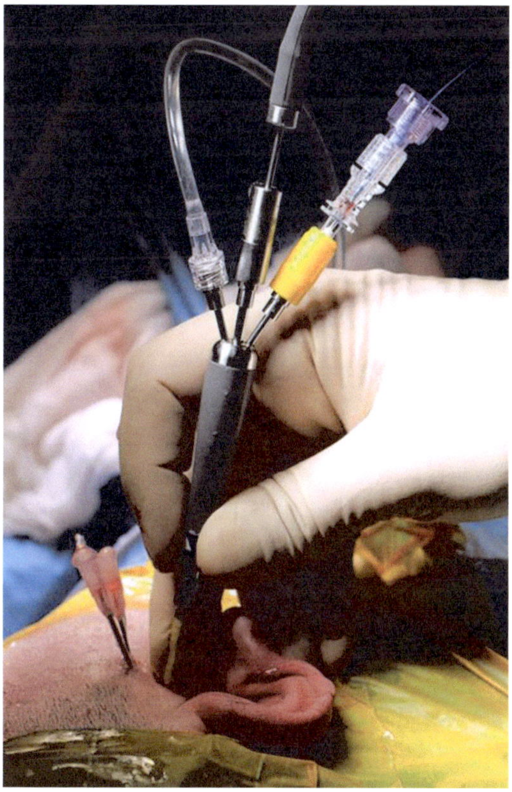

Fig. 2.31 Visually guided OSCA. Intraoperative setup of the Ho:YAG laser fiber

in the most medial aspect of the joint and then swept laterally along the disc-synovial junction with an inferoanterior maneuver. Then, by sweeping medially to laterally along the articular eminence, a superoanterior maneuver is executed to complete the lysis. These maneuvers are repeated until an adequate recess volume is restored. In many instances, anterior recess lysis is followed by posterior recess lysis. A marked increase in the range of movement (ROM) of the condyle is immediately achieved. For this procedure, the authors prefer the highly versatile Ho:YAG laser, set on cutting mode, over the probe.

2.5.4.2 Synovectomy

Effective reduction of a redundant synovium can be performed via Ho:YAG-assisted OSCA. A redundant synovium is most often observed in the posterior pouch, especially after disc reduction procedures. Occasionally, it can be encountered in the anterior recess. Hypervascularity and redundancy can effectively be reduced by Ho:YAG laser vaporization. The synovial clinical response is manifested by a change in color from bright red to off-white or even a light brown (Fig. 2.32).

2.5.4.3 Anterior Release

Conditions such as chronic disc dislocation, fibrosis, adhesive bands, or pseudowall formation can obliterate the disc-synovial crease. A blunt probe is used for the lysis procedure. If the anteroposterior disc dimension appears adequate and a relatively normal disc shape is ascertained, the release procedure is initiated in the medial half of the disc-synovial crease. Using an Ho:YAG laser in cutting mode, the synovial capsule is incised just anterior and parallel to the anterior margin of the disc. The surgeon observes the muscle fibers penetrating into the disc and capsule. Dissection should be performed to a depth no greater than 5 mm or until the anterior band is fully mobile, without tethering. Caution must be exercised when performing the myotomy at the most anteromedial corner. When the anteromedial synovial drape is incised at its junction with the disc, an artery, approximately 1–2 mm in diameter, can usually be found directly subjacent to the junction. Arthroscopically, it appears as a white tubular structure. If this vessel is inadvertently incised, copious intra-articular hemorrhaging will occur. This vessel cannot be cauterized or tied off by any current means. To tamponade the bleeder, all instruments must be removed and constant lateral pressure maintained

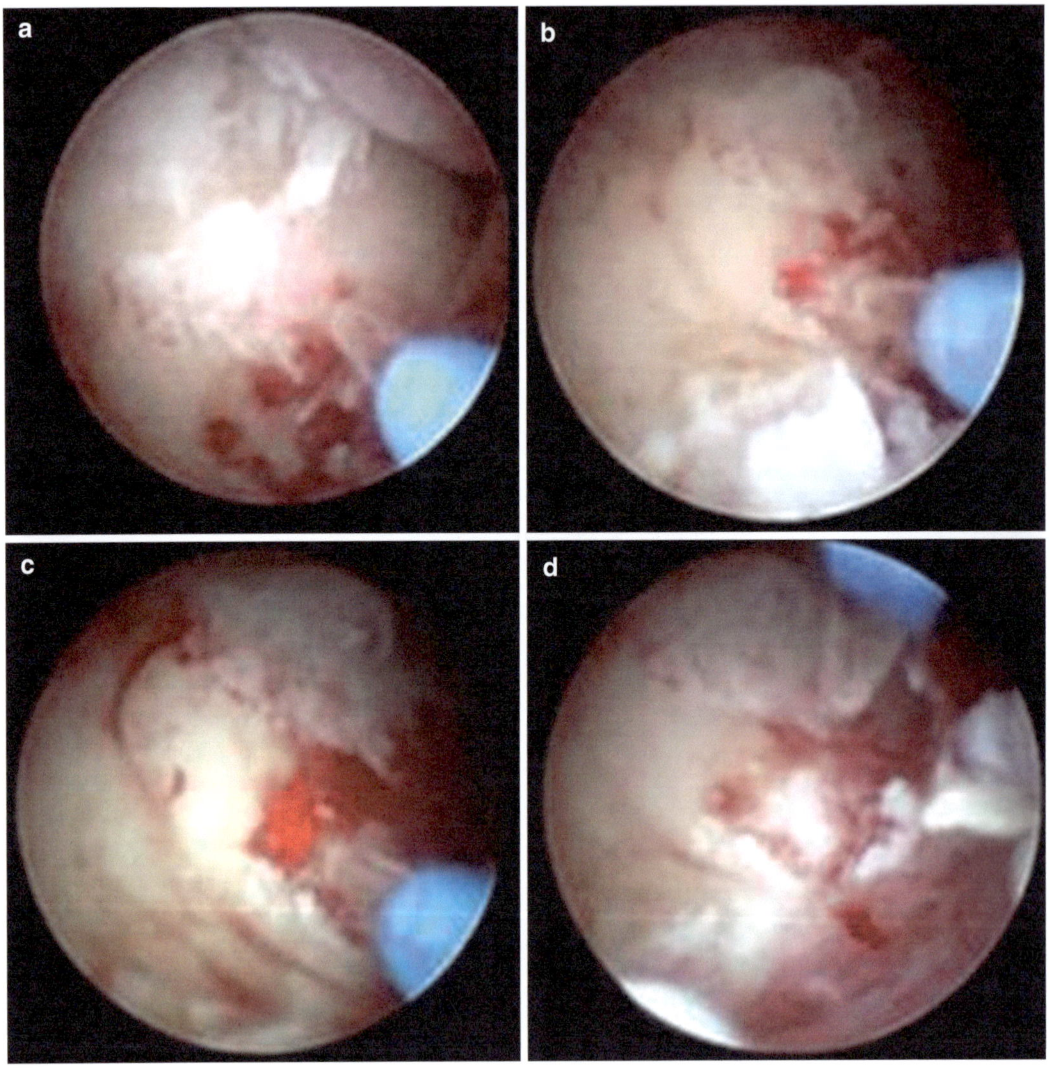

Fig. 2.32 (**a–d**) Adhesions, fibrillations, and synovitis treated intraoperatively using Ho:YAG-assisted OSCA

on the joint for 5 full minutes, while the condyle is held in a forward and contralateral position. The OSCA technique is then repeated and the joint is lavaged and suctioned free of clots. No further releasing is performed in the area and the release is completed laterally. Identification of this artery will avoid this problem and the myotomy can be carefully completed around the artery. The lateral one-third to two-thirds of the anterior release can be performed more expediently, with less concern for hemorrhage. Probing to assess anterior band mobility should be routinely performed during the anterior release.

2.5.4.4 Posterior Scarification/Contracture

Once disc reduction is achieved, an increased amount of redundant synovium is noted in the retrodiscal flexure. Even with minor disc repositioning and less evidence of redundancy of the posterior synovium, in the absence of discopexy, this procedure should be performed. Typically, "reefing," or bunching up, of the retrodiscal tissue occurs and requires bulk reduction using an Ho:YAG laser; otherwise, this fairly large amount of tissue can fibrose during healing, which can later displace the disc upon postoperative settling.

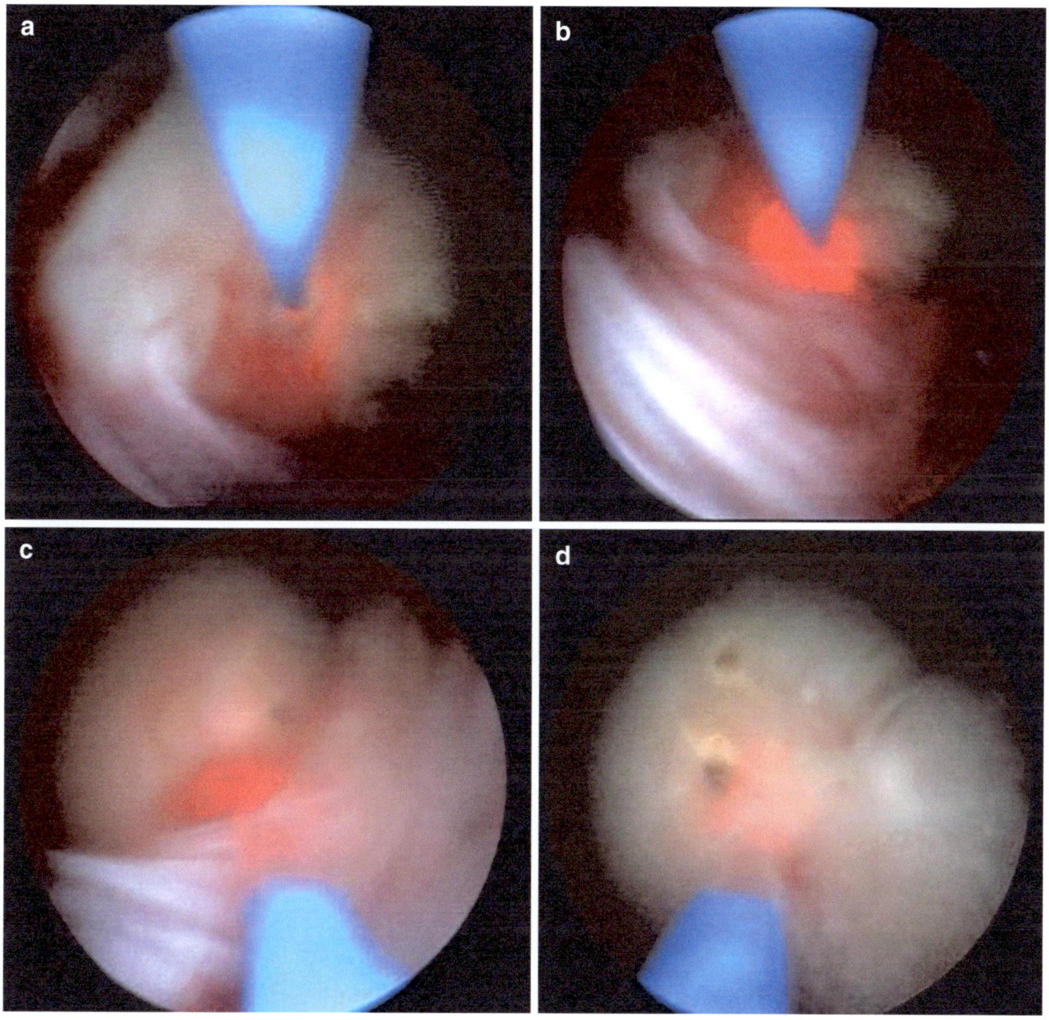

Fig. 2.33 (**a**–**d**) Contracture of retrodiscal synovium using Ho:YAG-assisted OSCA

Retrodiscal ablation should, therefore, be performed until a normal-shaped retrodiscal flexure is sculpted. The inflamed synovium and the areas of excess tissue bulk are ablated. Deep laser contracture of the oblique protuberance should then be performed. An examination of the anterior and posterior pouches is then performed (Fig. 2.33).

2.5.5 Advantages and Disadvantages of OSCA

The central advantage of the OSCA technique over the single-puncture technique lies in its provision for performance of advanced visually guided arthroscopy through a single cannula. In comparison to the traditional double-puncture arthroscopy technique, OSCA is relatively simple, requires less proficiency and less coordination from the surgeon, and is associated with a shorter learning curve. Its requirement for one working cannula only, without the need for a second puncture, decreases facial scaring and may reduce incidence of facial nerve injury. It is as effective as the traditional technique, with regard to pain relief and mouth opening improvements (Fig. 2.34a, b) [10]. Operative time is shorter, rendering the approach more cost effective (Fig. 2.34c) [10]. Another advantage of OSCA is the ability to inject medication to specific tissue

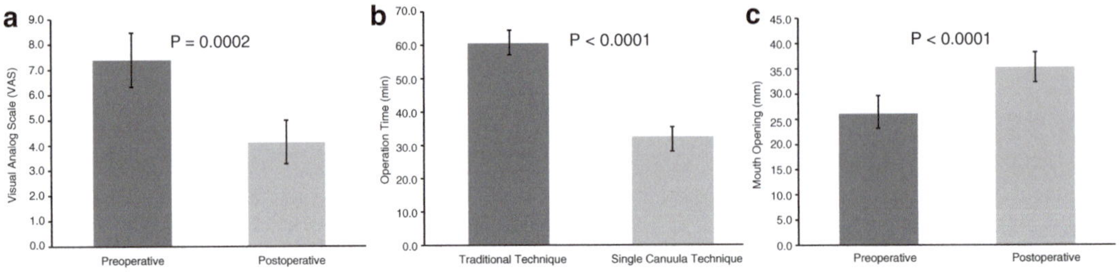

Fig. 2.34 (**a**) Pre-OSCA versus post-OSCA pain VAS scores (scale 0–10: 0 no pain, 10 severe pain), showing statistically significant (p value = 0.002) improvement in pain levels 3 months following the procedure. (**b**) Maximal mouth opening before versus 3 months after OSCA (p value <0.0001). (**c**) Surgery times for the OSCA versus traditional arthroscopy technique, showing a significantly (p value <0.0001) shorter mean operation time for the OSCA technique [10]

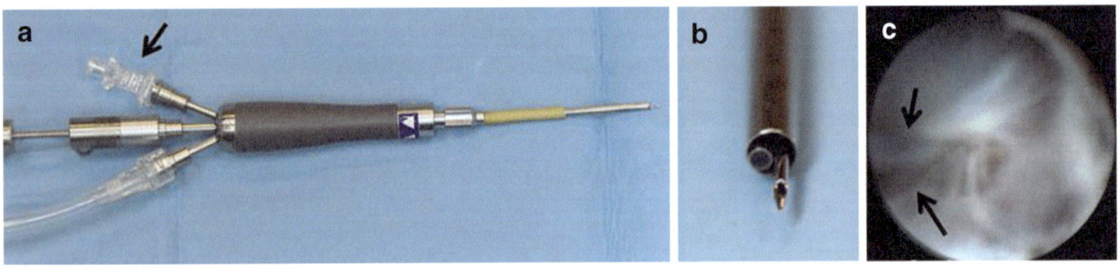

Fig. 2.35 Visually guided injection. (**a**) Spinal needle (150 mm length, 0.72 mm diameter) with an arthroscope. (**b**) Optic fiber and needle passing throw the cannula. (**c**) Injection of Depo-Medrol (white solution) into the joint space using a spinal needle (*arrows*)

regions under visual guidance. The main drawback of OSCA in comparison to the traditional technique is the relatively higher focal distance which may result in poorer image quality. However, to date, the image quality has proven satisfactory and all anatomical and pathological structures can be adequately observed.

2.5.6 Intra-articular Delivery of Medications via OSCA

Before the advent of arthroscopy, intra-articular medications were injected using a blind technique. The OSCA technique enables visually guided injection of medications, specifically targeting various anatomic articular sites.

2.5.6.1 Steroids

The authors' experience and research support the claimed benefit of steroid injection in the reduction of muscular irritation and spasm, consequently decreasing joint pain during function. The technique employs a 3 mL syringe with a 25-gauge spinal needle to intra-articularly inject methylprednisolone acetate (depo-medrol by Pfizer Inc.) or to perform visually guided injections into TMJ structures (Figs. 2.35 and 2.36).

2.5.6.2 Botulinum Toxin A

Local injection of Botox to treat chronic facial pain associated with hyperactivity of the masticatory muscles has been well documented. The efficacy of direct, arthroscopy-assisted injection of Botox into the superior head of the lateral pterygoid at the pterygoid shadow has very promising outcomes.

2.5.6.3 Hyaluronic Acid

Hyaluronic acid, a polysaccharide of the glycosaminoglycans family, is a component of many extracellular tissues, including the synovial fluid and cartilage, and is produced by the articular chondrocytes and synoviocytes. Hyaluronate

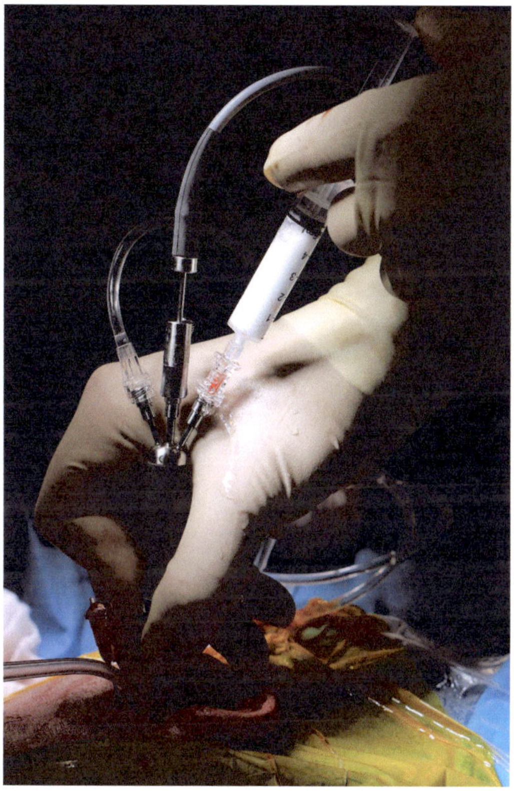

Fig. 2.36 Visually guided intraoperative injection of Depo-Medrol

injection into the TMJ aims to stimulate the endogenous synthesis of hyaluronic acid (HA) from the exogenously generated hyaluronic acid. Hyalgan is a 500–730 kDa fraction of highly purified avian sodium hyaluronate, buffered (pH 6.8–7.5) in physiologic saline. The authors believe that hyaluronate can serve as an excellent intra-articular lubricating agent to facilitate navigation while minimizing iatrogenic intra-articular injury.

2.5.6.4 Platelet Concentrates

Autologous platelet concentrates (PCs), derived from the patient's own blood, contain a highly concentrated cocktail of platelet-derived growth factors and endogenous fibrin scaffolds, which can be harnessed for regenerative purposes and other biological therapies [17]. They have been shown to accelerate healing and their transforming growth factor (TGF)-b component has been associated with chondrogenesis during cartilage repair [18]. Recent data support the application of platelet-rich plasma (PRP), a subtype of PC, to effectively and safely treat the initial stages of knee osteoarthritis (OA) [19, 20]. Furthermore, a number of randomized clinical studies have concluded that PCs provide for superior clinical results compared to hyaluronic acid (HA) in symptomatic alleviation of mild-to-moderate osteoarthritis of the knee [21, 22]. The content of the PC can vary according to preparation technique, and can be in a solution or a gel form. For TMJ purposes, PCs must be in solution form, as they are delivered via injection. The authors are currently conducting a study to assess the efficacy of post-OSCA injection of PCs into the TMJ, in comparison to other injectable medications, such as HA and steroids, in pain reduction and mouth opening improvement.

2.5.7 Post-OSCA Patient Management

2.5.7.1 General Anesthesia Considerations

The spastic perimandibular musculature contractions secondary to the gag reflex must be avoided, especially in patients who have undergone suture discopexies or posterior scarification procedures. Extubation in a semi-obtunded patient is ideal in such clinical situations. To ensure uneventful extubation, the surgeon passes a nasogastric tube and suctions all gastroesophagopharyngeal contents or secretions at the end of surgical procedure.

2.5.7.2 Anti-inflammatory and Pain Management

Patients receive tapered doses of intravenous/oral steroids for 18–24 h postoperatively. NSAIDs are also prescribed for no longer than 7 days.

2.5.7.3 Antibiotics

Notwithstanding the minimally invasive (MI) character of TMJ arthroscopic procedures and impeccable surgical technique, we have begun to routinely administer postoperative antibiotics;

ever since, our rate of postoperative infection has dropped to 0%. Every patient is bridged from intravenous to oral antibiotics such as cephalexin (Keflex) or amoxicillin and clavulanic acid (Augmentin) for no more than 7 days, conditional on absence of intolerance or allergic reactions.

2.5.7.4 Diet

A fully liquid diet is advanced to a strictly soft diet in a very gradual fashion. The expected transitional malocclusion, usually with posterior occlusion, is a period of intra-articular settling that should be allowed to progress in an undisturbed environment. This critical postoperative transition to norm occlusion should not be encroached upon by an accelerated return to function or parafunction.

2.5.8 Complications of Traditional Arthroscopy and OSCA

Owing to its minimally invasive nature, arthroscopy is usually associated with few complications. Use of a single cannula in the OSCA technique renders it even less invasive than the traditional double-puncture arthroscopy technique, and it is therefore expected to elicit an even lower percentage of complications.

2.5.8.1 Scuffing of Fibrocartilage

The cartilage covering the eminence and fossa is most prone to iatrogeny, this being the most common arthroscopic complication. At the time of insufflation, the needle point is directed toward the posterior slope of the eminence, making contact with the fibrocartilage. Also, examination sweeps of the joint cavity, involving translation of the arthroscope along with cannula, could also release pieces of cartilage into the superior joint space. If scuffing becomes significant, it impairs procedural visibility, to the point of misdiagnosis of chondromalacia by the inexperienced arthroscopist.

2.5.8.2 Damage to the VII Cranial Nerve

When using the OSCA technique and introducing the cannula 10 mm medially and 5 mm caudally along the cantho-tragal line, the temporal branch should be anterior to the entry point. Yet, injury to the temporal nerve and the adjacent zygomatic branch may occur, resulting in direct nerve damage arising from scarring of the nerve fibers or perineural tissue. Alternatively, the damage can be the consequence of extravasation, during which irrigation solution is forced beyond the joint capsule into adjacent tissues, resulting in compressive forces on the nerve, subsequent release of ischemic factors, localized nerve fiber changes, and segmental demyelinization. Extravasation of irrigation solution usually occurs upon blockage of the irrigation system or an excessively high-inflow current. While it is a common and self-limiting condition, quickly reabsorbed via the venous and lymphatic systems, it is imperative to visualize the soft palate and clear the airway before extubation. Injury to the temporal branch results in inability to elevate the eyebrow, while injury to the zygomatic branch results in inability to tightly close the eyes. Such assessments are made 24 h following surgery. Typically, the duration of nerve weakness varies from 1 week to 6 months.

2.5.8.3 Damage to the V Cranial Nerve

The auriculotemporal nerve is a branch of the mandibular nerve (V3) that runs along the superficial temporal artery and vein. It passes between the neck of the mandible and the sphenomandibular ligament in proximity to the fossa puncture site. Postoperative hypoesthesia in the area of the puncture site is quite common and usually spontaneously resolves within 2 weeks. Medial extravasation of the irrigation solution secondary to medial capsule perforation may result in compressive forces on the lingual and inferior alveolar nerves. Since the irrigation solution is quickly reabsorbed, symptoms resolve within a few days to weeks.

2.5.8.4 Damage to the VIII Cranial Nerve

The vestibulocochlear nerve transmits sound and equilibrium from the inner ear to the brain. Tympanic membrane perforation with subsequent hypoacousia may occur upon penetration into the middle ear via the osseous or soft-tissue external acoustic meatus. If perforation does occur, the procedure must be immediately discontinued and intraoperative consultation with an ear, nose, and throat specialist is required. A study by Park et al. indicated that perforation size and pneumatization of the middle ear influence the degree of conductive hearing loss in cases of tympanic membrane perforation [23]. Treatment include use of antibiotic ear drops (e.g., ciprofloxacin), a gelfoam plug, fibrin glue, a patch composed of a hyaluronic acid ester, and a dressing component or, in cases of large perforations, tympanoplasty. Following small perforations of the tympanic membrane, patients usually regain normal hearing levels within 2 months.

2.5.8.5 Damage to Vessels and Hamartosis

Injury to the superficial temporal artery and vein may occur, since it passes behind the neck of the condyle, superficially over the posterior root of the zygomatic process of the temporal bone, in close proximity to the point of entry. Applying controlled pressure is usually sufficient. Laceration of the medial pterygoid artery during myotomy may also occur, resulting in hamartosis. Hamartosis prolongs healing and increases postoperative discomfort. It also increases the risk for the formation of adhesions, scaring, and fibrous ankyloses, resulting in a limited range of mandibular movements.

2.5.8.6 Perforation of the Glenoid Fossa

Very rarely, the glenoid fossa is perforated. Such a complication can be easily prevented by marking the length of entry (25 mm) and directing the instruments toward the tubercle and away from the fossa. Perforation may result in cerebrospinal fluid leakage and require immediate cessation of surgery and neurosurgeon consultation.

2.5.8.7 Instrument Failure

Instrument failure can be the result of wearing of parts, manufacturing defects, or misuse, such as application of excessive force on the instrument. It is obligatory to have backup instruments, especially "golden retrievers" or graspers, to remove broken pieces. In case of a broken part within the TMJ space, it is mandatory to stop the operation, prepare the retriever, and maintain visibility while removing the fragment. If retrieval is not possible, a second attempt should be made as early as possible, i.e., within 6 weeks. It goes without saying that the patient must be informed of the possibilities of future osteoarthritis and infection.

Acknowledgment We would like to express our deepest gratitude to Dr. Daniel Oren and Dr. Adeeb Zoabi who were valuable contributors to the writing of this chapter. They both accompanied us and provided considerable support from the early initiation stages of the OSCA technique.

References

1. Onishi M. Arthroscopy of the temporomandibular joint. Kokubyo Gakkai Zasshi. 1975;42:207–13.
2. Murakami K, Hoshino K. Regional anatomical nomenclature and arthroscopic terminology in human temporomandibular joints. Okajimas Folia Anat Jpn. 1982;58:745–60.
3. McCain J. Arthroscopy of the human temporomandibular joint. J Oral Maxillofac Surg. 1988;46:648–55.
4. McCain JP. Principles and practice of temporomandibular joint arthroscopy. St. Louis: Mosby; 1996.
5. Sanders B. Arthroscopic surgery of the temporomandibular joint: treatment of internal derangement with persistent closed lock. Oral Surg Oral Med Oral Pathol. 1986;62:361–72.
6. Holmlund A, Hellsing G. Arthroscopy of the temporomandibular joint: an autopsy study. Int J Oral Maxillofac Surg. 1985;14:169–75.
7. Nitzan DW, Dolwick MF, Martinez GA. Temporomandibular joint arthrocentesis: a simplified treatment for severe, limited mouth opening. J Oral Maxillofac Surg. 1991;49:1163–7.
8. Koslin MG, Martin JA. TMJ arthroscopic surgery. Clinical results in 79 cases. J Ala Dent Assoc. 1990;74(1):26–31.
9. McCain JP, Hossameldin RH. Advanced arthroscopy of the temporomandibular joint. Atlas Oral Maxillofac Surg Clin North Am. 2011;19:145–67.
10. Srouji S, Oren D, Zoabi A, Ronen O, Zraik H. Temporomandibular joint arthroscopy technique using a single working cannula. Int J Oral Maxillofac Surg. 2016;45:1490–4.
11. González-García R, Gil-Díez Usandizaga JL, Rodríguez-Campo FJ. Arthroscopic anatomy and lysis and lavage of the temporomandibular joint. Atlas Oral Maxillofac Surg Clin North Am. 2011;19:131–44.

12. Wilkes CH. Internal derangements of the temporomandibular joint: pathological variations. Arch Otolaryngol Head Neck Surg. 1989;115:469–77.
13. Barkin S, Weinberg S. Internal derangements of the temporomandibular joint: the role of arthroscopic surgery and arthrocentesis. J Can Dent Assoc. 2000;66:199–203.
14. American Association of Oral and Maxillofacial Surgeons. Position paper on TMJ arthroscopy 1988. In: Thomas M, Bronstein S, editors. Arthroscopy of the temporomandibular joint. Philadelphia: WB Saunders; 1991. p. 347–50.
15. Israel H. Arthroscopy of the temporomandibular joint. In: Peterson L, Indresano T, Marciani R, et al., editors. Principles of oral and maxillofacial surgery. Philadelphia: JB Lippincott; 1992. p. 2015–40.
16. Murakami K, Ono T. Temporomandibular joint arthroscopy by inferolateral approach. J Oral Maxillofac Surg. 1986;15:410.
17. Fernández Sanromán J, Fernández Ferro M, Costas López A, Arenaz Bua J, López A. Does injection of plasma rich in growth factors after temporomandibular joint arthroscopy improve outcomes in patients with Wilkes stage IV internal derangement? A randomized prospective clinical study. Int J Oral Maxillofac Surg. 2016;45:828–35.
18. Everts PAM, Knape JTA, Weibrich G, et al. Platelet-rich plasma and platelet gel: a review. J Extra Corpor Technol. 2006;38:174.
19. Chang KV, Hung CY, Aliwarga F, Wang TG, Han DS, Chen WS. Comparative effectiveness of platelet-rich plasma injections for treating knee joint cartilage degenerative pathology: a systematic review and meta-analysis. Arch Phys Med Rehabil. 2014;95:562–75.
20. Khoshbin A, Leroux T, Wasserstein D, Marks P, Theodoropoulos J, Ogilvie-Harris D, et al. The efficacy of platelet-rich plasma in the treatment of symptomatic knee osteoarthritis: a systematic review with quantitative synthesis. Arthroscopy. 2013;29:2037–48.
21. Sánchez M, Fiz N, Azofra J, Usabiaga J, Aduriz Recalled E, Garcia Gutierrez A, et al. A randomized clinical trial evaluating plasma rich in growth factors (PRGF-Endoret) versus hyaluronic acid in the short-term treatment of symptomatic knee osteoarthritis. Arthroscopy. 2012;28:1070–8.
22. Vaquerizo V, Plasencia MÁ, Arribas I, Sei-jas R, Padilla S, Orive G, et al. Comparison of intra-articular injections of plasma rich in growth factors (PRGF-Endoret) versus Durolane hyaluronic acid in the treatment of patients with symptomatic osteoarthritis: a randomized controlled trial. Arthroscopy. 2013;29:1635–43.
23. Park H, Hong SN, Kim HS, et al. Determinants of conductive hearing loss in tympanic membrane perforation. Clin Exp Otorhinolaryngol. 2015;8(2):92–6.

3 Arthrocentesis: A Minimally Invasive Approach to the Temporomandibular Joint

Dorrit W. Nitzan and Hadas Lehman Naaman

Abstract

Arthrocentesis is traditionally defined as a procedure in which the fluid in a joint cavity is aspirated with a needle followed by injection of a therapeutic substance. Arthrocentesis of the temporomandibular joint (TMJ) is a non-arthroscopic lysis and lavage performed under local anesthesia with two needles that are introduced into the upper compartment of the joint. It is always performed in conjunction with joint load control and movement rehabilitation. When arthrocentesis fails, we can surmise that open surgery is needed. Thus, arthrocentesis should become a primary tool in the treatment of the TMJ disorders, successfully filling the gap between failed conservative treatments and complex surgical interventions.

3.1 Introduction

Arthrocentesis is traditionally defined as a procedure in which the fluid in a joint cavity is aspirated with a needle followed by injection of a therapeutic substance. The procedure is usually carried out under local anesthesia with or without sedation, under sterile conditions. Its simplicity enables repetitions as necessary [1–3].

Bernardino de Sahagun recorded that approximately five centuries ago the Aztec Indians realized that inflamed joints were potentially harmful, and performed therapeutic arthrocentesis, using an unspecified thorn. They noted that the aspirated fluid was similar to the viscid fluid from the leaves of the nopal cactus [1, 4, 5].

Arthrocentesis became a subject of interest in the medical literature in the 1960s. The method provides symptomatic relief, especially in cases of traumatic synovitis. Techniques have been developed for the performance of arthrocentesis in many joints, including the hip [6–8], knee [9–13], manubrium of the sternum [14], shoulder, tarsus, wrist, ankle, and even the first metatarsal and metacarpal phalangeal joints [15–21]. In order to master the technique and enhance reliability it has been recommended that physicians practice the procedure on cadavers, or simulate it on plastic models before they apply it to patients

D.W. Nitzan, DMD (✉) • H. Lehman Naaman, DMD, MASc
Oral and Maxillofacial Surgery Department, The Hebrew University—Hadassah School of Dental Medicine, Ein Karem, Jerusalem, Israel
e-mail: dorrit.nitzan@mail.huji.ac.il

O. Nahlieli (ed.), *Minimally Invasive Oral and Maxillofacial Surgery*,
http://doi.org/10.1007/978-3-662-54592-8_3

[22–25]. Three-way stopcock was suggested as a useful adjunct in the practice of arthrocentesis [26]. A microdialysis technique that allows collecting serial synovial fluid samples has been developed in dogs to be used instead of arthrocentesis [27].

Numerous studies have described the diagnostic and therapeutic value of arthrocentesis and emphasized the low incidence of complications. Complications include joint contamination and local irritation caused by the introduction of foreign materials [12, 28–32].

Arthrocentesis can also be used for macroscopic diagnosis and therapy of diseased joints in emergency situations [33–35]. For example, when hemarthrosis is suspected, aspiration of blood from the joint confirms the diagnosis, and simultaneously prevents the devastating damage caused by the buildup of pressure from the hemorrhage and its sequelae, such as fibro-adhesions [36]. The presence of numerous tiny globules floating in the blood aspirated from the joint may indicate intra-articular fracture [37]. Aspiration of pus from a symptomatic joint establishes the diagnosis of septic arthritis, an acute emergent condition requiring immediate care. In such cases, arthrocentesis provides not only rapid diagnosis and samples for culture and for antibiotic sensitivity testing, but also instantaneous symptomatic relief.

Culturing the fluid obtained from diseased joints can reveal the presence of a single or multiple strain infection [38–42], and facilitate identification of the pathogens such that appropriate antibiotics can be administered. Isolation of *Streptococcus* from a symptomatic joint has been described in a case of bacterial endocarditis, leading to the correct diagnosis and treatment [43].

The aspiration of relatively clear fluid from perfused joints is indicative of acute, nonspecific arthritis, such as pseudogout and lupus erythematosus [44–46]. Arthrocentesis is especially critical for immediate diagnosis in disputed cases, such as suspicion of septic arthritis in hemophilic patients [47] or in patients with rheumatoid arthritis (RA) controlled by cytotoxic drugs [48]. Microscopic analysis of the synovial fluid is a valuable diagnostic tool. Identification of crystals allows differentiation of innocuous effusion due to osteoarthritis (OA) from crystal-induced inflammation, and the significantly more dangerous septic arthritis [49–51]. The determination of total white blood cell count and the percentage of polymorphonuclear cells in synovial fluid may help distinguish between inflammatory and non-inflammatory disease, and it is essential for therapeutic success. The presence of succinic acid and to a lesser extent lactic acid or depressed glucose concentrations in the synovial fluid are useful in the diagnosis of septic arthritis [49]. Total protein, albumin, and individual immunoglobulin levels allow the clinician to differentiate between mechanical, acute inflammatory, and chronic inflammatory processes, especially when compared with serum values [50]. However, the value of biochemical studies of synovial fluid has often been challenged [51].

Other studies on substances aspirated by arthrocentesis have provided insight into the pathogenesis of diseases of the joint. For example, the role of kinins in pain in inflamed joints was determined from the analyses of synovial fluid [51], and the use of kinin agonists and kallikrein inhibitors is warranted. Other pain mediators, including prostaglandins and thromboxane B, have been detected in osteoarthritis. Another study found that IgE-containing immune complexes were produced intra-articulary, thus providing evidence of their role in rheumatoid synovitis [52]. Calpain, an intracellular proteinase that also has proteoglycan-degrading activity, together with its inhibitor calpastatin, contributes to the turnover of the cartilage matrix in osteoarthritic joints [53]. The concentration of cartilage proteoglycan components in the synovial fluid reflects the synthesis and degradation of the joint cartilage matrix, and as such has been used for diagnosis, grading, and prediction of outcome of various joint diseases, such as gout, pseudogout, and reactive arthritis. Interleukin (IL)-6 induces antibody activity when present in the synovial fluid of chronically and actively diseased joints, e.g., in rheumatoid arthritis and psoriatic arthritis. Matrix metalloproteinase (MMP)-1 is a biomarker for joint disease and prognosis, although its levels may be increased by repeated arthrocentesis procedures [54]. The presence of vascular endothelial growth factors (VEGF) in osteoarthritic joints suggests that they play a role in the pathogenesis of this condition, and indeed an animal model of VEGF-induced osteoarthritis has been developed [55, 56].

While these findings represent a respectable amount of information regarding the synovial fluid, much still remains unknown about it.

3.2 The Incentives for Using the Minimally Invasive Approach for Temporomandibular Disorders

Reports on the efficiency of arthrocentesis are often related to diagnoses such as temporomandibular disorders (TMD) or even internal derangement (ID). Regrettably, both these terms are "catch phrases," often used in a commitment-free manner by clinicians and researchers alike, avoiding well-defined, established diagnostic criteria for clinical research, and treatment. Pain and dysfunction of the temporomandibular joint (TMJ) itself only account for a small proportion of the conditions included under the umbrella of TMD. Furthermore, the effectiveness of TMJ arthrocentesis, i.e., non-arthroscopic lysis and lavage, in some disorders and ineffectiveness in others has led to a refinement of our understanding of TMJ function and dysfunction. The relatively simple nature of the procedure has dramatically decreased the need for surgical interventions for a variety of disorders [56, 57].

Displacement of the articular disc in the TMJ was described and identified as a potential clinical problem over 100 years ago [56]. However, the importance of the location of the disc in TMJ pathology has decreased and disc displacement can be considered "normal" in asymptomatic individuals [57, 58]. Lavage of the upper compartment of the TMJ using arthroscopic lavage and lysis, or arthrocentesis, is not expected to change the position of the disc, yet it improves function and alleviates pain [57–63]. Taken together, there has been a shift in the literature from focusing on disc position to researching the intra-articular biomechanical and biochemical events that underlie pain and disc displacement. Understanding TMJ function and risk factors for joint pain and dysfunction should be the basis for diagnosis and treatment.

3.2.1 TMJ Integrity

The location, function, and architecture of the TMJ are complex (Fig. 3.1a, b). Its impressive endurance is facilitated by an efficient lubrication system, load attenuation, and remodeling potential. The joint becomes vulnerable when these mechanisms are compromised.

3.2.2 TMJ Lubrication

In a healthy TMJ the articular surfaces are smooth with large contact areas and high surface energy [64]. When lubrication is adequate the friction coefficient between these surfaces is almost zero [65]. Conversely, inadequate lubrication enables the generation of various physical phenomena such as increased friction, generation of adhesive force, shear stress, and rupture of articular surfaces [66].

Despite the reliance of TMJ movements on free sliding of the disc down the slope of the eminence, interest in lubrication only began about 20 years ago. Additionally, of the plethora of studies published on internal derangement of the TMJ only ~5% deal with lubrication, mostly in the last 25 years. Due to the intimate relationship of joint lubrication with the outcome of arthrocentesis, we will now describe this system.

Although there is much debate regarding joint lubrication, it seems that the system includes hyaluronic acid (hyaluron; HA) and lubricin which includes surface-active phospholipids (SAPLs).

The major component of synovial fluid is *lubricin*, a glycoprotein encoded by the gene proteoglycan 4 (Prg4). Lubricin is synthesized by chondrocytes on the surface of the articular carti-

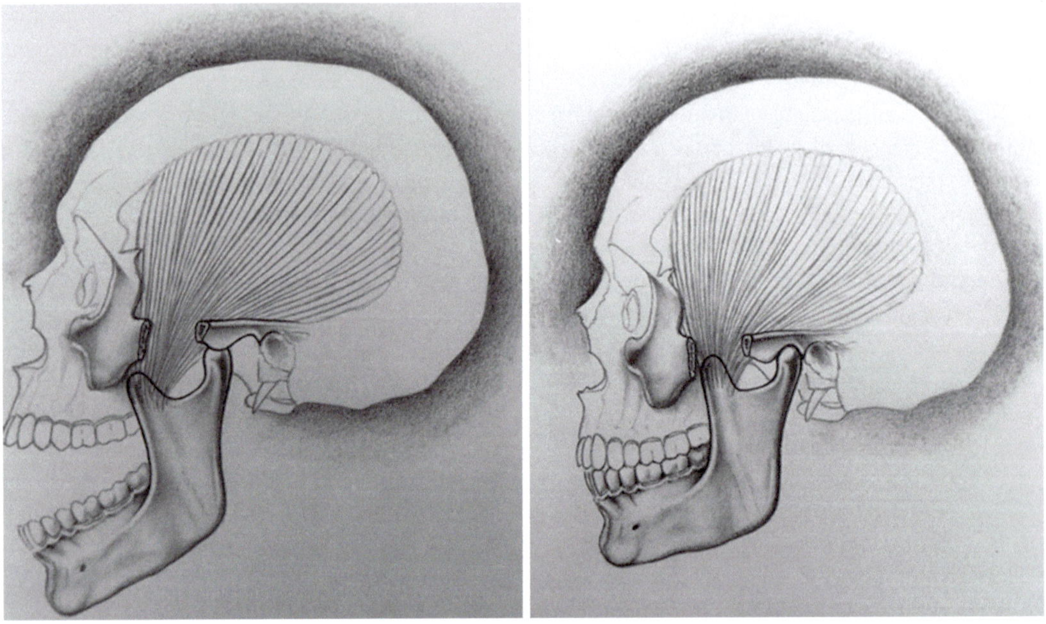

Fig. 3.1 Mandibular closed (*right*) and open (*left*) mouth position: note the unique movement which combines rotation and sliding of the mandible

lage and by synovial lining cells. It general it plays essential roles in boundary lubrication and movement in synovial joints and in the TMJ it helps preserve structural and cellular integrity [67]. Lack of lubricin in the TMJ causes osteoarthritis-like degeneration that affects the articular cartilage as well as the integrity of multiple joint tissues [68]. Chang et al. noted that the articular cartilage surface contains both hydrophilic and hydrophobic elements, and lubricin is able to mediate the frictional response between these surfaces equally, likely preventing direct surface-to-surface contact at sufficient concentrations, whereas HA provides considerably less boundary lubrication [69].

As for phospholipids (PLs), in 1997 Marchetti et al. noted that an electron-dense layer was not discernible in disordered joints, and postulated that this layer maintained joint function and prevented conditions conducive to adhesion [70]. Osmiophilic layers with embedded vesicular structures were later demonstrated using electron microscopy and were similar to the surface coating described [71–76]. Increased friction was documented following the addition of phospholipase to synovial fluid [77, 78].

Phospholipids are found in the lipid bilayer of membranes or in a free state. The unique characteristic of the "free" PLs is their high surface activity. Morphologic evidence suggests that SAPLs line the articular surface, significantly reducing friction [79–81] (Fig. 3.2a). Phospholipid bilayers enable the hydration and lubrication mechanisms that underlie low-friction sliding in biological systems. They are easily delaminated by pressure placed on opposing cartilage surfaces. The bilayers have highly hydrated head groups that act as nano-ball bearings, thereby facilitating extremely low friction [82] (Fig. 3.3).

Phospholipid composition and levels are altered by pathological processes [83]. Phospholipids are reactive oxygen species (ROS) scavengers and anti-inflammatory mediators. Thus they affect not only joint movement but also the inflammatory status of joint [2].

Hyaluronic acid (HA) is a high-molecular-weight mucopolysaccharide secreted by type B

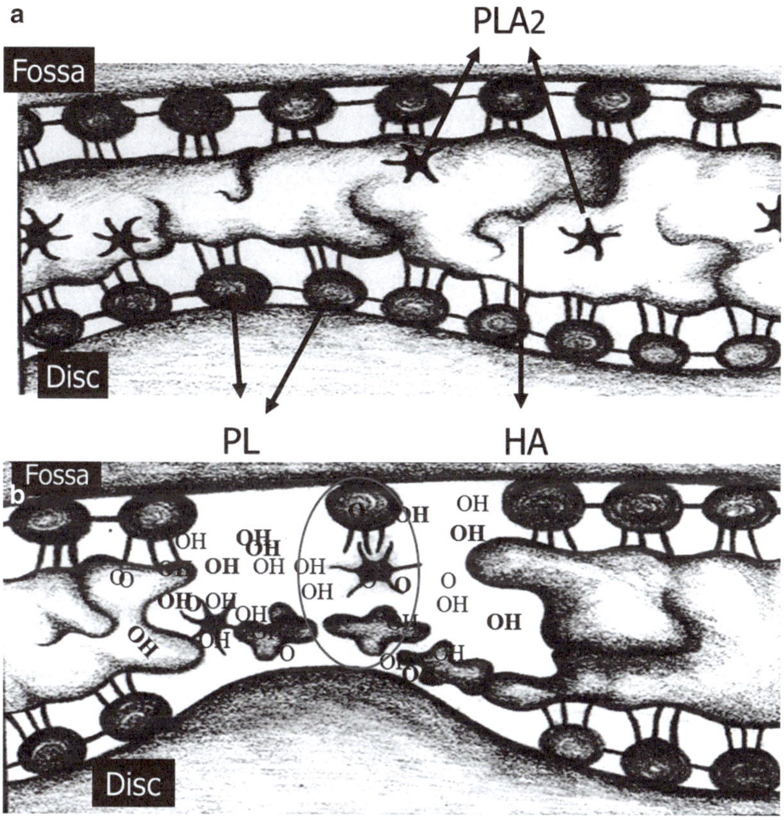

Fig. 3.2 (**a**) SAPLs line the articular surfaces (fossa and disc). They form dense boundary layers that efficiently reduce friction coefficients. Phospholipase A_2 (PLA2) is secreted by synoviocytes, chondrocytes, and osteoblasts into the synovial fluid. PLA2 specifically degrades PLs, is present in inflammatory processes, and is potentially harmful to the lubrication system. In vitro studies showed that the adhesion of HA to PL protects them from degradation by PLA2. (**b**) Among the outcomes of overloading is free radical generation that immediately degrades HA. As such, HA loses its characteristics including the protection of SAPL. Adhesive forces and friction are then generated between the uncovered high-energy articular surfaces

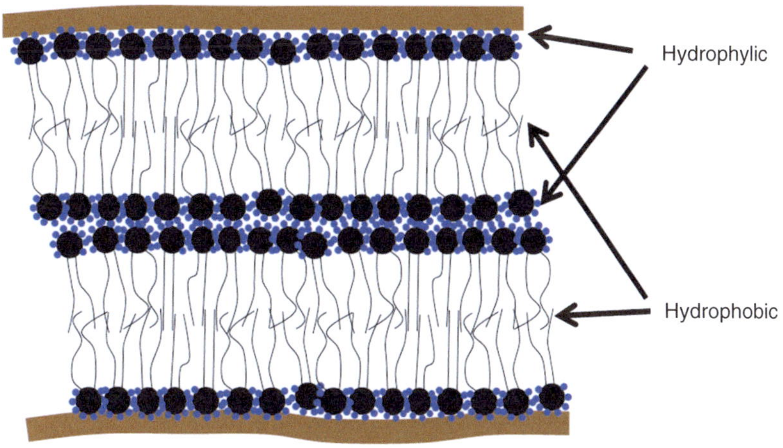

Fig. 3.3 Hydrophilic lubrication: The phospholipid bilayers are easily delaminated by pressure on opposing cartilage surfaces. These bilayers have highly hydrated head groups that act as nano-ball bearings, thereby facilitating extremely low friction

synovial cells; it is a polymer of D-glucuronic acid and *N*-acetyl-D-glucosamine comprising 0.14–0.36% of synovial fluid. The higher the molecular weight and concentration, the greater the improvement in lubrication; that is, the addition of HA to the synovial fluid reduces the coefficient of friction [84].

On the other hand, HA has a negligible load-bearing capacity and interestingly its degradation by hyaluronidase does not affect joint lubrication [85]. HA also plays an indirect role in joint lubrication by protecting PLs from being lysed by PLA2 [86] (Fig. 3.2a).

Studies on the effect of hyaluronic acid on TMJ disorders have produced controversial results [84, 85] showing no significant benefit of the HA over arthrocentesis alone. Therefore, the therapeutic value of HA injection is questionable. With its high molecular weight and high viscosity, HA acts as space filler, a wetting agent, a flow barrier within the synovium, and a protector of the cartilage surfaces [86]. In addition to its mechanical role in joint function, HA acts as a scavenger, an inhibitor of phagocytosis and chemotaxis, and an anti-inflammatory agent, and prevents angiogenesis and formation of scar tissue [86].

3.2.3 TMJ Load Attenuation

Load attenuation in synovial joints is shared by the articular cartilage, disc, and subchondral bone; 1–3% of forces are attenuated by cartilage and normal subchondral bone can attenuate about 30% of the load [87] (Fig. 3.4).

Thus, the porous subchondral bone protects the articular cartilage from damage caused by excessive loading. In addition, normal subchondral bone contains bone marrow and trabecular bone with many terminal arterial branches. The subchondral bone marrow is important for cartilage metabolism, providing more than 50% of its glucose, oxygen, and water requirements [87].

3.2.4 TMJ Condyle Remodeling Potential

In long bones, the growth plate closes at the end of the growth period. In contrast, the mesenchymal cells in the proliferative layer of the TMJ condyle have unlimited growth potential (Fig. 3.5). This unique potential is clearly demonstrated in the pathological condition of condylar hyperplasia where progressive, usually unilateral, exten-

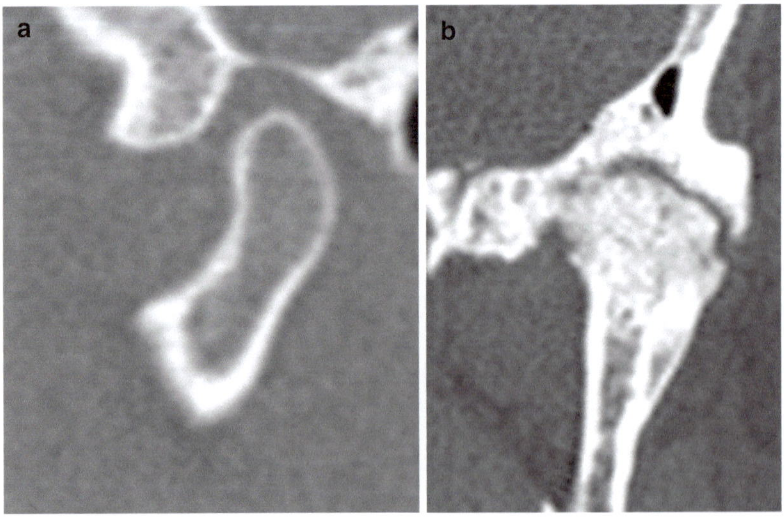

Fig. 3.4 (**a**) The normal subchondral bone attenuates 30% of the load. (**b**) With sclerosis, the subchondral bone does not attenuate load and does not provide blood supply to the articular cartilage which becomes highly vulnerable

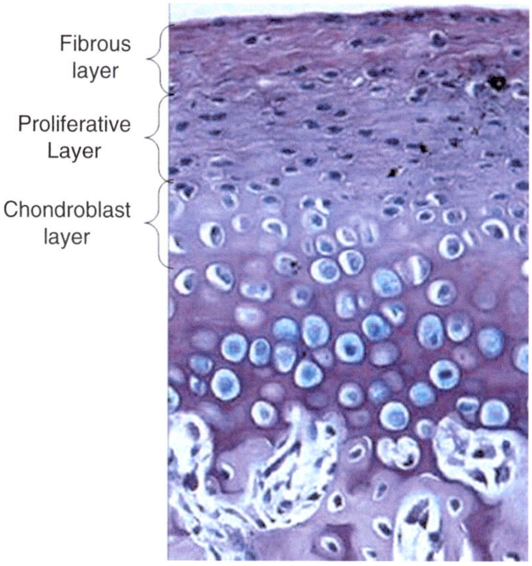

Fig. 3.5 As opposed to most synovial joints, the mesenchymal stromal cells (MSCs) constitute the proliferative layer, and are located in between the fibrous and the chondroblastic layers. The proliferative activity of the MSCs ceases around the age of 20, but retains their growth potential which allows them to respond to external stimuli throughout life (from: Li QF, Rabie AB. A new approach to control condylar growth by regulating angiogenesis. Arch Oral Biol. 2007;52(11):1009–17)

sive condylar growth occurs, resulting in facial asymmetry. This growth potential also allows the joint to remodel, rehabilitate, and adapt.

3.3 Mechanical Challenges to Joint Integrity

Joints continue to function normally for as long as their adaptive capacity is not compromised [88–91], and joint integrity remains when loading is controlled and normal movements are possible. Compromised movements and *overloading* due to both intrinsic (e.g., joint effusion, hemarthrosis) and extrinsic (e.g., parafunction, posterior bite collapse) factors, all challenge joint lubrication, load attenuation, and remodeling potential mechanically.

As the joint moves the changes in intra-articular pressure pump the synovial fluid, which supplies the nutrients and removes waste products. Lack of movement abolishes this pump-like metabolic exchange (Fig. 3.6). Controlled loading

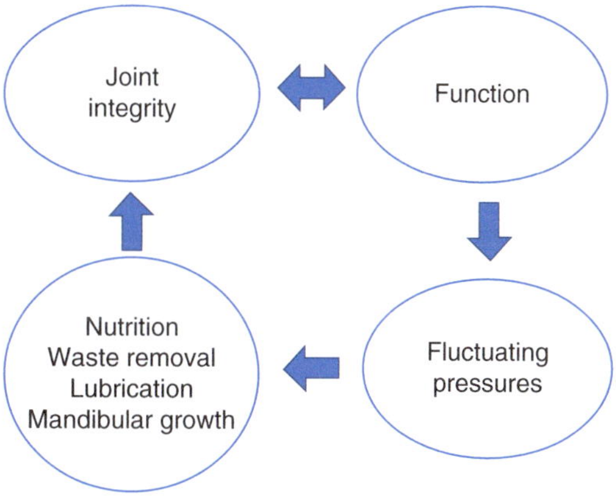

Fig. 3.6 Movement of the TMJ is associated with fluctuating intra-articular pressure, acting like a pump, enabling waste removal and the supply of oxygen and nutrition supply as well as the actual condylar growth. Therefore, immobilization is potentially harmful

is essential for the pumping effect. On the other hand, parafunctions, such as clenching, are a good example of repetitive jaw movements associated with high loading that may be harmful to synovial joints [92–97]. Parafunctions can harm all parts of the joint, e.g., (1) sclerosis of the subchondral bone which abolishes its load attenuation characteristics, (2) damage to the articular cartilage which limits remodeling, and (3) elimination of the lubrication system which prevents the disc sliding [70, 98, 99]. The generated hypoxia-reperfusion cycle in the joint evokes nonenzymatic release of ROS, such as superoxide and hydroxyl anions [100, 101]. ROS undergo rapid chemical reactions, and degraded hyaluronic acid decreases the viscosity of the synovial fluid [102]. In vitro studies had shown that the degraded form of hyaluronic acid indirectly affects joint lubrication. By failing to inhibit phospholipase A_2, which lyses SAPLs, the continuity of the SAPL layer is jeopardized (Fig. 3.2b). The lubrication system and subchondral bone constantly rebuild itself in adaptable condition unless joint loading (intrinsic or extrinsic) and immobilization exceed the joint's adaptive capacity [76].

For example, in the absence of lubricant the smooth articular surfaces imply large contact areas that together with the surface's elasticity (such as at the disc) and the high surface energy lead to increased adhesive forces, and friction up to shear and rupture of articular surfaces [64, 103–110]. We believe that the latter is associated with the pathogenesis of internal derangement. Various factors leading to internal derangement have been proposed. The suggestion that spasm of the superior head of the lateral pterygoid muscle is responsible for the displacement of the disc has been rejected [108, 109]. Joint laxity might be a contributing factor but is not prevalent in enough cases of disc displacement [110]. Trauma was thought to be involved; however, several studies have failed to confirm significant relationships between indirect trauma and disc displacement [111, 112] and the prevalence of disc displacement in patients with and without history of whiplash is similar [112]. Another possibility is interference in the free articular movements caused by impaired lubrication [113–115] (Fig. 3.7). It seems that as a result of repetitive disc hesitation the ligaments are gradually stretched [116], while the condyle is pulled freely forward by the lateral pterygoid muscle, increasing disc mobility and finally inducing its displacement. In support, TMJ arthrography in disc displacement with reduction (DDwR) demonstrates disfiguration of the lower compartment that proves that the condyle is sliding under the "hesitating" disc, thereby stretching the anterior wall of the capsule [115, 117, 118].

The joint may deteriorate when overloaded or when the lack of movement is associated with subchondral bone sclerosis, preventing delivery of the required nutrients to the articular cartilage. The load attenuation and the remodeling potential of the proliferative layer of the articular cartilage are also affected.

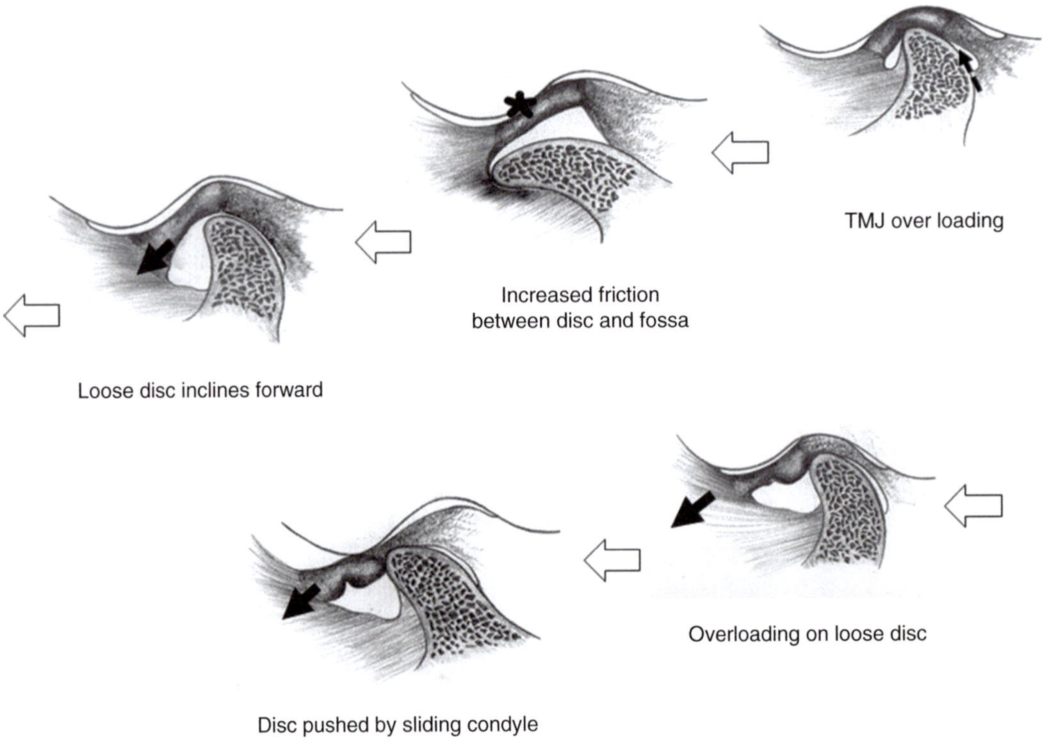

Fig. 3.7 Pathophysiology of the process disc displacement: Upon overloading (*arrow*) generation of free radicals disrupts the lubrication system associated with slow sliding of the healthy disc (*star*). The condyle is then pulled forward by the lateral pterygoid muscle away from the disc, against the anterior wall of the lower compartment (*arrow*), thus stretching the joints' ligaments. The now loose disc falls forward (*arrow*). When clenching the disc is now repetitively pushed forwards, causing further displacement (*arrow*). Opening is associated with further disc displacement (*arrow*)

3.4 Temporomandibular Joint Arthrocentesis: Technique

Before describing the technique, one must note that the procedure should always be performed in conjunction with the elimination of uncontrolled loading (such as parafunction, premature contacts, posterior bite collapse) (Fig. 3.8) and intra- or extra-articular causes of limited mandibular movements must also be corrected.

Murakami et al. were the first to offer a systematic description of (TMJ) arthrocentesis, which they termed *"manipulation technique followed by pumping and hydraulic pressure"* [119]. Arthrocentesis of the TMJ, as discussed in this chapter, is a modification of the traditional method, in which two needles are introduced into the upper joint space. This adaptation permits massive lavage of the joint, as well as aspiration and injection [120].

The seated patient is inclined at a 45° angle, with their head turned to the unaffected side to provide access to the affected joint. After proper preparation of the target site, the external auditory meatus is blocked with cotton soaked in mineral oil. The points of needle insertion are marked on the skin according to the method suggested by McCain for the performance of arthroscopy as follows: A line is drawn from the middle of the tragus to the outer canthus (Fig. 3.9a–c). The posterior entrance point is located along the canthotragal line, approximately 10 mm from the middle of the tragus and 2 mm below the line. Murakami et al. and Segami only used the posterior port for pumping fluid into the upper compartment in order to increase the hydraulic pressure within the joint [119, 121, 122]. The anterior point of entry is 10 mm further along the line and 10 mm below it. The markings on the skin indicate the location of the articular fossa and the eminence of the TMJ.

A local anesthetic is injected at the planned entrance points. A 19-gauge needle connected to a 1 mL syringe filled with lactated Ringer's solution

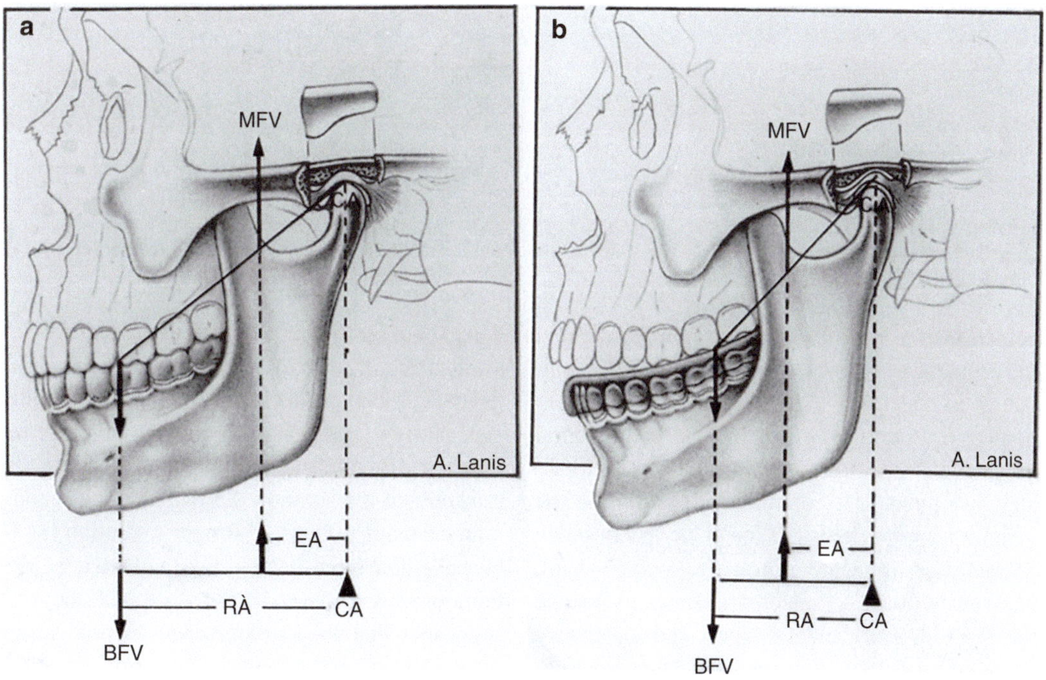

Fig. 3.8 The use of a simple interocclusal appliance (IOA): (**a**, **b**) Clenching on a uniformly elevated occlusal plane decreases the intra-articular pressure by 81.2% due to the reduction in the length of the resistance arm: the distance between the condyle and the bite force vector in a lever III system. *EA* effective arm, *RA* resistance arm, *CA* condylar axis, *BFV* bite force vector

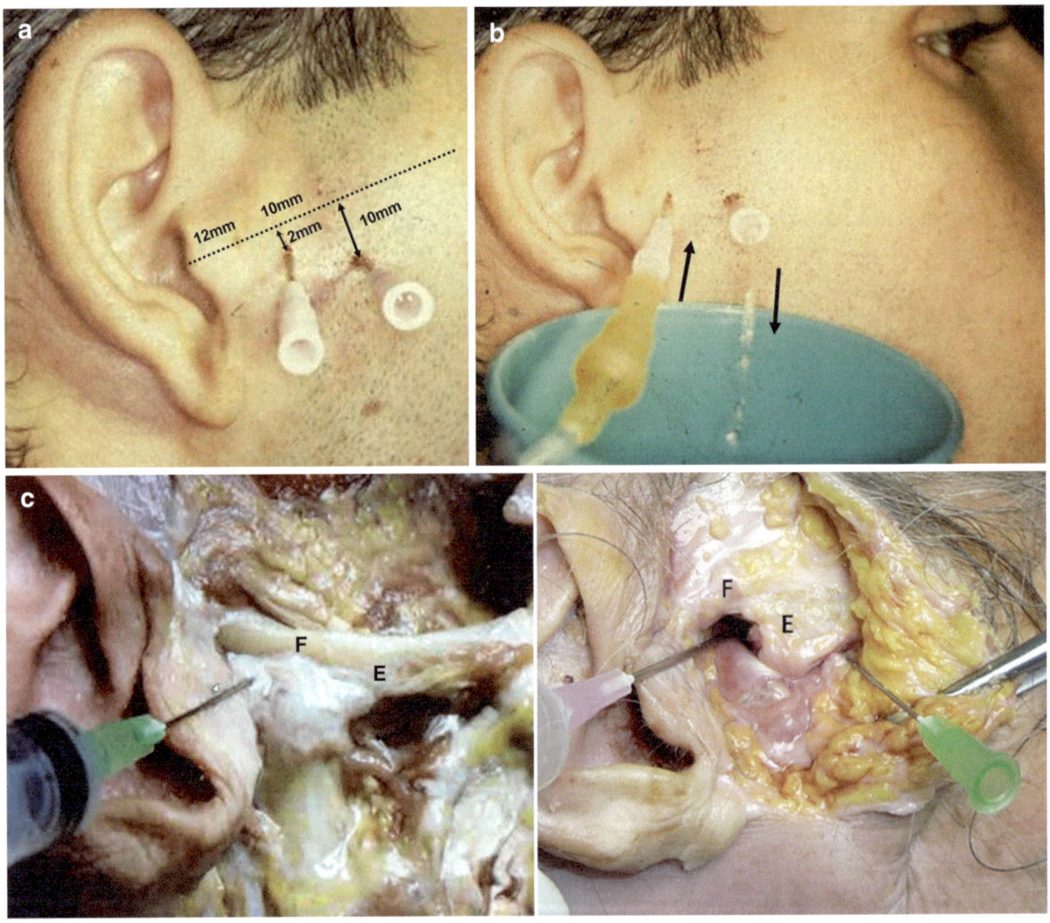

Fig. 3.9 Arthrocentesis of the temporomandibular joint (TMJ): (**a**) The two points of entrance into the superior compartment of the TMJ. (**b**) Flow through the superior compartment. (**c**) Exposed TMJ in a cadaver: *Left*: The joint capsule in relation to the tragus and the route of entrance into the fossa region in the upper compartment. *Right*: Exposed upper compartment. Two needles are located, left in the fossa and right in front of the eminence. *E* Eminence, *F* Fossa

is then inserted into the superior compartment at the articular fossa (posterior point) aided by palpation of the fossa and the patient opens their mouth or performs intermittent contralateral movements. The solution is injected and immediately aspirated. It is common for the fluid in the syringe to be sucked into the joint space which normally has a negative pressure. Next, 2–3 mL bupivacaine 0.5% is injected in order to distend the upper distended anterior space and anesthetize the adjacent tissues. A second 19-gauge needle is then inserted into the compartment in the area of the articular eminence to enable the Ringer's solution to flow freely through the superior compartment (Fig. 3.9a–c). The amount of flow depends upon the purpose of the procedure such as releasing the disc in ADP compared to washing away degraded products in OA. In cases of sluggish outflow, additional needles may be inserted into the distended compartment to enhance the transport of the solution. Zardeneta et al. recommended using 100 mL of Ringer's solution [123], because denatured hemoglobin and various proteinases were recovered in this fraction. Kaneyama suggested that the concentration of bradykinin, interleukin-6, and protein during arthrocentesis is only effectively reduced by more than 200 mL of lavage, and when a perfusate volume of 300–400 mL was used the protein and bradykinin were no longer detectable [121, 124]. A simplified procedure can be performed, whereby the second needle is inserted next to the first one, in the posterior rather than the anterior recess, and saline is then flushed through the upper compartment.

A single-needle cannula method, in which inflow and outflow are through the same cannula and lumens, as first described by Guarda-Nardini [125] is also acceptable. Another variation is the double- or dual-needle cannula method, in which inflow and outflow are through the same cannula but at different ports and lumens [124]. Usually a single session is used, although more intensive protocols such as five weekly sessions have been described [85, 125]. During the lavage, the mandible is guided through opening, excursive, and protrusive movements to facilitate free sliding of the disc [74]. Upon termination of the procedure and following the removal of one needle, medication, such as hyaluronic acid (HA), can be injected into the joint space [126–128]. The molecular weight at which HA should be injected and its effectiveness are still being debated [125, 129, 130]. Inflammatory products should be removed by arthrocentesis prior to injection because HA is instantly degraded by free radicals. Other medications that can be injected into the joint include (1) steroids—Depo-Medrol (methylprednisolone acetate), betamethasone, or Kenalog (triamcinolone acetonide) and (2) opioids (usually morphine or fentanyl). Opioids are used to reduce postoperative pain and facilitate movement; they seem to improve pain relief more than simple arthrocentesis alone [17]. Recently, and controversially, platelet-rich plasma (PRP) has been injected into the TMJ in combination with arthrocentesis or as a solo treatment due to its potential healing properties via recruitment, proliferation, and differentiation of cells [131]. More long-term controlled trials are needed as is verification or dismissal of the concern that PRP promotes extensive bone growth or ankylosis.

Contraindications for arthrocentesis include:

- Regional or systemic infectious diseases such as cellulitis overlying the injection site (unless the diagnosis is septic arthritis)
- Regional neoplastic disease
- Incontinuity of the base of skull in the area of the glenoid fossa
- Former open joint surgery or discectomy
- Fibrous and/or osseous ankylosis

Complications are rare and mostly transient. Temporary facial paresis or paralysis from the local anesthetic agent may be seen. Swelling of the neighboring tissues caused by perfusion of Ringer's solution might also follow arthrocentesis [132]. Both signs disappear within a few hours.

Penetration into the brain and inner ear and damage to the facial nerve have been reported. However, if the guidelines are followed these complications do not occur.

3.5 Mode of Action

Lavage of the upper compartment by TMJ arthrocentesis forces separation of the flexible disc from the fossa, washes away degraded particles and inflammatory components, and reduces effusion hemarthrosis, inflammation, or infection that may cause significant damage when associated with increased intrinsic loading.

The literature describes the elimination of numerous inflammatory products. The levels of cytokines in TMJ synovial fluid, following successful and unsuccessful arthrocentesis, reflect the effect of the procedure on pain [133]. Eliav et al. found that the mean electrical detection threshold ratios in areas surrounding the auriculotemporal nerve were significantly elevated after arthrocentesis, indicating a resolution of hypersensitivity [134]. The released disc and the elimination of inflammatory products and pain enable the joint to be rehabilitated and return to the normal range of movement (ROM), which is the hallmark of joint health.

When arthrocentesis fails important diagnostic information is revealed. Failure of lavage implies that surgical means are required for diagnostic and/or treatment purposes and are legitimate to release the joint and rehabilitate its movement. Indeed, arthrocentesis or arthroscopy is a prerequisite for most surgical interventions.

3.6 Patient Evaluation

3.6.1 Patient Self-Assessment and Clinical Examination

A detailed and thorough patient evaluation is essential for an accurate diagnosis which is the key to appropriate treatment. Each patient should be evaluated as if assembling a new puzzle. A conclusion can only be drawn when all pieces are collected and properly assessed; missing pieces must be searched for and misleading pieces of information should be recognized and discarded.

A useful diagnostic aid is a patient-completed questionnaire including details about the chief complaint and its history in the patient's own words, the initial symptoms, their characteristics, onset and duration, triggering, modifying or aggravating factors, and the presence of oral habits (Table 3.1). Location of pain should be illustrated by the patient on a diagram of the head and neck region. Patients with intra-articular pain usually locate pain accurately around the joint and ear. Pain characteristics and timing are noted: on forced opening, on biting and/or chewing, on the contralateral side, and upon joint loading. A joint-loading test is performed by biting asking the patient to bite on a wooden stick placed on the canines and molars on both sides and to point to the painful area and score its intensity. Following the lever class III system, intra-articular inflammation is associated with localized joint pain when the patient bites contralaterally, while mus-

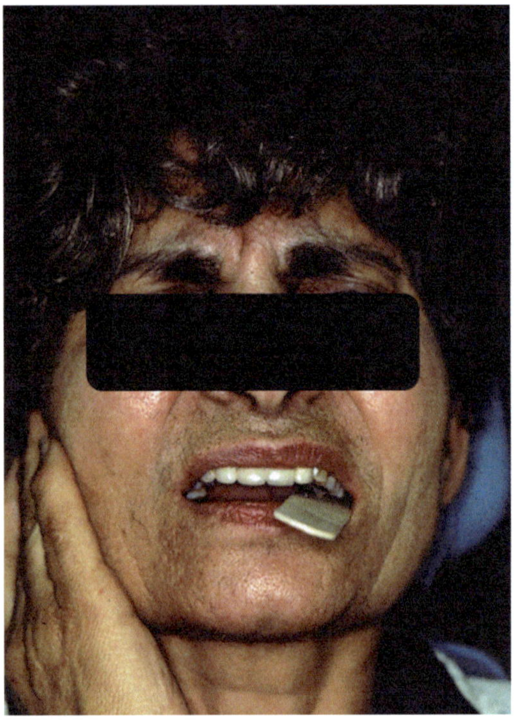

Fig. 3.10 *Loading test* based upon lever III system. The longer the resistance arm (see also Fig. 3.8) the higher the load on the joint. Pain is initiated when the joint is inflamed. On the other hand biting on the ipsilateral side unloads the joint

Table 3.1 Comparison between the common clinical signs and symptoms and imaging of the anchored disc phenomenon, disc displacement without reduction, and osteoarthritis (MMO Maximal Mouth Opening, CLM Contra Lateral Movement, ILM Ipsi- Lateral Movement)

Characteristics	Anchored disc phenomenon	Disc displacement without reduction	Osteoarthritis
Occurrence	Sudden	Gradual	Sudden/gradual
Past clicks	No (30%)	Yes	Yes or no
MMO	15–25 mm	30–45 mm	10–30 mm
CLM	Limited	Limited	Limited
ILM	Normal	Normal	Limited
Pain (self-assessment)	−/+	+/−	None to severe
Dysfunction (self-assessment)	+	−	− to +++
Magnetic resonance imaging (open-mouth position)	Anchored disc to fossa	Nonreduced displaced disc	Effusion, adhesion displaced/deformed perforated disc +/− Bone erosion, sclerosis +/−
Effect of arthrocentesis	Excellent	Moderate	Very good (80%)

cle disorders usually result in pain ipsilateral to the loading (Fig. 3.10). The severity of pain at rest and during function as well as the extent of any dysfunction should be assessed using a visual analogue scale (VAS) that enables objective assessment of changes over time and response to treatment. A thorough dental history and examination are essential to exclude relevant primary or secondary occlusal problems such as deviation of the dental midline, premature contact, and collapsed or open bites. Previous treatments for the presenting problem and the result obtained should be recorded. General health problems and current or past medications need to be recorded as they are highly relevant to diagnosis and treatment.

Clinical examination of the TMJ should begin with the clinician becoming familiar with the patient's behavior, relative sensitivity, and their primary complaint, e.g., limited function, pain with function and/or joint sounds, and changes in occlusion. The examination and interview should be performed facing the patient so that responses can be assessed and asymmetry of form or movement can be observed. The joint should then be carefully palpated with uniform pressure from its lateral aspect and posteriorly both in the open and closed positions. The degree of resultant tenderness and pain may be recorded on a simple ordinal scale (0 = no pain, 1 = mild pain, 2 = moderate pain, and 3 = very painful) or employing a 10 cm VAS scale.

The presence and characteristics of joint sounds should be recorded. This may be performed digitally via light palpation or via stethoscopic auscultation. Joint sounds may be present continuously throughout movement or at particular positions. Maximal unassisted and assisted interincisal mouth opening should be accurately measured; the presence and pattern of deviation should be recorded. For example, persistent deviation to one side is usually characteristic of ipsilateral limited joint movements due to disorders such as in osteoarthritis anchored disc phenomenon or disc derangement without reduction. Diagnosis is based upon the location of pain when the mandible is forced to the midline. Deviation during opening that corrects itself following a joint sound (the classic "S"-shaped mouth opening) is characteristic of ipsilateral DDwR. Pain produced on assisted opening, its severity, and very importantly its location should be carefully noted taking into account proximity of the posterior part of the masseter and the pterygoid muscles to the joint. Other characteristics associated with limitation in jaw movement should be recorded when present. The anchored disc phenomenon is usually associated with a sudden limited mouth opening while muscle disorders or disc displacement without reduction (DDwoR) may allow increased opening with manual assistance. In ankylosis limited mouth opening has a history and is persistent and inflexible. Other jaw movements such as protrusion and lateral excursions should be accurately assessed and measured on a mm scale, and the exact location of resultant pain recorded. These measurements are important for differentiating TMJ origin from extra-articular causes such as muscles and coronoid hyperplasia [2, 135–137].

If the signs and symptoms do not yield a comprehensive diagnosis the patient should be carefully reevaluated. Figure 3.11 demonstrates such patient with final diagnosis of nasopharyngeal carcinoma (Fig. 3.12).

3.6.2 Imaging

Imaging of the TMJ is complementary to the clinical examination and is used to confirm a diagnosis, aid in treatment planning, and assess disease severity. For routine screening or evaluation, panoramic radiographs are adequate. For the basic evaluation of the TMJ, transpharyngeal and transcranial radiographs in the closed and open-mouth positions provide information on the hard tissue structures and ROM [3].

Other imaging modalities of the TMJ, such as computerized tomography (CT), magnetic resonance imaging (MRI), cone-beam CT (CBCT), or bone scan, should only be considered when the diagnostic process indicates their need; they may also be essential prior to surgical intervention. MRI has greatly improved our understanding of TMJ disorders and indeed clinical examination and occurrence of certain signs may accurately predict the abnormalities seen on MRI [138].

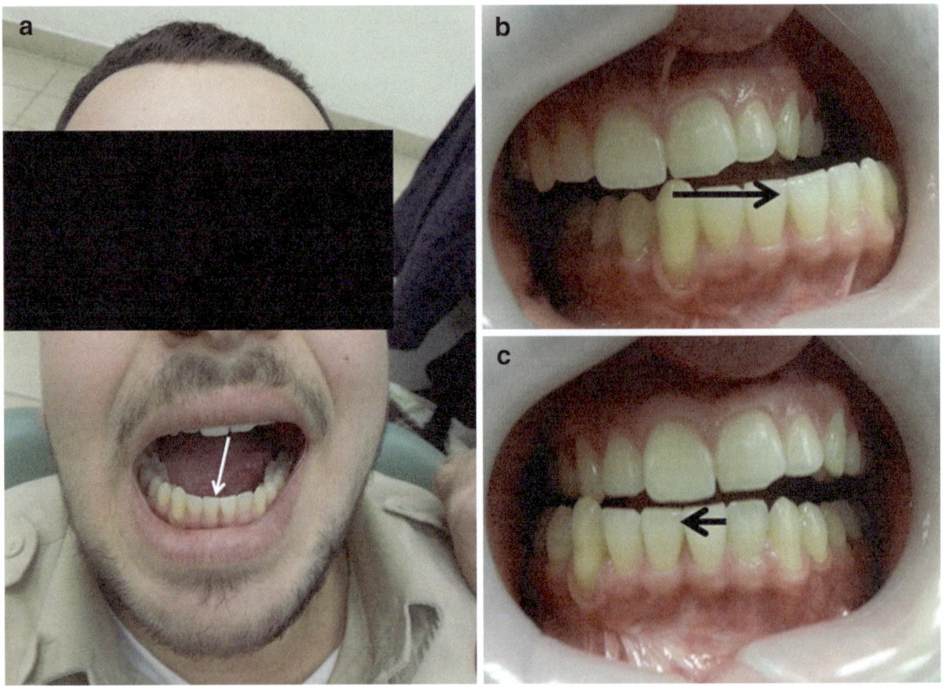

Fig. 3.11 Contradicting signs and symptoms should call for further investigation: (**a**) A 20-year-old man, presented with limited mouth opening and a persistent deviation to the right 1 year after left mandibular fracture. Sounds obvious? However, the lateral movements to the left are normal and limited to the right (**b**, **c**)

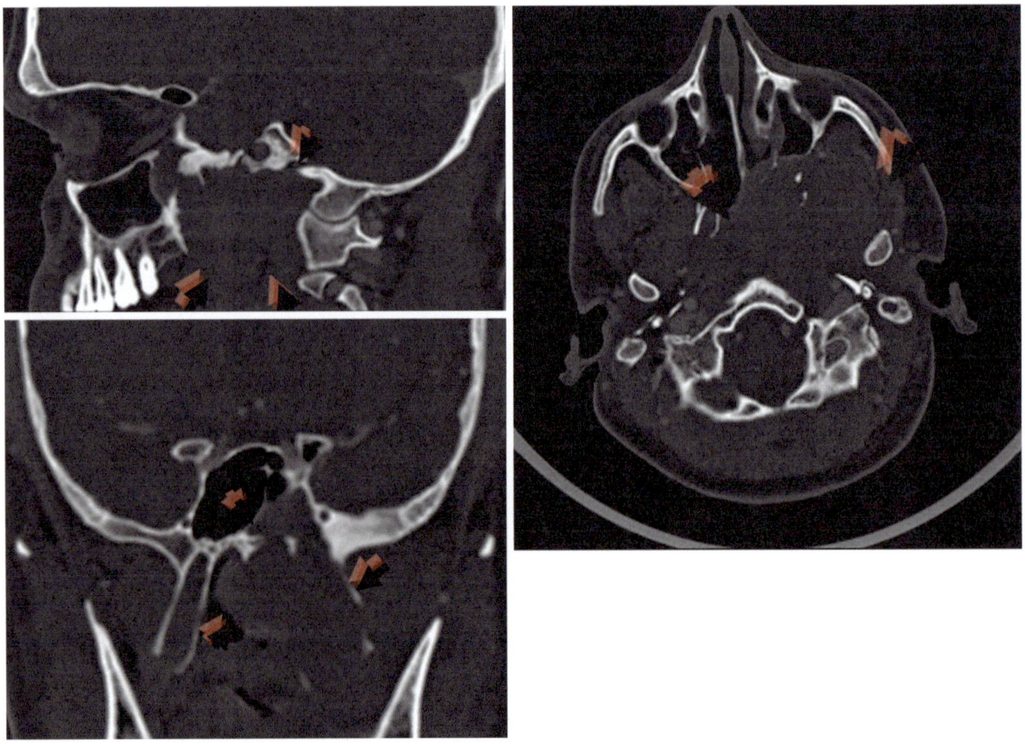

Fig. 3.12 Further evaluation revealed nasopharyngeal carcinoma as demonstrated on the left side (*arrows*)

Consecutive MRI images may be performed to create a dynamic representation of joint movement and this clearly shows the causes of limited movement, such as anchored disc or disc displacements without reduction. Additionally, joint effusions and mandibular condyle marrow abnormalities can be detected using MRI [139, 140].

Bone scanning (scintigraphy or radionuclide studies) provides information on the metabolic activity of bone, showing increased activity in osteoarthritic joints, even in the absence of radiographic changes [141]. Severe osteoarthritic joint degeneration associated with a negative bone scan indicates inactive disease, making scintigraphy an invaluable tool.

3.7 The Role of Arthrocentesis in Various TMJ Disorders

Although arthrocentesis has been widely used and researched, the reports often describe results obtained for diagnoses such as TMJ disorders (TMD) or TMJ internal derangement, and lack information about signs and symptoms of the patients [142–148]. Arthrocentesis is effective for localized TMJ pain limited function and is able to reduce the severity of clicking and disc displacement [76, 113, 114, 134, 145, 149, 150]. There are studies confirming the long-term effectiveness of arthrocentesis [120, 126, 142–145, 151–153], yet the need for high-quality long-term prospective studies is clear [154–156]. However in order to study the efficacy of arthrocentesis, clear definitions of the disorders are required. Conversely, studying the effects of arthrocentesis will also increase our understanding of TMJ disorders as happened following the introduction of arthrography and MRI.

3.7.1 The Clicking Joint

Clicking could be either intermittent or constant. The first occurs due to sudden separation of the adhered disc from the fossa. The latter appears upon mouth opening and closing as a result of disc displacement. Upon opening the displaced disc is reduced to the proper position relative to the condoyle. The reduction is associated with the clicking noise followed by the disc sliding down the slope of the eminence. Upon closing, the disc returns to the displaced position, and this may also be associated with a clicking sound. Clinical examination usually reveals a normal range of motion. The clicking noise might be associated with an intolerable noise, and/or severe joint pain mostly due to overloading of the retrodiscal tissue.

The pathogenesis of disc adherence and disc displacement suggests that joint loading should be considered among the contributing factors [114, 115]. Short-term studies support this theory [157, 158]. Prospective long-term studies are warranted. The lavage of the upper joint compartment, either by arthroscopic lavage and lysis or by arthrocentesis, allows free disc sliding without events of adherence in intermittent clicking [60, 120]. In constant clicking it provides better disc sliding and any changes in disc location are due to the release of adhesions and not because of changes in the anatomical position of the displaced disc [62, 63]. This explains the debatable efficiency of arthrocentesis for treating clicking caused by disc displacement.

Arthrocentesis may soften the severity of the noise and reduced localized joint pain upon release of the adhered disc to the fossa and eliminate joint effusion [3, 159]. Pain associated with overloading of the retrodiscal tissue is eliminated by an IOA. Intermittent clicking, on the other hand, is reversible. Lavage of the upper compartment releases the disc and enables both the condyle with the disc to move simultaneously.

3.7.2 Limited Mouth Opening

Many studies have described the effectiveness of arthrocentesis in resolving limited mouth opening but have not been suitably detailed [126, 140, 143–145]. Diagnoses such as DDwoR [126, 142, 160, 161] or closed lock [25, 162, 163] might be insufficient if not based on clear criteria. For example, a diagnosis of "closed lock" may include patients with DDwoR, anchored disc phenomenon, or osteoarthritis, each reacting differently to arthrocentesis [163, 164].

3.7.2.1 Disc Displacement Without Reduction

DDwoR describes the situation in which the disc becomes displaced and non-reducible condylar sliding becomes partially obstructed, and consequently mouth opening is partially limited. Unless painful, this disorder can remain unnoticed by the affected individual.

Symptomatic DDwoR is characterized by relatively limited mouth opening (ranging between 35 and 40 mm) that develops gradually with a history of clicking. Pain may occur on forced mouth opening and on loading. Stretching of the innervated retrodiscal tissue causes it to become a pseudodisc under adaptable conditions. In plain open-mouth radiographs and computerized tomography scans, the TMJ always shows evidence of condylar sliding; however it is limited. In arthrography and MRI, the disc appears to be located in front of the condyle in both closed- and open-mouth positions without signs that typify degenerative joint disease.

Many studies confirm that arthrocentesis improved limited mouth movements and decreased the pain caused by disc displacement [142, 147, 160, 164]. A study of 19 patients (15 females, 4 males, 41.4 ± 15.64 years of age) with DDwoR, with a mean maximal mouth opening of 31.9 ± 7.1 mm and contralateral movements of 8.2 ± 2.9 mm at presentation, showed marginal improvement after arthrocentesis (reaching 36.44 ± 6.82 mm and 8.44 ± 2.35 mm, respectively). Pain and dysfunction levels, as assessed by the patients, were slightly reduced from 8.4 ± 3.5 to 5.0 ± 3.9, and 6.0 ± 3.2 to 5.3 ± 4.3, respectively, on a 1 to 10 visual analogue scale (unpublished data). It is not surprising that arthrocentesis, which cannot change the disc shape or position [62, 63], only provides limited relief for these patients. The improvements described by other authors were probably in patients less strictly diagnosed, thus including other disorders [163, 164] as discussed below.

3.7.2.2 Anchored Disc Phenomenon (Figs. 3.13 and 3.14)

Anchored disc phenomenon is characterized by sudden severe and persistent limited mouth opening, ranging from 10 to 30 mm (considerably less than in DDwoR), with deviation to the affected side. Contralateral movements are limited, and on protrusion the mandible deviates toward the affected side. A history of clicking is not obligatory. While there is usually no pain in the TMJ upon loading, forced mouth opening evokes pain in the affected joint. In long-standing anchored disc phenomena, the clinical characteristics become less apparent. In plain open-mouth radiographs and computerized tomography scans, the TMJ shows evidence of a non-sliding, rotated, normally structured condyle [164–167]. In MRI, the disc appears attached to the articular eminence and the condoyle slides underneath it [165, 168]. It was suggested that a "suction-cup effect," whereby the disc clings to the articular eminence, is responsible for the limitation of disc movement [60]. However, the introduction of a needle into the upper joint space abolishes the vacuum and does not cure this limitation; therefore adhesive forces between the disc and fossa have been implicated [163, 165, 167].

Overloading of the joint is considered damaging to the normal lubrication of the joint. Adhesive forces may be generated between the pressed, denuded, smooth, elastic wet disc and the eminence and even a small area of adhesion between the two opposing surfaces is capable of suddenly preventing the disc from sliding down the slope of the eminence [163, 165, 167]. Forced opening is not recommended, as it pulls away the adhered disc and the ligaments are stretched, thus disrupting the tight relationship between the condyle and the disc. Arthrocentesis neutralizes these adhesive forces and separates the flexible disc from the surface of the eminence, thus enabling normal disc sliding [61, 120, 166]. Physical therapy, which is not indicated while the disc is stuck, should be intensively used following release. Under these circumstances recurrence is extremely rare [61]. Failure of the procedure means that the diagnosis needs to be reevaluated.

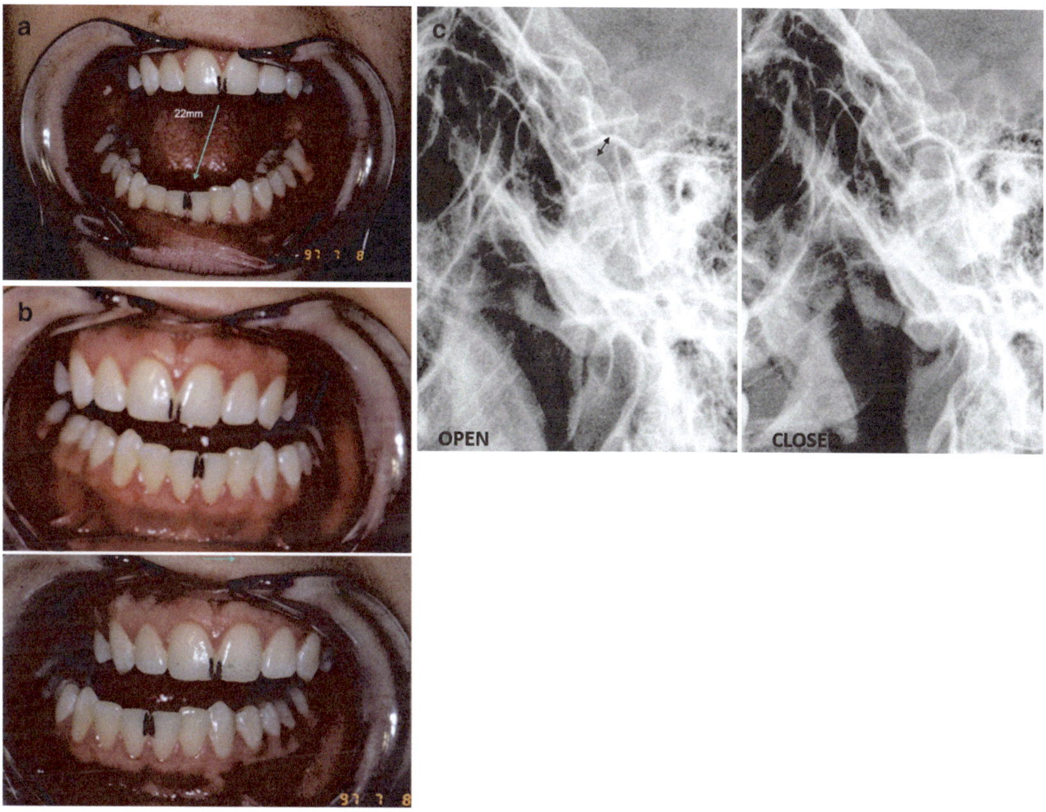

Fig. 3.13 Anchored disc phenomenon (ADP) in the Rt TMJ: (**a**) Limited mouth opening with deviation to the right. Localized arthralgia of the right joint upon forced opening. (**b**) Limited lateral movement to the left and normal to the right. (**c**) Transcranial radiograph in closed- and open-mouth positions. Note the lack of condylar sliding down the slope of the eminence

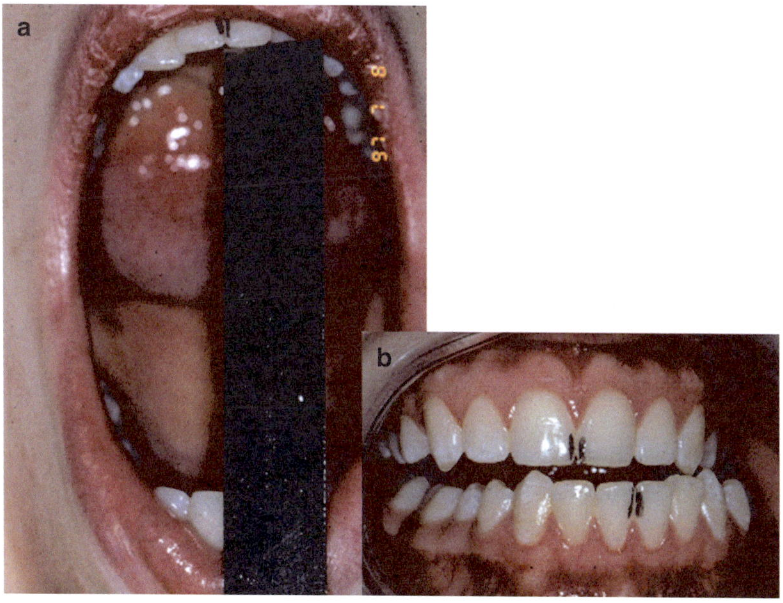

Fig. 3.14 Immediate response to arthrocentesis of right temporomandibular joint: (**a**) Normal mouth opening. (**b**) Normal lateral movements to the left

3.7.3 Symptomatic Osteoarthritis

Temporomandibular joint osteoarthritis (TMJOA) is characterized by chronic inflammation in the synovial tissue, progressive cartilage degradation, subchondral bone sclerosis, and cysts; however the pathogenesis is controversial [169] (Figs. 3.15 and 3.16).

The TMJ is an adaptable organ and therefore patients with osteoarthritic changes can remain symptom free. Symptoms begin when the joint is unable to adapt. At this stage, the patient typically reports at least one of the following complaints: joint pain both at rest and upon movement in all directions, limited mouth opening, pain on biting and chewing (usually on the contra lateral side), early-morning joint stiffness and swelling, and changes in occlusion, such as anterior, ipsi, or contralateral open bite depending on the cause. Some occlusal changes contribute to OA such as posterior bite collapse, premature contact, or absence of leeway space. Clinical examination reveals localized pain on palpation and on loading of the affected joint, associated with variable pain in the masticatory muscles. Crepitation in the arthritic joint, with or without clicking, may occur during movement. The history of clicking is variable [170]. Limited mouth opening may or may not be accompanied by pain in the affected joint and is noted upon attempting to open the mouth or to force the jaw laterally in either direction.

The inconstant presentation of osteoarthritis is probably a result of the variety of factors associated with the disease. It is essential to study each patient in order to gain insight into the origin of their signs and symptoms and then select the appropriate treatment approach. Extrinsic (parafunction, posterior bite collapse) or intrinsic (joint effusion, hemarthrosis) overloading increases intra-articular pressure and disrupts the lubrication system, gradually causing fatigue and wear of joint elements [105, 171–174].

Overloading is also associated with subchondral bone sclerosis and affects load attenuation and blood supply to the articular cartilage. It also allows cytokines, growth factors, and prostaglandins produced by the subchondral bone tissue to cross through the bone-cartilage interface [87, 175]. The restricted movement further compromises the blood supply and the elimination of the inflammatory products [176]. Arthrocentesis washes away the “inflamed” synovial fluid, removes degradation products, forces apart the joint surfaces enabling movement, decreases joint loading and pain, and is highly effective in bringing the joint back to its adaptable state [177–179]. Of course, in addition to the procedure other interventions such as IOA, soft diet, medication, frequent and intensive physiotherapy, and when required correction of occlusion should be used. Our recent analysis of 79 TMJOA patients, 67 (84.8%) females and 12 (15.2%) males with age range of 13–70 years (mean 36.9 ± 1.7 years), and follow-up of 56.9 ± 6.7 month showed that 64 patients (81%) reacted favorably to arthrocentesis; therefore surgical intervention was unnecessary. For these patients, maximal mouth opening increased from 26.25 ± 0.8 mm to 39.24 ± 0.9 mm ($p < 0.001$). Pain and dysfunction scores were reduced from 6.92 ± 0.2 to 2.36 ± 0.3, and from 7.37 ± 0.2 to 2.24 ± 0.4 (on a scale of 0–to–10), respectively ($p < 0.001$). Overall patient satisfaction with arthrocentesis was 8.78 ± 0.3 (on a scale of 0–10). No permanent complications were observed. Interestingly, there were no correlations between the clinical signs and symptoms and the severity of the radiographic changes or the response to arthrocentesis. Thus these elements cannot be used to predict the outcome of arthrocentesis. In other words, in symptomatic osteoarthritis the doctor cannot predict the efficiency of arthrocentesis based upon the individual clinical and/or radiological findings. However, the clinician can clarify that the chance of success is about 82%. Furthermore arthrocentesis is a reliable diagnostic tool that will determine the need for further surgical intervention or further evaluation (Figs. 3.17 and 3.18).

It is important to note that the Wilkes classification is based upon the assumption that the clinical signs and symptoms progress with the radiographic changes [179]. Therefore the lack of correlation between the clinical and the radiologic findings calls for reassessment of this

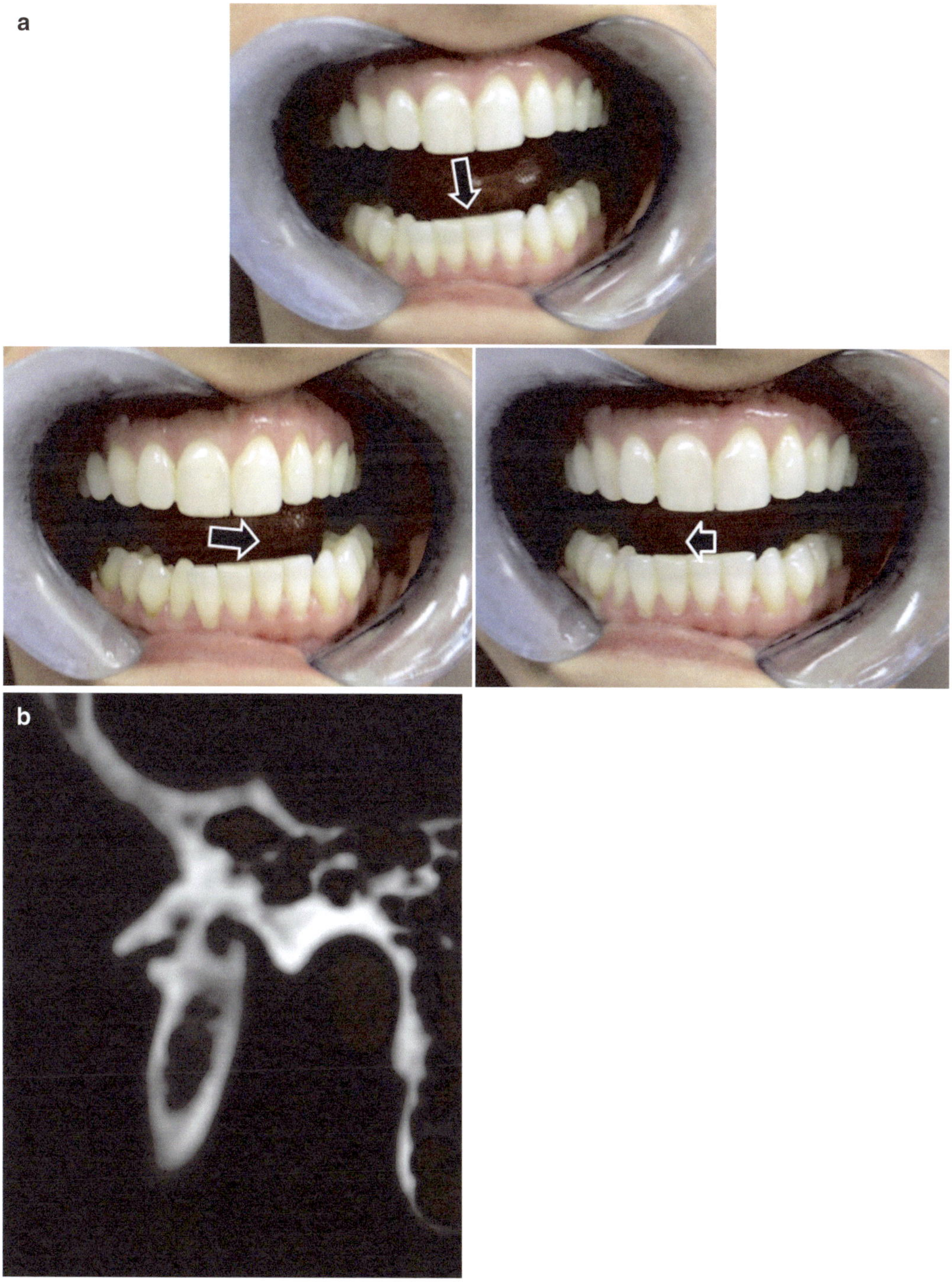

Fig. 3.15 45-year-old lady with symptomatic left TMJOA, not responding to non-surgical treatment for 6 weeks: (**a**) LMO with slight deviation to the left with severe pain upon loading. (**b**) Severe degenerative changes

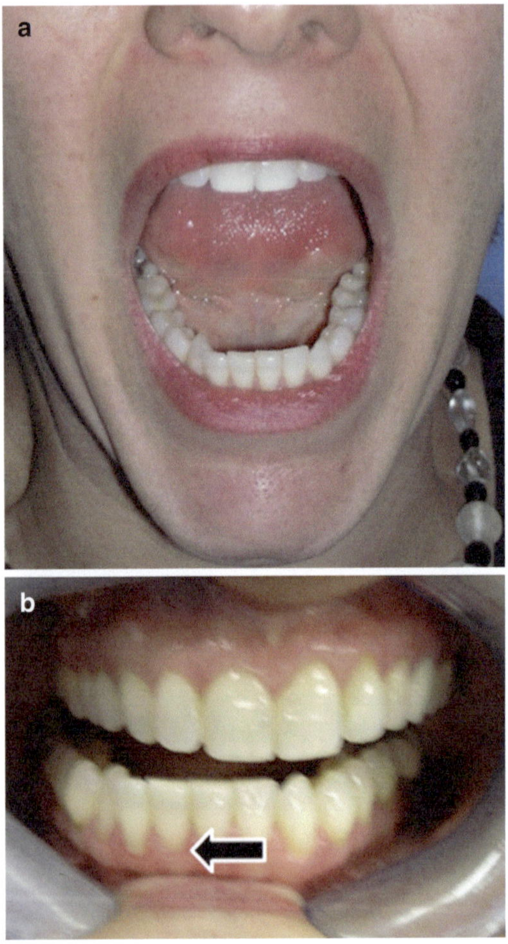

Fig. 3.16 Two years after arthrocentesis: (**a**) Normal MMO. (**b**) Normal lateral movements to the right

classification, which needs to be reevaluated and modified. The clinical and radiologic findings should be introduced into the classification separately because mild symptoms may appear with severe radiological changes and vice versa.

3.7.4 Open Lock

Open lock is characterized by a sudden inability to close the mouth, and is usually released by self-manipulation. Mouth opening during open lock is usually not as extreme as in condylar dislocation [114]. In plain radiographs and computerized tomography scans, the condoyle in "open lock" is located under the eminence (unlike condylar dislocation). MRIs show that the condoyle is locked in front of the lagging disc. The etiology of open lock is probably related to diminished lubrication; thus friction between the disc and the eminence increases. The disc, which normally moves together with the condoyle, lags behind it, and consequently the condoyle slides under and in front of the disc and cannot return to its former position in the fossa; hence, the mouth remains open. Lavage of the upper compartment can restore sliding of the disc, allowing it and the condoyle to move simultaneously. Preventing the condoyle from moving in front of the disc provides relief, with rare long-term recurrence [114].

3.7.5 Hemarthrosis

Another indication for arthrocentesis is hemarthrosis. Hemarthrosis of the TMJ is characterized by painful swelling in the affected joint and occlusal inconvenience. Mouth opening is usually limited and characterized by deviation to the affected side, lateral movements to both sides are limited, and protrusion is also limited with deviation toward the affected side. Open bite is usually noted on the affected side. Transcranial radiography in closed-mouth position usually shows widening of the intra-articular space.

The most common cause for hemarthrosis is trauma. This condition should be treated immediately to eliminate the blood and reduce intra-articular pressure either by arthrocentesis or intensive physiotherapy and joint unloading in order to prevent articular damage and functional sequelae. Analgesics, anti-inflammatory agents, and antibiotics should be considered. One should bear in mind that trauma to the joint without fracture still has the same harmful potential.

Undiagnosed TMJ hemarthrosis may lead to the development of severe fibro-adhesions. Hemarthrosis can also be associated with acquired coagulation deficiencies such as leukemia, thrombopenia, and uncontrolled anticoagulant treatment and inherited coagulation diseases such as hemophilia, von Willebrand disease, and congenital thrombopathies [180, 181]. Hemoglobinopathies, particularly sickle cell dis-

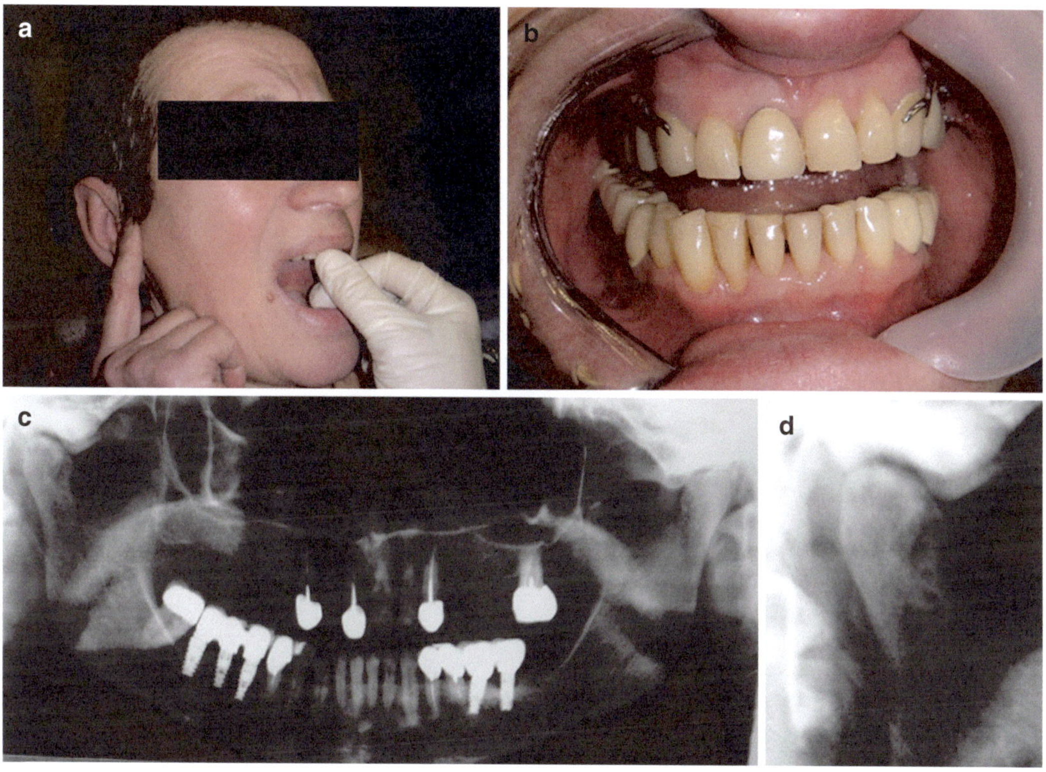

Fig. 3.17 Diagnostic arthrocentesis: 62-year-old lady presented severe Rt TMJ pain associated with LMO)**a**, **b**(. Panoramic and transpharyngeal radiographs revealed mild changes in the Rt TMJ. Missing teeth in the right upper quadrant)**c**, **d**)

ease, have been documented as the cause for hemarthrosis in a few patients. One can include tumors, pigmented villonodular synovitis, and degenerative and metabolic diseases among local or regional disorders of the joints. A complete anamnesis is crucial.

3.7.6 Autoimmune Inflammatory Arthritis

There are vast number of autoimmune inflammatory diseases that can jeopardize the integrity of the TMJ and thus cause pain and dysfunction. The disease most commonly affecting the TMJ is rheumatoid arthritis (RA) in adults or juvenile rheumatoid arthritis (JRA) in pediatric populations.

RA is a chronic disease of unknown etiology, characterized by synovitis of the diarthrodial joints, gradual bone erosion, and cartilage destruction.

The reported incidence of TMJ involvement secondary to RA varies from 2 to 86% because of ambiguous clinical and radiologic criteria. The TMJ is seldom the first joint to be affected. This diversity exists because TMJ osteoarthritis in a patient with RA was often considered as the presentation of the systemic disease. Therefore the literature on TMJ RA is often misleading. Patients with certain JRA subtypes, a higher ESR at disease onset, involvement of upper extremity joints, and younger age at diagnosis were found to be more likely to develop TMJ arthritis [182, 183]. The presence of HLA-B27 seems to be protective.

The clinical findings in the TMJ affected with RA are similar to those described for other joints, i.e. pain, swelling, movement impairment, and crepitation. Condylar resorption is associated with

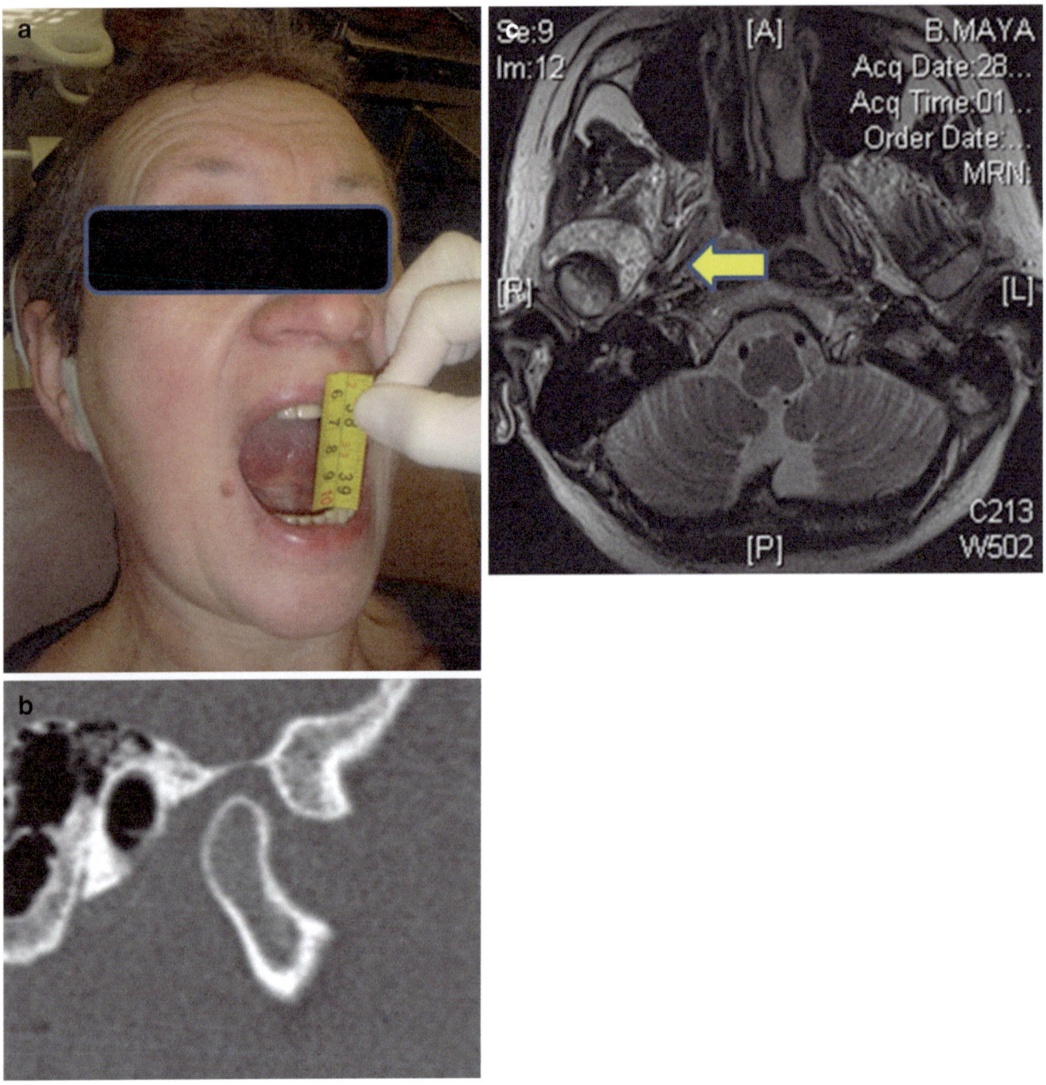

Fig. 3.18 Following the splint therapy and arthrocentesis: (**a**) Normal MMO with persistent unexplained Rt TMJ pain. Further evaluation revealed: (**b**) Normal CT. (**c**) On MRI extended SOL interpreted as synovial chondromatosis

malocclusion and anterior open bite may occur at advanced stages. Total protein in the synovial fluid of RA patient is increased and includes proteins involved in inflammation. These protein and lipid moieties act on nerve endings of the synovial membrane causing pain. Arthrocentesis and controlled joint loading in patients with an intra-articular steroid injection increase opening and provide pain relief. The most important role of arthrocentesis is to control active disease in the joint. This is particularly important before orthognathic surgery [184–186].

Conclusions

1. TMJ arthrocentesis is a non-arthroscopic lysis and lavage performed under local anesthesia with two needles that are introduced into the upper compartment of the joint. It is always performed in conjunction with joint load control and movement rehabilitation.
2. The modes of action of arthrocentesis include releasing the disc by eradicating adhesive forces, eliminating joint effusions,

and removing degradation products. Thus, it is particularly effective in the relief of localized joint pain and improves mandibular movements. Therefore arthrocentesis is indicated for releasing the anchored disc in ADP, open lock, and has satisfactory results in more than 80% of cases of TMJ osteoarthritis. Arthrocentesis is inefficient when dysfunction is caused by factors that cannot be eliminated by lavage, such as disc displacement or fibrous adhesions. Therefore, in cases of disc displacement with or without reduction (DDwR/DDwoR) arthrocentesis reduces pain but other effects are debatable. When effective, arthrocentesis negates the need for other surgical interventions.

3. When arthrocentesis fails, we can surmise that open surgery is needed. Thus, arthrocentesis should become a primary tool in the treatment of TMJ disorders, successfully filling the gap between failed conservative treatments and complex surgical interventions.
4. Remarkably, the severity of preoperative pain, dysfunction, and restricted range of motion and the radiographic changes do not correlate with the outcome of arthrocentesis.
5. The aspirated fluid can be used for diagnostic, therapeutic, and research purposes.

References

1. Aceves-Avila FJ, Delgadillo-Ruano MA, Ramos-Remus C, Gomez-Vargas A, Gutierrez-Urena S. The first descriptions of therapeutic arthrocentesis: a historical note. Rheumatology (Oxford). 2003;42(1):180–3.
2. Brown PW. Arthrocentesis for diagnosis and therapy. Surg Clin North Am. 1969;49(6):1269–78.
3. Manadan AM, Block JA. Daily needle aspiration versus surgical lavage for the treatment of bacterial septic arthritis in adults. Am J Ther. 2004;11(5):412–5.
4. Alarcon-Segovia D. Descriptions of therapeutic arthrocenthesis and of synovial fluid in a Nahuatl text from prehispanic Mexico. Ann Rheum Dis. 1980;39(3):291–3.
5. Hansen SE. Arthrocentesis in the past. Comment on an article by Aceves-Avila et al. Rheumatology (Oxford). 2003;42(12):1569–70.
6. Luhmann SJ, Jones A, Schootman M, Gordon JE, Schoenecker PL, Luhmann JD. Differentiation between septic arthritis and transient synovitis of the hip in children with clinical prediction algorithms. J Bone Joint Surg Am. 2004;86-A(5):956–62.
7. Smith SW. Emergency physician-performed ultrasonography-guided hip arthrocentesis. Acad Emerg Med. 1999;6(1):84–6.
8. Wu YG, Li XG, Zhang KN, Ren YJ, Li SF, Lu MY. Perioperative management of orthopedic patients with hemophilia A. Zhonghua Wai Ke Za Zhi. 2004;42(23):1430–3.
9. Jay GD, Elsaid KA, Zack J, Robinson K, Trespalacios F, Cha CJ, et al. Lubricating ability of aspirated synovial fluid from emergency department patients with knee joint synovitis. J Rheumatol. 2004;31(3):557–64.
10. Raynauld JP, Goldsmith CH, Bellamy N, Torrance GW, Polisson R, Belovich D, et al. Effectiveness and safety of repeat courses of hylan G-F 20 in patients with knee osteoarthritis. Osteoarthr Cartil. 2005;13(2):111–9.
11. Tanaka N, Sakahashi H, Hirose K, Ishima T, Ishii S. Volume of a wash and the other conditions for maximum therapeutic effect of arthroscopic lavage in rheumatoid knees. Clin Rheumatol. 2006;25(1):65–9.
12. Vachal J, Kriz J, Jehlicka D, Novak P. Infectious complications after arthroscopic replacement of the cruciate ligaments. Acta Chir Orthop Traumatol Cech. 2005;72(1):28–31.
13. Senolt L, Braun M, Olejarova M, Forejtova S, Gatterova J, Pavelka K. Increased pentosidine, an advanced glycation end product, in serum and synovial fluid from patients with knee osteoarthritis and its relation with cartilage oligomeric matrix protein. Ann Rheum Dis. 2005;64(6):886–90.
14. Kernodle GW Jr, Allen NB. Acute gout presenting in the manubriosternal joint. Arthritis Rheum. 1986;29(4):570–2.
15. Epis O, Viola E, Bruschi E, Benazzo F, Montecucco C. Milwaukee shoulder syndrome (apatite associated destructive arthritis): therapeutic aspects. Reumatismo. 2005;57(2):69–77.
16. Wang Y, Dong S, Li Z. Clinical study on double contrast CT diagnosis of traumatic anterior shoulder instability. Zhongguo Xiu Fu Chong Jian Wai Ke Za Zhi. 2005;19(7):551–3.
17. van Den BR, van de Lest CH, Bull S, Brama RA, van Weeren PR, Barneveld A. Influence of repeated arthrocentesis and exercise on synovial fluid concentrations of nitric oxide, prostaglandin E2 and glycosaminoglycans in healthy equine joints. Equine Vet J. 2005;37(3):250–6.
18. Utsinger PD, Resnick D, Zvaifler NJ. Wrist arthropathy in calcium pyrophosphate dihydrate deposition disease. Arthritis Rheum. 1975;18(5):485–91.
19. Roy S, Dewitz A, Paul I. Ultrasound-assisted ankle arthrocentesis. Am J Emerg Med. 1999;17(3):300–1.

20. Scott PM. Arthrocentesis to diagnose and treat acute gouty arthritis in the great toe. JAAPA. 2000;13(10):93–6.
21. Vazquez de Mercado R, Stover SM, Taylor KT, Zarucco L, Willits NH. Lateral approach for arthrocentesis of the distal interphalangeal joint in horses. J Am Vet Med Assoc. 1998;212(9):1413–8.
22. Oxentenko AS, Ebbert JO, Ward LE, Pankratz VS, Wood KE. A multidimensional workshop using human cadavers to teach bedside procedures. Teach Learn Med. 2003;15(2):127–30.
23. Dooley P, Martin R. Corticosteroid injections and arthrocentesis. Can Fam Physician. 2002;48:285–92.
24. Vogelgesang SA, Karplus TM, Kreiter CD. An instructional program to facilitate teaching joint/soft-tissue injection and aspiration. J Gen Intern Med. 2002;17(6):441–5.
25. Waikakul S, Vanadurongwan B, Chumtup W, Assawamongkolgul A, Chotivichit A, Rojanawanich V. A knee model for arthrocentesis simulation. J Med Assoc Thail. 2003;86(3):282–7.
26. Simkin PA, Gardner GC. The 3-way stopcock: a useful adjunct in the practice of arthrocentesis. Arthritis Rheum. 2005;53(4):627–8.
27. Qian M, West W, Wu JT, Lu B, Christ DD. Development of a dog microdialysis model for determining synovial fluid pharmacokinetics of antiarthritis compounds exemplified by methotrexate. Pharm Res. 2003;20(4):605–10.
28. MacGregor RR, Schimmer BM, Steinberg ME. Results of combined amphotericin B-5-fluorcytosine therapy for prosthetic knee joint infected with Candida parapsilosis. J Rheumatol. 1979;6(4):451–5.
29. Good AE, Hague JM, Kauffman CA. Streptococcal endocarditis initially seen as septic arthritis. Arch Intern Med. 1978;138(5):805–6.
30. Ostensson A, Geborek P. Septic arthritis as a nonsurgical complication in rheumatoid arthritis: relation to disease severity and therapy. Br J Rheumatol. 1991;30(1):35–8.
31. Atilola MA, Lumsden JH, Hulland TJ, Pennock PW. Intra-articular tissue response to analytical grade metrizamide in dogs. Am J Vet Res. 1984;45(12):2651–7.
32. Stover SM, Pool RR. Effect of intra-articular gentamicin sulfate on normal equine synovial membrane. Am J Vet Res. 1985;46(12):2485–91.
33. Israel HA, Saed-Nejad F, Ratcliffe A. Early diagnosis of osteoarthrosis of the temporomandibular joint: correlation between arthroscopic diagnosis and keratan sulfate levels in the synovial fluid. J Oral Maxillofac Surg. 1991;49(7):708–11.
34. Pacchiana PD, Gilley RS, Wallace LJ, Hayden DW, Feeney DA, Jessen CR, et al. Absolute and relative cell counts for synovial fluid from clinically normal shoulder and stifle joints in cats. J Am Vet Med Assoc. 2004;225(12):1866–70.
35. Samuelson CO Jr, Cannon GW, Ward JR. Arthrocentesis. J Fam Pract. 1985;20(2):179–84.
36. Gerster JC, Wauters JP, Waldburger M, Saudan Y. Hemarthroses complicating anticoagulant therapy (heparin, oral anticoagulants). Schweiz Med Wochenschr. 1977;107(33):1170–2.
37. Horowitz MD, Abbey L, Sirota DK, Spiera H. Intraarticular noninflammatory free urate suspension (urate milk) in 3 patients with painful joints. J Rheumatol. 1990;17(5):712–4.
38. Phupong V, Sittisomwong T, Wisawasukmongchol W. Disseminated gonococcal infection during pregnancy. Arch Gynecol Obstet. 2005;273(3):185–6.
39. Sun HY, Chang IC, Chen MJ, Hung CC, Chang SC. Acute urethritis and arthritis-dermatitis syndrome due to Neisseria meningitidis. J Formos Med Assoc. 2004;103(11):858–9.
40. Ross JJ, Saltzman CL, Carling P, Shapiro DS. Pneumococcal septic arthritis: review of 190 cases. Clin Infect Dis. 2003;36(3):319–27.
41. Li SF, Henderson J, Dickman E, Darzynkiewicz R. Laboratory tests in adults with monoarticular arthritis: can they rule out a septic joint? Acad Emerg Med. 2004;11(3):276–80.
42. Baerwald C, Krause A, Goebel KM. Septic arthritis as an initial manifestation of endocarditis. Z Rheumatol. 1990;49(3):165–8.
43. Albrecht HU, Saxer U. Diagnosis of latent late infections following total hip replacement. Schweiz Med Wochenschr. 1978;108(33):1262–70.
44. Rothschild BM, Round MJ. Subcutaneous crystal deposition in pseudogout. JAMA. 1980;244(18):2079–80.
45. Hartmann LC, Nauseef WM. Group B streptococcal polyarthritis complicating hemophilia B. Acta Haematol. 1990;84(2):95–7.
46. Palella TD, Kelley WN. An approach to hyperuricemia and gout. Geriatrics. 1984;39(11):89–6, 101.
47. Shmerling RH, Delbanco TL, Tosteson AN, Trentham DE. Synovial fluid tests. What should be ordered? JAMA. 1990;264(8):1009–14.
48. Stiehl P, Hantzschel H, Herz G. Cytodiagnosis of the synovial fluid. Z Gesamte Inn Med. 1976;31(16):615–23.
49. Borenstein DG, Gibbs CA, Jacobs RP. Gas-liquid chromatographic analysis of synovial fluid. Succinic acid and lactic acid as markers for septic arthritis. Arthritis Rheum. 1982;25(8):947–53.
50. Ringelmann R, Amin SM. Laboratory diagnosis and antibacterial therapy in joint diseases. Z Orthop Ihre Grenzgeb. 1990;128(4):391–5.
51. Bhoola KD, Elson CJ, Dieppe PA. Kinins—key mediators in inflammatory arthritis? Br J Rheumatol. 1992;31(8):509–18.
52. De Clerck LS, Struyf NJ, Bridts CH, Breedveld FC, Westedt ML, Cats A, et al. IgE-containing immune complexes in synovial fluid of patients with rheumatoid arthritis. Clin Rheumatol. 1990;9(2):176–81.
53. Suzuki K, Shimizu K, Hamamoto T, Nakagawa Y, Hamakubo T, Yamamuro T. Biochemical demonstration of calpains and calpastatin in osteoarthritic synovial fluid. Arthritis Rheum. 1990;33(5):728–32.

54. Ludin A, Sela JJ, Schroeder A, Samuni Y, Nitzan DW, Amir G. Injection of vascular endothelial growth factor into knee joints induces osteoarthritis in mice. Osteoarthr Cartil. 2013;21(3):491–7.
55. Jansen H, Meffert RH, Birkenfeld F, Petersen W, Pufe T. Detection of vascular endothelial growth factor (VEGF) in moderate osteoarthritis in a rabbit model. Ann Anat. 2012;194(5):452–6.
56. Greene CS. The etiology of temporomandibular disorders: implications for treatment. J Orofac Pain. 2001;15(2):93–105.
57. Carlsson GE. Epidemiology and treatment need for temporomandibular disorders. J Orofac Pain. 1999;13(4):232–7.
58. Kircos LT, Ortendahl DA, Mark AS, Arakawa M. Magnetic resonance imaging of the TMJ disc in asymptomatic volunteers. J Oral Maxillofac Surg. 1987;45(10):852–4.
59. Kaplan PA, Tu HK, Sleder PR, Lydiatt DD, Laney TJ. Inferior joint space arthrography of normal temporomandibular joints: reassessment of diagnostic criteria. Radiology. 1986;159(3):585–9.
60. Sanders B. Arthroscopic surgery of the temporomandibular joint: treatment of internal derangement with persistent closed lock. Oral Surg Oral Med Oral Pathol. 1986;62(4):361–72.
61. Nitzan DW, Samson B, Better H. Long-term outcome of arthrocentesis for sudden-onset, persistent, severe closed lock of the temporomandibular joint. J Oral Maxillofac Surg. 1997;55(2):151–7.
62. Montgomery MT, Van Sickels JE, Harms SE, Thrash WJ. Arthroscopic TMJ surgery: effects on signs, symptoms, and disc position. J Oral Maxillofac Surg. 1989;47(12):1263–71.
63. Moses JJ, Sartoris D, Glass R, Tanaka T, Poker I. The effect of arthroscopic surgical lysis and lavage of the superior joint space on TMJ disc position and mobility. J Oral Maxillofac Surg. 1989;47(7):674–8.
64. Bloebaum RD, Radley KM. Three-dimensional surface analysis of young adult human articular cartilage. J Anat. 1995;187(Pt 2):293–301.
65. Nickel JC, Iwasaki LR, Beatty MW, Moss MA, Marx DB. Static and dynamic loading effects on temporomandibular joint disc tractional forces. J Dent Res. 2006;85(9):809–13.
66. Rahamim E, Better H, Dagan A, Nitzan DW. Electron microscope and biochemical observations of the surface active phospholipids on the articular surfaces and in the synovial fluid of the temporomandibular joint: a preliminary investigation. J Oral Maxillofac Surg. 2001;59(11):1326–32.
67. Koyama E, Saunders C, Salhab I, Decker RS, Chen I, Um H, et al. Lubricin is required for the structural integrity and post-natal maintenance of TMJ. J Dent Res. 2014;93(7):663–70.
68. Hill A, Duran J, Purcell P. Lubricin protects the temporomandibular joint surfaces from degeneration. PLoS One. 2014;9(9):e106497.
69. Chang DP, Abu-Lail NI, Coles JM, Guilak F, Jay GD, Zauscher S. Friction force microscopy of Lubricin and hyaluronic acid between hydrophobic and hydrophilic surfaces. Soft Matter. 2009;5(18):3438–45.
70. Marchetti C, Bernasconi G, Reguzzoni M, Farina A. The articular disc surface in different functional conditions of the human temporo-mandibular joint. J Oral Pathol Med. 1997;26(6):278–82.
71. Hills BA. Synovial surfactant and the hydrophobic articular surface. J Rheumatol. 1996;23(8):1323–5.
72. Schwarz IM, Hills BA. Synovial surfactant: lamellar bodies in type B synoviocytes and proteolipid in synovial fluid and the articular lining. Br J Rheumatol. 1996;35(9):821–7.
73. Ghadially FN, Yong NK, Lalonde JM. A transmission electron microscopic comparison of the articular surface of cartilage processed attached to bone and detached from bone. J Anat. 1982;135(Pt 4):685–706.
74. Forster H, Fisher J. The influence of continuous sliding and subsequent surface wear on the friction of articular cartilage. Proc Inst Mech Eng H. 1999;213(4):329–45.
75. Hills BA, Monds MK. Enzymatic identification of the load-bearing boundary lubricant in the joint. Br J Rheumatol. 1998;37(2):137–42.
76. Nitzan DW, Nitzan U, Dan P, Yedgar S. The role of hyaluronic acid in protecting surface-active phospholipids from lysis by exogenous phospholipase A(2). Rheumatology (Oxford). 2001;40(3):336–40.
77. Hills BA. Surface-active phospholipid: a Pandora's box of clinical applications. Part II. Barrier and lubricating properties. Intern Med J. 2002;32(5–6):242–51.
78. Sivan S, Schroeder A, Verberne G, Merkher Y, Diminsky D, Priev A, et al. Liposomes act as effective biolubricants for friction reduction in human synovial joints. Langmuir. 2010;26(2):1107–16.
79. Goldberg R, Schroeder A, Silbert G, Turjeman K, Barenholz Y, Klein J. Boundary lubricants with exceptionally low friction coefficients based on 2D close-packed phosphatidylcholine liposomes. Adv Mater. 2011;23(31):3517–21.
80. Gaisinskaya A, Ma L, Silbert G, Sorkin R, Tairy O, Goldberg R, et al. Hydration lubrication: exploring a new paradigm. Faraday Discuss. 2012;156:217–33.
81. Kosinska MK, Liebisch G, Lochnit G, Wilhelm J, Klein H, Kaesser U, et al. A lipidomic study of phospholipid classes and species in human synovial fluid. Arthritis Rheum. 2013;65(9):2323–33.
82. Kawai N, Tanaka E, Takata T, Miyauchi M, Tanaka M, Todoh M, et al. Influence of additive hyaluronic acid on the lubricating ability in the temporomandibular joint. J Biomed Mater Res A. 2004;70(1):149–53.
83. Volpi N, Schiller J, Stern R, Soltes L. Role, metabolism, chemical modifications and applications of hyaluronan. Curr Med Chem. 2009;16(14):1718–45.
84. Manfredini D, Rancitelli D, Ferronato G, Guarda-Nardini L. Arthrocentesis with or without additional drugs in temporomandibular joint inflammatory-

degenerative disease: comparison of six treatment protocols. J Oral Rehabil. 2012;39(4):245–51.
85. Guarda-Nardini L, Ferronato G, Favero L, Manfredini D. Predictive factors of hyaluronic acid injections short-term effectiveness for TMJ degenerative joint disease. J Oral Rehabil. 2011;38(5):315–20.
86. Laurent TC, Laurent UB, Fraser JR. The structure and function of hyaluronan: an overview. Immunol Cell Biol. 1996;74(2):A1–7.
87. Imhof H, Sulzbacher I, Grampp S, Czerny C, Youssefzadeh S, Kainberger F. Subchondral bone and cartilage disease: a rediscovered functional unit. Investig Radiol. 2000;35(10):581–8.
88. Milam SB, Schmitz JP. Molecular biology of temporomandibular joint disorders: proposed mechanisms of disease. J Oral Maxillofac Surg. 1995;53(12):1448–54.
89. Haskin CL, Milam SB, Cameron IL. Pathogenesis of degenerative joint disease in the human temporomandibular joint. Crit Rev Oral Biol Med. 1995;6(3):248–77.
90. de Bont LG, Stegenga B. Pathology of temporomandibular joint internal derangement and osteoarthrosis. Int J Oral Maxillofac Surg. 1993;22(2):71–4.
91. Solberg WK. Temporomandibular disorders: management of internal derangement. Br Dent J. 1986;160(11):379–85.
92. Wright V, Dowson D, Longfied MD. Joint stiffness—its characterisation and significance. Biomed Eng. 1969;4(1):8–14.
93. Dowson D, Wright V, Longfield MD. Human joint lubrication. Biomed Eng. 1969;4(4):160–5.
94. Walker PS, Dowson D, Longfield MD, Wright V. Lubrication of human joints. Ann Rheum Dis. 1969;28(2):194.
95. Walker PS, Sikorski J, Dowson D, Longfield MD, Wright V, Buckley T. Behaviour of synovial fluid on surfaces of articular cartilage. A scanning electron microscope study. Ann Rheum Dis. 1969;28(1):1–14.
96. Walker PS, Sikorski J, Dowson D, Longfield D, Wright V. Behaviour of synovial fluid on articular cartilage. Ann Rheum Dis. 1969;28(3):326.
97. Mow VC. Lubrication and wear of diarthrodial joints. In: Mow VC, Hayes WC, editors. Basic orthopedic biomechanics. New York: Lippincott-Raven; 1997.
98. Merry P, Winyard PG, Morris CJ, Grootveld M, Blake DR. Oxygen free radicals, inflammation, and synovitis: and synovitis: the current status. Ann Rheum Dis. 1989;48(10):864–70.
99. Mapp PI, Grootveld MC, Blake DR. Hypoxia, oxidative stress and rheumatoid arthritis. Br Med Bull. 1995;51(2):419–36.
100. Merry P, Grootveld M, Lunec J, Blake DR. Oxidative damage to lipids within the inflamed human joint provides evidence of radical-mediated hypoxic-reperfusion injury. Am J Clin Nutr. 1991;53(1 Suppl):362S–9S.
101. Blake DR, Merry P, Unsworth J, Kidd BL, Outhwaite JM, Ballard R, et al. Hypoxic-reperfusion injury in the inflamed human joint. Lancet. 1989;1(8633):289–93.
102. Grootveld M, Henderson EB, Farrell A, Blake DR, Parkes HG, Haycock P. Oxidative damage to hyaluronate and glucose in synovial fluid during exercise of the inflamed rheumatoid joint. Detection of abnormal low-molecular-mass metabolites by proton-n.m.r. spectroscopy. Biochem J. 1991;273(Pt 2):459–67.
103. Takahashi I, Mizoguchi I, Sasano Y, Saitoh S, Ishida M, Kagayama M, et al. Age-related changes in the localization of glycosaminoglycans in condylar cartilage of the mandible in rats. Anat Embryol (Berl). 1996;194(5):489–500.
104. Tabor D. Friction—The present state of our understanding. J Lubr Technol. 1981;103:169–79.
105. AAOS Symposium on Sports Medicine: The knee. In: Finerman GAM, editor. Biomechanics of impact induced micro damage to articular surface—a possible genesis for chondromalacia patella. 1985.
106. Etzion I, Amit M. The effect of small normal loads on the static friction coefficient for very smooth surfaces. J Tribol. 1992;11(100):1524–25.
107. Stanley HM, Etzion I. Adhesion of contacting rough surfaces in the presence of sub-boundary lubrication. J Tribol. 1990;112:98.
108. Mao J, Stein RB, Osborn JW. The size and distribution of fiber types in jaw muscles: a review. J Craniomandib Disord. 1992;6(3):192–201.
109. Ericson S, Lundberg M. Structural changes in the finger, wrist and temporomandibular joints. A comparative radiologic study. Acta Odontol Scand. 1968;26(2):111–26.
110. Westling L, Holm S, Wallentin I. Temporomandibular joint dysfunction. Connective tissue variations in skin biopsy and mitral valve function. Oral Surg Oral Med Oral Pathol. 1992;74(6):709–18.
111. Isacsson G, Linde C, Isberg A. Subjective symptoms in patients with temporomandibular joint disk displacement versus patients with myogenic craniomandibular disorders. J Prosthet Dent. 1989;61(1):70–7.
112. Katzberg RW, Westesson PL, Tallents RH, Drake CM. Anatomic disorders of the temporomandibular joint disc in asymptomatic subjects. J Oral Maxillofac Surg. 1996;54(2):147–53.
113. Stegenga B. Osteoarthritis of the temporomandibular joint organ and its relationship to disc displacement. J Orofac Pain. 2001;15(3):193–205.
114. Nitzan DW. Temporomandibular joint "open lock" versus condylar dislocation: signs and symptoms, imaging, treatment, and pathogenesis. J Oral Maxillofac Surg. 2002;60(5):506–11.
115. Nitzan DW. The process of lubrication impairment and its involvement in temporomandibular joint disc displacement: a theoretical concept. J Oral Maxillofac Surg. 2001;59(1):36–45.

116. Ogus H. Common disorders of the temporomandibular joint. Bristol: Wright; 1981.
117. Ogus H. The mandibular joint: internal rearrangement. Br J Oral Maxillofac Surg. 1987;25(3):218–26.
118. Nitzan DW, Etsion I. Adhesive force: the underlying cause of the disc anchorage to the fossa and/or eminence in the temporomandibular joint—a new concept. Int J Oral Maxillofac Surg. 2002;31(1):94–9.
119. Murakami KI, Iizuka T, Matsuki M, Ono T. Recapturing the persistent anteriorly displaced disk by mandibular manipulation after pumping and hydraulic pressure to the upper joint cavity of the temporomandibular joint. Cranio. 1987;5(1):17–24.
120. Nitzan DW, Dolwick MF, Martinez GA. Temporomandibular joint arthrocentesis: a simplified treatment for severe, limited mouth opening. J Oral Maxillofac Surg. 1991;49(11):1163–7.
121. Kaneyama K, Segami N, Nishimura M, Sato J, Fujimura K, Yoshimura H. The ideal lavage volume for removing bradykinin, interleukin-6, and protein from the temporomandibular joint by arthrocentesis. J Oral Maxillofac Surg. 2004;62(6):657–61.
122. Segami N, Murakami K, Iizuka T. Arthrographic evaluation of disk position following mandibular manipulation technique for internal derangement with closed lock of the temporomandibular joint. J Craniomandib Disord. 1990;4(2):99–108.
123. Zardeneta G, Milam SB, Schmitz JP. Elution of proteins by continuous temporomandibular joint arthrocentesis. J Oral Maxillofac Surg. 1997;55(7):709–16.
124. Senturk MF, Cambazoglu M. A new classification for temporomandibular joint arthrocentesis techniques. Int J Oral Maxillofac Surg. 2015;44(3):417–8.
125. Guarda-Nardini L, Tito R, Staffieri A, Beltrame A. Treatment of patients with arthrosis of the temporomandibular joint by infiltration of sodium hyaluronate: a preliminary study. Eur Arch Otorhinolaryngol. 2002;259(5):279–84.
126. Alpaslan C, Bilgihan A, Alpaslan GH, Guner B, Ozgur YM, Erbas D. Effect of arthrocentesis and sodium hyaluronate injection on nitrite, nitrate, and thiobarbituric acid-reactive substance levels in the synovial fluid. Oral Surg Oral Med Oral Pathol Oral Radiol Endod. 2000;89(6):686–90.
127. Zhong WQ, Zhou G. Intraarticular injection-dilatation and later lavage plus viscosupplementation of TMJ for the treatment of anterior disc displacement without reduction. Shanghai Kou Qiang Yi Xue. 2004;13(1):23–6.
128. Xinmin Y, Jian H. Treatment of temporomandibular joint osteoarthritis with viscosupplementation and arthrocentesis on rabbit model. Oral Surg Oral Med Oral Pathol Oral Radiol Endod. 2005;100(3):e35–8.
129. Guarda-Nardini L, Rossi A, Arboretti R, Bonnini S, Stellini E, Manfredini D. Single- or multiple-session viscosupplementation protocols for temporomandibular joint degenerative disorders: a randomized clinical trial. J Oral Rehabil. 2015;42(7):521–8.
130. Arinci A, Ademoglu E, Aslan A, Mutlu-Turkoglu U, Karabulut AB, Karan A. Molecular correlates of temporomandibular joint disease. Oral Surg Oral Med Oral Pathol Oral Radiol Endod. 2005;99(6):666–70.
131. Hanci M, Karamese M, Tosun Z, Aktan TM, Duman S, Savaci N. Intra-articular platelet-rich plasma injection for the treatment of temporomandibular disorders and a comparison with arthrocentesis. J Craniomaxillofac Surg. 2015;43(1):162–6.
132. Carroll TA, Smith K, Jakubowski J. Extradural haematoma following temporomandibular joint arthrocentesis and lavage. Br J Neurosurg. 2000;14(2):152–4.
133. Nishimura M, Segami N, Kaneyama K, Sato J, Fujimura K. Comparison of cytokine level in synovial fluid between successful and unsuccessful cases in arthrocentesis of the temporomandibular joint. J Oral Maxillofac Surg. 2004;62(3):284–7.
134. Eliav E, Teich S, Nitzan D, El Raziq DA, Nahlieli O, Tal M, et al. Facial arthralgia and myalgia: can they be differentiated by trigeminal sensory assessment? Pain. 2003;104(3):481–90.
135. LeResche L, Dworkin SF, Wilson L, Ehrlich KJ. Effect of temporomandibular disorder pain duration on facial expressions and verbal report of pain. Pain. 1992;51(3):289–95.
136. Dworkin SF, Sherman J, Mancl L, Ohrbach R, LeResche L, Truelove E. Reliability, validity, and clinical utility of the research diagnostic criteria for Temporomandibular Disorders Axis II Scales: depression, non-specific physical symptoms, and graded chronic pain. J Orofac Pain. 2002;16(3):207–20.
137. Celic R, Jerolimov V, Knezovic ZD, Klaic B. Measurement of mandibular movements in patients with temporomandibular disorders and in asymptomatic subjects. Coll Antropol. 2003;27 (Suppl 2):43–9.
138. Manfredini D, Tognini F, Zampa V, Bosco M. Predictive value of clinical findings for temporomandibular joint effusion. Oral Surg Oral Med Oral Pathol Oral Radiol Endod. 2003;96(5):521–6.
139. Takahashi T, Nagai H, Seki H, Fukuda M. Relationship between joint effusion, joint pain, and protein levels in joint lavage fluid of patients with internal derangement and osteoarthritis of the temporomandibular joint. J Oral Maxillofac Surg. 1999;57(10):1187–93.
140. Guler N, Uckan S, Imirzalioglu P, Acikgozoglu S. Temporomandibular joint internal derangement: relationship between joint pain and MR grading of effusion and total protein concentration in the joint fluid. Dentomaxillofac Radiol. 2005;34(3):175–81.
141. Epstein JB, Rea A, Chahal O. The use of bone scintigraphy in temporomandibular joint disorders. Oral Dis. 2002;8(1):47–53.
142. Carvajal WA, Laskin DM. Long-term evaluation of arthrocentesis for the treatment of internal derange-

ments of the temporomandibular joint. J Oral Maxillofac Surg. 2000;58(8):852–5.
143. Alpaslan GH, Alpaslan C. Efficacy of temporomandibular joint arthrocentesis with and without injection of sodium hyaluronate in treatment of internal derangements. J Oral Maxillofac Surg. 2001;59(6):613–8.
144. Fridrich KL, Wise JM, Zeitler DL. Prospective comparison of arthroscopy and arthrocentesis for temporomandibular joint disorders. J Oral Maxillofac Surg. 1996;54(7):816–20.
145. Spallaccia F, Rivaroli A, Cascone P. Temporomandibular joint arthrocentesis: long-term results. Bull Group Int Rech Sci Stomatol Odontol. 2000;42(1):31–7.
146. Goudot P. Articular surgery in the treatment of temporomandibular dysfunction. Orthod Fr. 1998;69(1):61–7.
147. Yura S, Ooi K, Izumiyama Y. Relationship between the effectiveness of arthrocentesis under sufficient pressure and conditions of the temporomandibular joint. ISRN Dent. 2011;2011:376475.
148. Guarda-Nardini L, Cadorin C, Frizziero A, Ferronato G, Manfredini D. Comparison of 2 hyaluronic acid drugs for the treatment of temporomandibular joint osteoarthritis. J Oral Maxillofac Surg. 2012;70(11):2522–30.
149. Goudot P, Jaquinet AR, Hugonnet S, Haefliger W, Richter M. Improvement of pain and function after arthroscopy and arthrocentesis of the temporomandibular joint: a comparative study. J Craniomaxillofac Surg. 2000;28(1):39–43.
150. Nishimura M, Segami N, Kaneyama K, Suzuki T. Prognostic factors in arthrocentesis of the temporomandibular joint: evaluation of 100 patients with internal derangement. J Oral Maxillofac Surg. 2001;59(8):874–7.
151. Emshoff R, Rudisch A. Determining predictor variables for treatment outcomes of arthrocentesis and hydraulic distention of the temporomandibular joint. J Oral Maxillofac Surg. 2004;62(7):816–23.
152. Kunjur J, Anand R, Brennan PA, Ilankovan V. An audit of 405 temporomandibular joint arthrocentesis with intra-articular morphine infusion. Br J Oral Maxillofac Surg. 2003;41(1):29–31.
153. Alpaslan C, Dolwick MF, Heft MW. Five-year retrospective evaluation of temporomandibular joint arthrocentesis. Int J Oral Maxillofac Surg. 2003;32(3):263–7.
154. Sorel B, Piecuch JF. Long-term evaluation following temporomandibular joint arthroscopy with lysis and lavage. Int J Oral Maxillofac Surg. 2000;29(4):259–63.
155. Hosaka H, Murakami K, Goto K, Iizuka T. Outcome of arthrocentesis for temporomandibular joint with closed lock at 3 years follow-up. Oral Surg Oral Med Oral Pathol Oral Radiol Endod. 1996;82(5):501–4.
156. Barkin S, Weinberg S. Internal derangements of the temporomandibular joint: the role of arthroscopic surgery and arthrocentesis. J Can Dent Assoc. 2000;66(4):199–203.
157. Kropmans TJ, Dijkstra PU, Stegenga B, de Bont LG. Therapeutic outcome assessment in permanent temporomandibular joint disc displacement. J Oral Rehabil. 1999;26(5):357–63.
158. Yoda T, Imai H, Shinjyo Y, Sakamoto I, Abe M, Enomoto S. Effect of arthrocentesis on TMJ disturbance of mouth closure with loud clicking: a preliminary study. Cranio. 2002;20(1):18–22.
159. Okeson JP. Management of temporomandibular disorders and occlusion. New York: Mosby; 2012.
160. Han Z, Ha Q, Yang C. Arthrocentesis and lavage of TMJ for the treatment of anterior disc displacement without reduction. Zhonghua Kou Qiang Yi Xue Za Zhi. 1999;34(5):269–71.
161. Reston JT, Turkelson CM. Meta-analysis of surgical treatments for temporomandibular articular disorders. J Oral Maxillofac Surg. 2003;61(1):3–10.
162. Emshoff R, Puffer P, Strobl H, Gassner R. Effect of temporomandibular joint arthrocentesis on synovial fluid mediator level of tumor necrosis factor-alpha: implications for treatment outcome. Int J Oral Maxillofac Surg. 2000;29(3):176–82.
163. Nitzan DW, Dolwick MF. An alternative explanation for the genesis of closed-lock symptoms in the internal derangement process. J Oral Maxillofac Surg. 1991;49(8):810–5.
164. Emshoff R, Rudisch A, Bosch R, Strobl H. Prognostic indicators of the outcome of arthrocentesis: a short-term follow-up study. Oral Surg Oral Med Oral Pathol Oral Radiol Endod. 2003;96(1):12–8.
165. Sanroman JF. Closed lock (MRI fixed disc): a comparison of arthrocentesis and arthroscopy. Int J Oral Maxillofac Surg. 2004;33(4):344–8.
166. Cascone P, Spallaccia F, Rivaroli A. Arthrocentesis of the temporomandibular joint. Long-term results. Minerva Stomatol. 1998;47(4):149–57.
167. Nitzan DW. 'Friction and adhesive forces'—possible underlying causes for temporomandibular joint internal derangement. Cells Tissues Organs. 2003;174(1–2):6–16.
168. Rao VM, Babaria A, Manoharan A, Mandel S, Gottehrer N, Wank H, et al. Altered condylar morphology associated with disc displacement in TMJ dysfunction: observations by MRI. Magn Reson Imaging. 1990;8(3):231–5.
169. Wang XD, Zhang JN, Gan YH, Zhou YH. Current understanding of pathogenesis and treatment of TMJ osteoarthritis. J Dent Res. 2015;94(5):666–73.
170. Kopp S. Temporomandibular disorders and related pain conditions (progress in pain research and management series). Seattle: IASP Press; 1995.
171. Nitzan DW. Intraarticular pressure in the functioning human temporomandibular joint and its alteration by uniform elevation of the occlusal plane. J Oral Maxillofac Surg. 1994;52(7):671–9.
172. Malemud CJ, Islam N, Haqqi TM. Pathophysiological mechanisms in osteoarthritis lead to novel

therapeutic strategies. Cells Tissues Organs. 2003;174(1–2):34–48.
173. Dan P, Nitzan DW, Dagan A, Ginsburg I, Yedgar S. H2O2 renders cells accessible to lysis by exogenous phospholipase A2: a novel mechanism for cell damage in inflammatory processes. FEBS Lett. 1996;383(1–2):75–8.
174. Zarb GA, Carlsson GE. Temporomandibular disorders: osteoarthritis. J Orofac Pain. 1999;13(4): 295–306.
175. Lajeunesse D. The role of bone in the treatment of osteoarthritis. Osteoarthritis Cartilage. 2004;12(Suppl A):S34–8.
176. Alexander CJ. Idiopathic osteoarthritis: time to change paradigms? Skelet Radiol. 2004;33(6): 321–4.
177. Nitzan DW, Price A. The use of arthrocentesis for the treatment of osteoarthritic temporomandibular joints. J Oral Maxillofac Surg. 2001;59(10): 1154–9.
178. Emshoff R. Clinical factors affecting the outcome of arthrocentesis and hydraulic distension of the temporomandibular joint. Oral Surg Oral Med Oral Pathol Oral Radiol Endod. 2005;100(4):409–14.
179. Wilkes CH. Internal derangements of the temporomandibular joint. Pathological variations. Arch Otolaryngol Head Neck Surg. 1989;115(4):469–77.
180. Gallardo A, Gallego JC, Enero J, Barambio M, Dominguez P, Aguilera M. Hemarthrosis as a hemorrhagic complication after thrombolytic treatment. Rev Esp Cardiol. 2001;54(10):1230–2.
181. Salvati G, Punzi L, Pianon M, Valvason C, Schiavon F, Noal N, et al. Frequency of the bleeding risk in patients receiving warfarin submitted to arthrocentesis of the knee. Reumatismo. 2003;55(3):159–63.
182. Trieger N, Hoffman CH, Rodriguez E. The effect of arthrocentesis of the temporomandibular joint in patients with rheumatoid arthritis. J Oral Maxillofac Surg. 1999;57(5):537–40.
183. Malliari M, Bakopoulou A, Koidis P. First diagnosis of rheumatoid arthritis in a patient with temporomandibular disorder: a case report. Int J Prosthodont. 2015;28(2):124–6.
184. Cannizzaro E, Schroeder S, Muller LM, Kellenberger CJ, Saurenmann RK. Temporomandibular joint involvement in children with juvenile idiopathic arthritis. J Rheumatol. 2011;38(3):510–5.
185. Sodhi A, Naik S, Pai A, Anuradha A. Rheumatoid arthritis affecting temporomandibular joint. Contemp Clin Dent. 2015;6(1):124–7.
186. Quinn JH, Bazan NG. Identification of prostaglandin E2 and leukotriene B4 in the synovial fluid of painful, dysfunctional temporomandibular joints. J Oral Maxillofac Surg. 1990;48(9):968–71.

4 Endoscopic Approach to Temporomandibular Fractures

Michael D. Turner

Abstract

Treatment of condylar fractures has been fraught with controversy regarding open reduction and internal fixation (ORIF) versus closed treatment. At this time, both the benefits and the risks are well known and can be summarized as improved function versus the risk of injury to the facial nerve and facial scarring. The minimally invasive techniques were developed to attempt to decrease the incidences of these complications. In this chapter, the instrumentation that is necessary, as well as the transoral and transcervical surgical approaches will be described. The history of the approaches, case selection, and reported complications will also be discussed.

4.1 Introduction

Treatment of condylar fractures has been fraught with controversy regarding open reduction and internal fixation (ORIF) versus closed treatment [1–3]. At this time, both the benefits and the risks are well known and can be distilled down to the following: Improved function versus the risk of injury to the facial nerve and facial scarring.

Many studies have been performed showing that the open repair, regardless of the approach, leads to an improvement in long-term function. A meta-analysis of the various studies on the treatment of condylar fractures concluded that there was a significant improvement in maximal interincisal opening, laterotrusive and protrusive movements, and chin deviation on mouth opening in patients who underwent ORIF as compared to closed treatment [4].

There are risks associated with the traditional approaches for ORIF, namely damage to the facial nerve, injury to the adjacent salivary glands, facial scarring, and infection. The minimally invasive techniques were developed to attempt to decrease the incidences of these complications. These techniques, for the purpose of this chapter, are divided into two approaches, the transoral and the transcervical. The adoption of either of these approaches, and the technique as a whole, is still very low as compared to both the standard open technique, and even more so the closed reduction/maxilla-mandibular fixation (CR/MMF). The reason for this is because of the extremely steep, and time consuming, learning curve that is encountered.

M.D. Turner, DDS, MD, FACS
Division of Oral and Maxillofacial Surgery, Icahn Mount Sinai School of Medicine, New York, NY, USA
e-mail: mturnerddsmd@gmail.com

O. Nahlieli (ed.), *Minimally Invasive Oral and Maxillofacial Surgery*,
http://doi.org/10.1007/978-3-662-54592-8_4

Initial attempts at endoscopic condylar repairs are typically frustrating. Loukota found that initially, the endoscopic approach took 2.5 times longer than the Endoscopic condylar repairs than the transparotid approach until about the 5th case, when the time scale equalized [5]. Anecdotally, the learning curve is much longer for the following reasons. Loukota, in his study, controlled multiple variables, particularly the operating room team, including the assistant surgeons, who were all familiar with the instrumentation associated with this technique. Realistically, unless there are a consistent number of these types of fractures encountered, it is very difficult to (1) consistently duplicate the surgical team, and (2) regularly perform this surgery so as to develop technical competence.

This is not to say that the endoscopic condylar fracture repair should not be attempted, just the opposite. The benefit of the return to function from the repair in conjunction with the decrease in risk to the facial nerve and facial scarring should necessitate that this procedure be performed. To become competent in the endoscopic condylar repair, three concepts should be considered: (1) Knowledge and familiarity with the appropriate instrumentation, (2) Familiarity with endoscopic surgery, and (3) The understanding that it will take persistence and patience to achieve technical proficiency.

4.2 History

In the English literature, the first reported case of an endoscopic repair of a condylar fracture was reported in February 1998, when a patient was treated successfully utilizing the transoral technique [6]. This was then followed by the same authors who reported a case series of 20 patients with 22 repaired condylar fractures with the transoral technique. They reported one complication consisting of a transient facial nerve palsy secondary to retraction which resolved over time [7].

Troulis, in 2001 reported the use of an transcervical endoscopic technique, in which five cases were repaired with no reported complications [8]. There have been other case series, some by other authors as well as the authors previously discussed, further expanding their case series (Table 4.1).

Table 4.1 Reported cases of endoscopically repaired condylar fractures

Authors	Year	Case #	Technique	Journal
Lee C, Jacobovicz J, Mueller RV	1997	1	Transoral	The Journal of craniofacial Surgery
Jacobovicz J, Lee C, Trabulsy PP	1998	1	Transoral	Plastic and Reconstructive Surgery
Lee C, Mueller RV, Lee K, Mathes SJ	1998	20	Transoral	Plastic and Reconstructive Surgery
Sandler NA, Andreasen KH, Johns FR	1999	7	Transoral	Oral Surg Oral Med Oral Pathol Oral Radiol Endod.
Lauer G, Schmelzeisen R	1999	3	Transcervical	J Oral Maxillofac Surgery
Chen CT, Lai JP, Tung TC, Chen YR	1999	8	Transoral	Plastic and Reconstructive Surgery
Schon R, Gutwald R, Schramm A, Gellrich NC, Schmelzeisen	2002	17	Transoral/ transcervical	Int J Oral Maxillofac Surgery
Kellman RM	2003	43	Transoral	Archives of Facial Plastic Surgery.
Schon R, Schramm A, Gellrich NC, Schmelzeisen R	2003	8	Transoral/ transcervical	J Oral Maxillofac Surgery
Miloro M	2003	6	Transcervical	Oral Surg Oral Med Oral Pathol Oral Radiol Endod.
Troulis MJ, Kaban LB	2004	22	Transcervical	J Oral Maxillofac Surg.
Schoen R, Gellrich NC, Schmelzeisen R	2005	58	Transoral	The British Journal of Oral & Maxillofacial Surgery
Loukota RA	2006	5	Transoral	The British Journal of Oral & Maxillofacial Surgery
Schoen R, Fakler O, Metzger MC, Weyer N, Schmelzeisen R	2008	26	Transoral	Int J Oral Maxillofac Surgery
Gonzalez-Garcia R, Sanroman JF, Goizueta-Adame C, Rodriguez-Campo FJ, Cho-Lee GY	2009	17	Transoral	Int J Oral Maxillofac Surgery

4.3 Technique

As with the treatment of any mandibular fracture, the patient should be placed into MMF. If there is another mandibular fracture in a tooth bearing region, this should be treated first before managing the condylar fractures. When placing the patient into MMF, elastics instead of wire should be utilized, since the mandible will need to be mobilized when caudal traction is applied during the reduction phase.

4.3.1 Transoral Approach

The intraoral incision should be placed along the external oblique ridge, lateral to the mandibular second molar, extending up the anterior border of the ramus. The periosteum should be reflected with the surgical pocket encompassing the condylar ramus complex. During flap reflection, extra care should be given in the posterior region so as not to further displace the proximal fracture segment. The angle of the mandible, sigmoid notch, the coronoid process, and as much of the extracapsular portion of the condylar process should be visible. All tissue fragments should be removed from the lateral ramus. Hemostasis should be achieved prior to proceeding to the fracture repair [9].

If the proximal portion of the fractured mandible has been displaced medially, and the head of the condyle is still within the fossa, a curved angular elevator should be placed into the sigmoid notch and the fracture segment should be brought laterally (Fig. 4.1). Once the lateral portion of the proximal segment is accessible, reduction of the fracture should be attempted. The muscles, particularly the masseteric sling, pull the distal portion of the fracture (the ramus) superiorly and create an overlap of the segments. To counteract this, caudally directed force is applied to reduce the fracture. As mentioned above, the patient must be in MMF elastics and not wires because wires will not allow the mandible to be manipulated caudally.

The easiest way to exert this forces is to press down on the posterior mandibular molars [10]. The difficulty in attempting to reduce the fracture in this way is that it limits the ability to place other instruments into the surgical field, so unless the segments reduce and lock into position, this technique is typically not an efficient way to generate an inferior force. Another option, which this author uses, is to make a small incision at the angle of the mandible and expose the bone. A bicortical bone screw is then placed in the angle and a stainless steel wire is looped around the screw and then clamped. Pulling on the clamp brings the distal segment caudally, without interfering with the transoral portion of the fracture repair.

At this point in the surgery, the endoscope and its associated sheath/retractors (Depuy Synthes© Paoli PA) is placed into the surgical site, and the retractor is hooked around the posterior border of the ramus on the distal segment (Fig. 4.2). This instrument, for the purpose of this chapter, will be termed the notch retractor (Fig. 4.3). Another type of retractor that can be used is a camera sheath with a soft-tissue retractor on the tip that prevents the soft tissue from falling onto the lens of the endoscope. This retractor was initially developed for endoscopic brow lift procedures so for the purpose of this chapter, will be termed a brow retractor (Fig. 4.4).

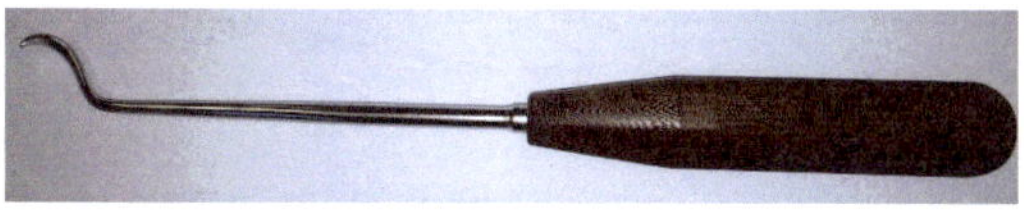

Fig. 4.1 Subcondylar curved elevator (Courtesy of Depuy Synthes©, Paoli PA)

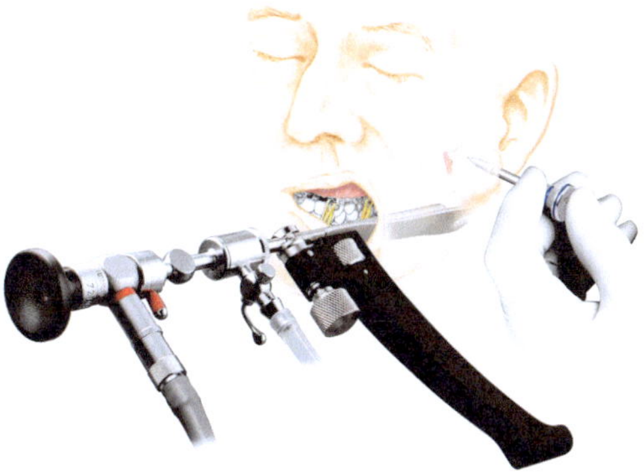

Fig. 4.2 Transoral introduction of endoscopic instrumentation (Courtesy of Depuy Synthes©)

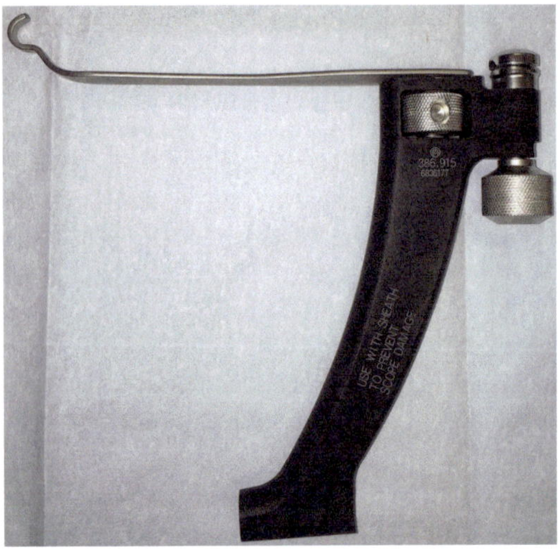

Fig. 4.3 Notch retractor (Courtesy of Depuy Synthes©, Paoli PA)

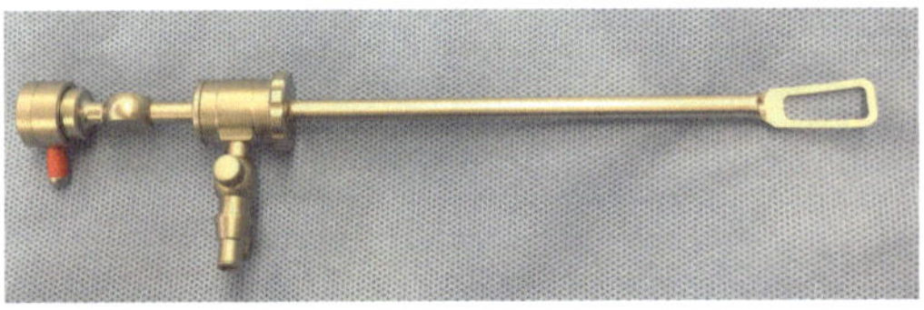

Fig. 4.4 Brow retractor (Courtesy of Karl Storz Endoscopy©, Tuttlingen, Germany)

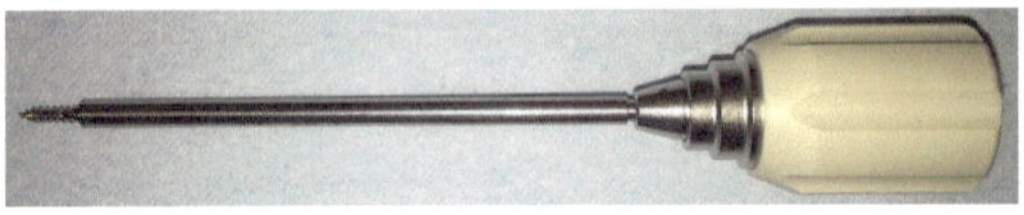

Fig. 4.5 Threaded fragment manipulator (Courtesy of Depuy Synthes©, Paoli PA)

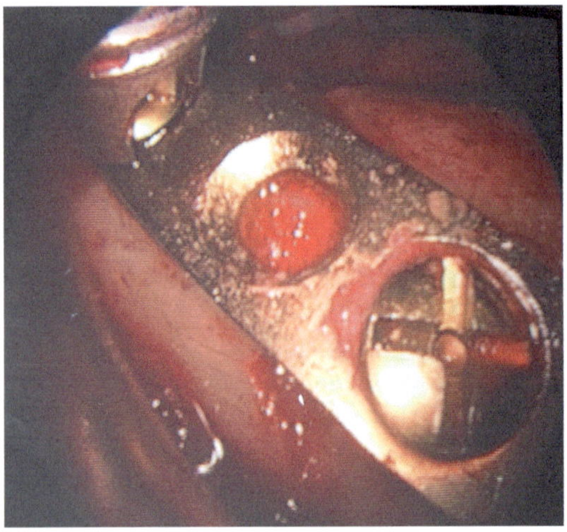

Fig. 4.6 Endoscopic view of a screw placement

Regardless of the retractor that is used, the endoscope should always be protected with an irrigation sheath. The endoscope used should have a 30° or 45° angulation. A plate is then introduced into the region, typically a 2.0 plate. Different sizes and number of bone plates have been described but no consensus has been formulated at this time [7, 11–13]. The plate is then introduced and placed overlying the fracture. If a transcervical trocar is placed, a screw hole can be drilled into the proximal segment. Multiple authors have described the placement of a threaded fragment manipulator (Fig. 4.5). This works like a Caroll-Girard screw, enabling the surgeon to guide and stabilize the proximal fragment into a reduced position. If a right angle drill and/or screw driver is available, the screws can be placed without a trocar, although obviously the threaded fragment manipulator cannot be used. Once the fragment is in reduced, a screw should then be placed into the distal segment. The next screws are then placed into the proximal and then distal segments respectfully (Fig. 4.6). If a fragment manipulator is being used, it is then removed and replaced with an emergency screw. Additional plates can be placed in other locations along the fracture [14].

4.3.2 Transcervical Technique

The transcervical technique is also termed the modified Risdon or modified submandibular approach. As above the patient should be placed into MMF with elastics. A 2–3 cm incision should be made 2 cm inferior to the angle of the mandible (Fig. 4.7). If the incision is made to posterior, difficulties in visualization and manipulation of the fracture can occur. Dissection is performed through the platysma down to the angle of the mandible. The pterygomasseteric attachment is then incised along the inferior border of the mandible. A retractor

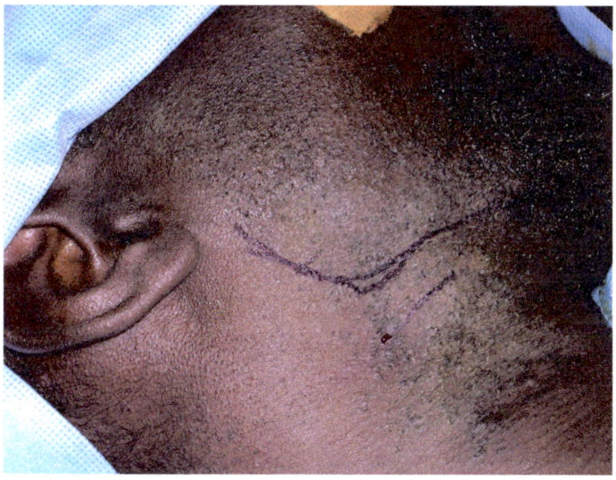

Fig. 4.7 Transcervical incision location

should then be placed, and the masseter is dissected off the lateral ramus. As the dissection moves superiorly, the endoscope should be introduced for visualization purposes. The muscle should be completely separated from the ramus and any muscle fragments should be removed. The dissection must extend as superior as possible along the neck of the condyle although violation of the temporomandibular joint capsule should be avoided. The sigmoid notch should be fully exposed as well as part of the coronoid process.

Like the transoral technique, a bicortical bone screw can be placed on the angle of the mandible and the distal segment is pulled caudally. Another technique is to place a large clamp on the angle to pull caudally although the clamp can interfere with placement of the other instruments into the surgical pocket. The endoscope is then introduced with a brow or notch retractor (Fig. 4.8). If the notch retractor is used, it should be placed into the sigmoid notch. Although the notch retractor keeps the pocket elevated, the hook portion that is in the sigmoid notch, if it tips laterally, can displace the proximal fragment from its reduced position. The brow retractor, because it is smaller, does not retract the soft tissue envelope as effectively as the notch retractor. An advantage of the brow retractor is that it does not displace the fragments and allows for the endoscope to be manipulated past the posterior border of the ramus.

Pulling caudally the fragments hopefully will be reduced into a stable position and the plate can

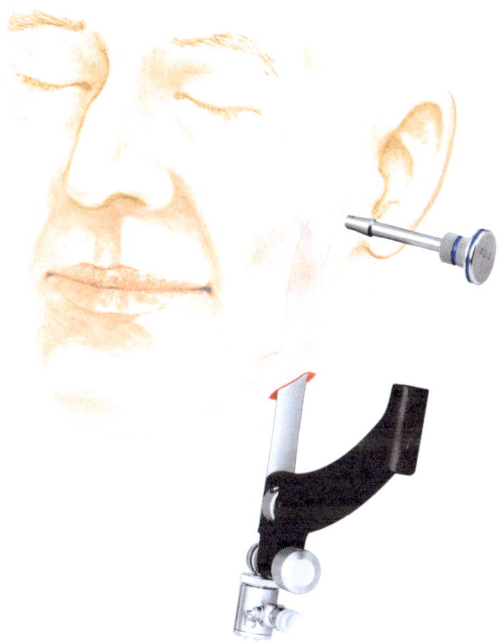

Fig. 4.8 Transcervical introduction of endoscopic instrumentation (Courtesy of Depuy Synthes©)

then be introduced. Similar to the transoral technique, a trocar can be introduced and a threaded fragment manipulator placed. In the transcervical technique, utilization of the threaded fragment manipulator can prove challenging. The presence of the threaded fragment manipulator seems to collapse the superior portion of the surgical pocket somewhat, creating visualization problems of the second screw hole on the proximal segment. A second trocar is placed and the remaining screws are either placed through the trocar or are placed through the incision site and the surgery is completed (Fig. 4.9).

4.3.3 Transoral vs. Transcervical Approaches: Technical Advantages and Disadvantages

Both approaches, as discussed in the introduction, do have a steep learning curve, and need to be performed on a regular basis to achieve competency

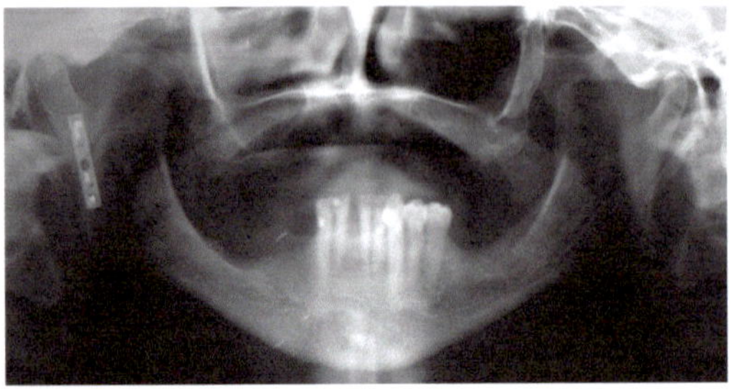

Fig. 4.9 Postoperative Panorex image

and efficiency. Both approaches have advantages and disadvantages when compared to each other. The transoral technique is esthetically superior to the extra-oral technique, because the incisions, for the most part, are in the mouth and are therefore not seen. The incision and the surgical pocket are generally larger than the extra-oral technique and because of this, the instruments are less likely to interfere with one another. Typically, with the proper case selection, it is less time consuming [11].

The major disadvantage is that even with a 45°, ideal visibility of the posterior portion of the fracture segment and the condylar neck, can be challenging. Because of this, the plate can sometimes be placed in a non-ideal location. In fractures where the condylar head is dislocated, it is very difficult to reduce it back into the fossa with this approach. A minor disadvantage is that a second incision, although small, needs to be made at the angle to facilitate the caudal traction.

The major advantage of the extra-oral technique, is complete visibility of the ramus condylar complex. The fracture from the notch to the posterior border of the ramus can be clearly seen. Also, the more posterior holes can be placed under direct visualization through the incision. There are two major disadvantages to the extra-oral approach. Because of the small size (2–3 cm) of the incision, there is a limit of the number of instruments that can be placed into the surgical pocket. This makes it sometimes difficult to have the suction, retractor, endoscope and manipulators present all at the same time without interfering with each other. Because of this, the incision sometimes needs to be extended into a formal submandibular incision length, which, as commented in the transoral section, is not cosmetic in nature.

4.4 Case Selection

Determining the whether to use the transoral or extra-oral approach in general, is based upon: (1) displacement of the fracture, (2) the anatomic location of the fracture, (3) and dislocation of the condylar head. Most fracture, other than the comminuted fractures, can be treated with a transoral approach. They can normally be reduced with caudal traction, and once they are reduced, remain stable, allowing for the plate to be fixated without displacing the fracture.

Dislocated condylar heads are the most technically challenging fractures to treat by the endoscopic method. These should generally be treated extra-orally, unless the experience level of the surgeon is of a high enough level where a transoral approach is even feasible. If the condyle cannot be reduced into the fossa, consideration should be given to converting the approach utilizing the "traditional" standard retromandibular incision or the combination of both the submandibular and preauricular incisions.

4.4.1 Complications

Although the number of fractures reported in the literature is relatively low, almost all the authors reported postoperative trismus that either resolved over time or following physiotherapy. Patient's postoperative occlusion returned to their normal pre-injury state in all reported cases. Both Troulis and Mueller reported one patient each with transient facial nerve weakness and Schon reported two cases [7, 11, 15]. Gonzalez-Garcia reported three cases of transient hypoesthesia [16]. Shoen reported one patient that had loosening of a screw on 3-month follow-up, necessitating plate removal and two fractured plates, that also needed to be removed [9, 14].

Conclusion

Surgical management of condylar fractures continues to be a contentious topic. The clinical evidence clearly states that open reduction with internal fixation results in significantly better functional results when compared to maxilla-mandibular fixation. That being said, surgeons are still hesitant to repair these fractures because of the potential risk of facial nerve injury and scarring. The development of endoscopic techniques has either eliminated or reduced these risks although the associated steep "learning curve" continues to curtail the adoption of this surgery.

References

1. Singh V, Bhagol A, Goel M, Kumar I, Verma A. Outcomes of open versus closed treatment of mandibular subcondylar fractures: a prospective randomized study. J Oral Maxillofac Surg. 2010;68(6):1304–9.
2. Undt G, Kermer C, Rasse M, Sinko K, Ewers R. Transoral miniplate osteosynthesis of condylar neck fractures. Oral Surg Oral Med Oral Pathol Oral Radiol Endod. 1999;88(5):534–43.
3. Yang WG, Chen CT, Tsay PK, Chen YR. Functional results of unilateral mandibular condylar process fractures after open and closed treatment. J Trauma. 2002;52(3):498–503.
4. Al-Moraissi EA, Ellis E 3rd. Surgical treatment of adult mandibular condylar fractures provides better outcomes than closed treatment: a systematic review and meta-analysis. J Oral Maxillofac Surg. 2015;73(3):482–93.
5. Loukota RA. Endoscopically assisted reduction and fixation of condylar neck/base fractures—the learning curve. Br J Oral Maxillofac Surg. 2006;44(6):480–1.
6. Jacobovicz J, Lee C, Trabulsy PP. Endoscopic repair of mandibular subcondylar fractures. Plast Reconstr Surg. 1998;101(2):437–41.
7. Lee C, Mueller RV, Lee K, Mathes SJ. Endoscopic subcondylar fracture repair: functional, aesthetic, and radiographic outcomes. Plast Reconstr Surg. 1998;102(5):1434–43; discussion 44–5.
8. Troulis MJ, Kaban LB. Endoscopic approach to the ramus/condyle unit: clinical applications. J Oral Maxillofac Surg. 2001;59(5):503–9.
9. Schon R, Fakler O, Gellrich NC, Schmelzeisen R. Five-year experience with the transoral endoscopically assisted treatment of displaced condylar mandible fractures. Plast Reconstr Surg. 2005;116(1):44–50.
10. Kellman RM. Endoscopically assisted repair of subcondylar fractures of the mandible: an evolving technique. Arch Facial Plast Surg. 2003;5(3):244–50.
11. Schon R, Gutwald R, Schramm A, Gellrich NC, Schmelzeisen R. Endoscopy-assisted open treatment of condylar fractures of the mandible: transcervical vs intraoral approach. Int J Oral Maxillofac Surg. 2002;31(3):237–43.
12. Schon R, Schramm A, Gellrich NC, Schmelzeisen R. Follow-up of condylar fractures of the mandible in 8 patients at 18 months after transoral endoscopic-assisted open treatment. J Oral Maxillofac Surg. 2003;61(1):49–54.
13. Cho-Lee GY, Rodriguez Campo FJ, Gonzalez Garcia R, Munoz Guerra MF, Sastre Perez J, Naval Gias L. Endoscopically-assisted transoral approach for the treatment of subcondylar fractures of the mandible. Med Oral Patol Oral Cir Bucal. 2008;13(8):E511–5.
14. Schoen R, Fakler O, Metzger MC, Weyer N, Schmelzeisen R. Preliminary functional results of endoscope-assisted transoral treatment of displaced bilateral condylar mandible fractures. Int J Oral Maxillofac Surg. 2008;37(2):111–6.
15. Troulis MJ. Endoscopic open reduction and internal rigid fixation of subcondylar fractures. J Oral Maxillofac Surg. 2004;62(10):1269–71.
16. Gonzalez-Garcia R, Sanroman JF, Goizueta-Adame C, Rodriguez-Campo FJ, Cho-Lee GY. Transoral endoscopic-assisted management of subcondylar fractures in 17 patients: an alternative to open reduction with rigid internal fixation and closed reduction with maxillomandibular fixation. Int J Oral Maxillofac Surg. 2009;38(1):19–25.

5 Minimally Invasive Approach to Orbital Trauma

Oded Nahlieli and Michael Abba

Abstract

With the equipment advances, the minimal invasive techniques can be applied in new surgical fields and have more applications. In this chapter, we would like to present a minimally invasive technique for treating orbital blowout fractures. The technique described has been practiced by two medical centers, The Barzilai medical center, Israel and The Jacobi Medical Center, NY, USA since 2007. Our results presented a high success rate with minimal rate of complications, thus our technique is a safe way with minimal morbidity for treating orbital floor fractures.

5.1 Introduction

Minimally invasive techniques have an increasing role in all surgical fields because they result in improved morbidity rates and better esthetic outcomes. The advantage of these techniques is that they involve smaller access incisions and thus less postoperative scaring. However, these techniques also have their drawbacks since they are usually more technique sensitive, require the use of specialized equipment, in most cases an indirect vision of the surgical field is used (endoscopes and monitor surgery) and have a longer learning curve.

In this chapter, we would like to present a minimally invasive technique for treating orbital blowout fractures (OBFs). The term orbital floor "blow out" fracture was first introduced in 1957 by Smith [1]. In the past, there was a tendency for operating on almost all of these type of fractures until 1972 when Crikelair and colleagues raised the claim that orbital fractures are being operated on too frequently [2]. These authors proposed a theory stating that an orbital floor fracture should be operated on only if diplopia and enophthalmos are persistent for a 2-week period. This approach further evolved when in 1974 Putterman and

O. Nahlieli, DMD (✉)
Department of Oral and Maxillofacial Surgery, Barzilai Medical Center, Ashkelon, Israel

Faculty of Medicine, Ben Gurion University of the Negev, Beer Sheva, Israel

Department of Oral and Maxillofacial Surgery, Eastman Institute for Oral Health University of Rochester, Rochester, NY, USA

Department of Oral and Maxillofacial Surgery, University of Michigan Health System, Ann Arbor, Michigan, USA
e-mail: nahlieli@yahoo.com

M. Abba, DMD
Department of Oral and Maxillofacial Surgery, Barzilai Medical Center, Ashkelon, Israel

O. Nahlieli (ed.), *Minimally Invasive Oral and Maxillofacial Surgery*,
http://doi.org/10.1007/978-3-662-54592-8_5

colleagues noticed that only a small percentage of blowout fractures had persistent symptoms for more than 3 weeks [3]. These findings caused a digression in the decision towards surgical intervention while a more conservative non-surgical treatment was adopted. This extreme shift in treatment decision of these fractures was followed with further work by different authors that suggested new and more case-specific parameters. For example, Dulley and Fells introduced new criteria for surgical intervention, including the following signs and only if they were persistent for over 2 weeks: enophthalmos >3 mm, large herniation of tissue into the antrum, entrapment with limited motion and diplopia [4].

Isolated orbital fractures consists 4–16% of facial fractures enrolled to the emergency room [5, 6]. These facial injuries have a distinct impact on the patient's life due to esthetic considerations. Facial appearance has a major impact on the well-being of these patients which further results in psychological and social consequences. Thus, the decision for surgical treatment of facial fractures is not as clear-cut as in many other skeletal fractures since the decision to operate or not is based not only on functional considerations, the esthetic considerations are sometimes no less important. Many facial fractures will have acceptable functional surgical outcomes following healing but may not have equally acceptable esthetic outcomes. When considering indications for treatment of facial fractures, we have to take into consideration these esthetic factors thus surgical treatment of certain facial injuries can be considered as esthetic surgery. The significance of understanding this point requires the surgeon to consider the surgical access in treating certain injuries not only as bone reductions but also taking into consideration the balance between the detriments and benefits of the trans-facial incisions.

Orbital fractures account for up to 40% of craniofacial injuries. Orbital involvement as a sole fracture site consists of up to 16% of cases [7–9]. The most frequently encountered orbital fractures involve the floor and medial wall. Medial wall fractures rarely require treatment while orbital floor fractures are operated on more frequently. The decision to treat these fractures is based on functional and esthetic factors. Usually, the diagnostic step is of the utmost importance and consists of the Computed Tomography (CT) Scan as the gold standard.

5.2 Surgical Anatomy of the Orbit

The orbital cavity has a conical shape with complex anatomic structures in a very limited space. It consists of seven bones and has four boundaries: the medial, the lateral, the floor, and the ceiling (Fig. 5.1). The orbital apex is of special consideration since it hosts the optic nerve. The optic nerve leaves the orbit through the bony canal (the optic canal) in the sphenoid bone (Fig. 5.2); CSF enters the intraorbital subarachnoidal space by the same route. The lumen varies in shape, but is practically oval. It runs between the body and the two roots of the lesser wing of the sphenoid bone. The anterior opening is oval in outline and measures 5–6 mm in longer diameter; the central part is circular, with an average diameter of 5.5 mm; the posterior portion is generally considered to be flattened from above downwards. If the canal is pathologically narrow because of congenital

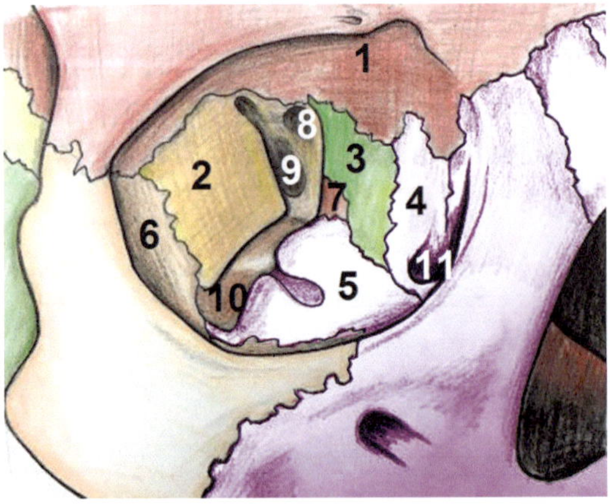

Fig. 5.1 The bones of the orbit. 1—the frontal bone, 2—the sphenoid bone, 3—the ethmoid bone, 4—the lacrimal bone, 5—the maxilla, 6—the zygomatic bone, 7—the palatine bone, 8—the optic canal in the sphenoid bone, 9—the superior orbital fissure, 10—the inferior orbital fissure, 11—the lacrimal groove

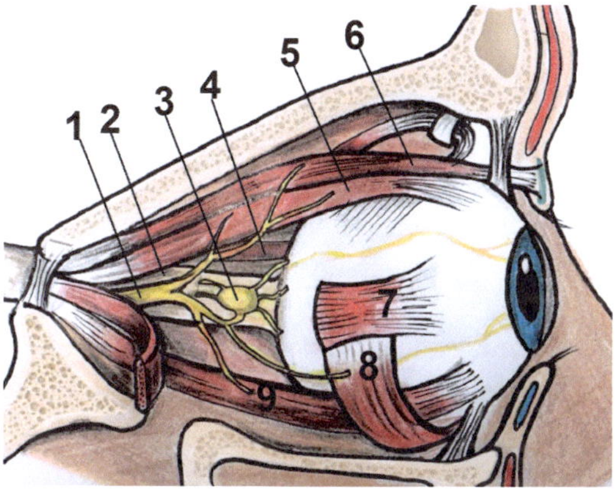

Fig. 5.2 The muscles and nerves of the orbit. 1—the oculomotor nerve (CN III), 2—the optic nerve, 3—the ciliary ganglion, 4, 7—the medial rectus muscle, 5—the superior rectus muscle, 6—the levator palbebrae superior muscle, 8—the inferior oblique muscle, 9—the inferior rectus muscle

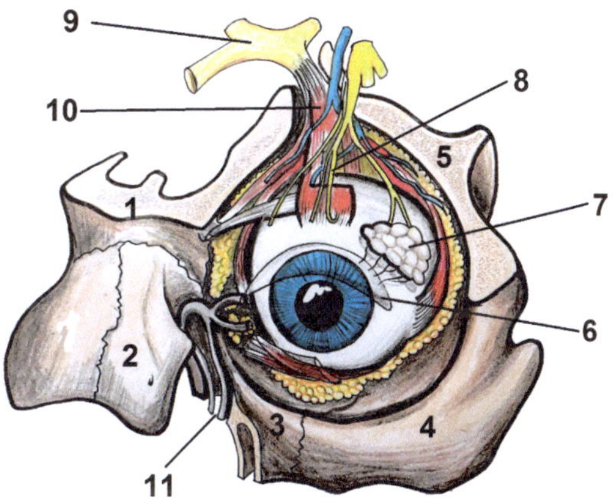

Fig. 5.3 Anatomical elements of the orbit. 1—the frontal bone, 2—the nasal bone, 3—maxilla, 4—the zygomatic bone, 5—the temporal bone, 6—the tarsal plate, 7—the lacrimal gland, 8—the supraorbital nerve, 9—the optic nerve, 10—the rectus muscles, 11—the nasolacrimal duct

anomalies or tumor, or became narrow because of the trauma, the optic nerve atrophy can occur and no CSF will pass through.

The medial side of the orbital cavity neighbors the nasal cavity and the lamina papyracea as a thin layer of bone usually <1 mm. Because of the neighboring ethmoidal sinus bony mesh, the medial part of the orbital cavity is less involved in traumatic events if compared to the floor [9, 10]. However, while this wall is very thin a trauma may create a dehiscence of it, and surgically, the two walls, which are easy to destroy when performing orbital decompression, are the inferior and the medial walls [11].

On the lateral side, the bone is much thicker and comprises the greater wing of the sphenoid and the zygomatic bones. The zygomatic bone is located close to the anterior rim, the Whitnall's orbital tubercle (lateral orbital tubercle) (Fig. 5.3). Posteriorly, the lateral orbital wall consists of the greater wing of the sphenoid. The floor of the orbit neighbors the maxillary sinus. This proximity makes the maxillary sinus a good option for accessing the orbital floor. Three bones participate in its formation: the orbital face of the zygomatic bone at the front and laterally, the orbital face of the maxillary bone at the front and medially, and posteriorly a very small bony area consisting of the orbital process of the palatine bone.

The orbital floor is usually 0.5 mm thick and does not serve as a protection mechanism against the globe injury. The orbital floor is most frequently fragmented in "blow out" fractures. The infraorbital sulcus runs over the posterior part of the floor. It arises from the anterior part of the inferior orbital fissure, goes forward, and penetrates the bone to form the infraorbital canal, which opens 5–6 mm under the infraorbital rim as the infraorbital foramen [11].

Attention Surgeons These structures contain the infraorbital nerve, the terminal branch of the maxillary nerve, and the infraorbital vessels. The infraorbital nerve provides branches for the teeth and the upper lip and it may be injured during orbital decompression.

The anterior antral wall is easily accessible for transantral approach for exploration of the orbital floor fracture. The most complex area to reach is the posterior medial wall since it is beyond the orbital axis. This area is much more accessible from outside the orbital cavity as will be described in this chapter.

5.3 Indications for Surgery After the Orbital Trauma

Clinical features of blowout fracture of the orbit are well known and are as follows:

- **Intraocular and intraorbital pain**
- **Diplopia**
- **Blindness** of the affected eye
- **Enophthalmos** (the posterior displacement of the eyeball within the orbit)
- **The eyeball displacement**
- **Local edema**
- **Local hematoma**
- **Infraorbital anesthesia and/or numbness of certain regions of face**
- **Restricted ocular mobility** up to complete **inability to move the eye**
- **Epistaxis**

The most common findings in blowout fractures are enophthalmos, diplopia, restricted eye movement, and infraorbital paraesthesia. Each of these findings is not an absolute indication for surgery. The decision to operate or not on orbital floor fractures is based on a combination of the clinical presentation of the patient and the radiologic findings. These fractures usually present a dilemma for the practitioner because of possible comorbidity due to the surgery performed through the conventional approaches and the fact that many cases resolve without the need of operation and without any residual symptoms. The clinical challenge is to identify the cases that require surgical intervention and especially those cases in need of emergency treatment. These patients usually present themselves with a severe periorbital swelling and hematoma and with different degrees of restriction of eye movement and diplopia. The most frequent esthetic presentations are the enophthalmos, hypoglobus (downward displacement of the eye in the orbit), and the functional disturbances such as the restriction of eye movement and related diplopia. The challenge is to identify and distinguish those cases that will resolve spontaneously from those that require treatment. To that end, many authors suggested key clinical signs and radiological findings that indicate the need for surgery [5, 6, 12–14].

In summary, the most common indications for surgical intervention are as follows:

- Eesthetic considerations
- Enophthalmos >2 mm
- Fuŋctional problems
- Diplopia at central gaze or up to 30° angle of view
- Alarming data of radiological evaluation
- Entrapment of extra-ocular muscles or a fracture of more than 50% of the orbital floor with significant orbital content prolapse.

These indications as aforementioned have been extensively published and are accepted as a rule of thumb in decision-making. As clinical experience and data collection continues to evolve, the physiology may show to be more complex as understanding of this crowded anatomic space develops more parameters to consider. Leo Koornneef [15] described a complex sheath of fibrous tissue septa covering the inferior rectus muscle. This tissue can be entrapped between bone fragment and cause restriction, even if not presented immediately, fibrosis of this tissue if entrapped can cause long-term restriction. Harris et al. proposed a radiographic CT correlation between the component of the soft tissue and bone displacement [16]. He suggested that fractures with proportionate soft-hard tissue displacement can be managed according to size, meaning that if the extent of tissue prolapse is severe enough to cause enophthalmos then the resultant future esthetic result is the indication for surgery [17]. It is worthy to emphasize that these cases are not considered emergency cases and surgical intervention can be delayed for up to 2 weeks. However, in cases with a disproportionate component of soft tissue involvement to the bone displacement, a trap door fracture can be assumed. Initial displacement of bone causes prolapse of tissue and consequently due to the elastic properties of the orbital bone these bone fragments readapt and cause entrapment of the prolapsed tissue. In these cases, ischemia is anticipated and if combined with clinical restriction and diplopia is an indication for immediate surgery. The shape of the inferior rectus muscle is another indicative radiologic finding. If its oval anatomic shape is kept, we can assume there is no entrapment of muscle but if an elongated vertical shape is observed and the muscle's position is outside the orbital volume the assumption is that surgery is inevitable.

Additional radiological findings have been described and further add to the complex decision-making in these cases. Following our experience, we suggest a decision algorithm that easily summarizes all clinical and radiographic findings. We call it "Two-week algorithm":

Two-Week Algorithm

Enophthalmos Present

- Severe prolapse → ***surgery***
- Moderate prolapse → wait for 2 weeks → surgery/no surgery decision
- Mild prolapse → observation

Dyplopia Present

- Soft > hard → ***surgery***
- Soft = hard → severe prolapse ± enophthalmos → ***surgery***
- Soft = hard → mild/moderate prolapse → wait for 2 weeks → surgery/no surgery decision

5.4 Surgical Approaches and Reconstruction Materials

There are several generally accepted surgical techniques in management of the orbital trauma that can be divided into transantral and transcutaneous approaches. Of them, the transantral approach includes transnasal and transmaxillary techniques and the transcutaneous approach includes subcilliary, transconjunctival, midtarsal, and infraorbital coronal techniques. The transnasal and transantral decompression leaves no external incision, but can provide only a limited decompression of the medial wall of the orbit and medial part of the floor.

The *transconjunctival approach* consists of a conjunctival incision without any cutaneous incisions. With this technique, there is no visible scarring and a decreased risk of entropion formation given that the orbital septal plane is not violated [18]. The transconjunctival incision also provides good access for medial wall decompression, but can present some surgical difficulty due to the presence of unrestrained orbital fat in the operative field. In a review of 400 cases, Mullins et al. showed the complication rate of this technique is between 2 and 42% [19]. The *subciliary approach* to the orbital floor also allows for broad access, but can cause lower lid retraction and malposition [20]. Following this approach, the post-orbicularis plane is reached through a subciliary incision. Better exposure can be gained with the *midtarsal incision* which causes minimal or no ectropion. **The midtarsal incision is sited between the edge of the eyelid and the orbital rim.**

Coronal incision or more specifically, *infraorbital coronal approach* provides the best exposure to the roof of the orbit. It is usually placed remotely to avoid visible facial scars. The subperiosteal or subgaleal planes are used for coronal flap dissection. The scalp incision is extended lateroinferiorly into the preauricular region to gain access to the zygomatic arch and the orbit. In fact, not only the floor of the orbit but the lateral and the medial walls also can be accessed by this approach. Danger: the temporal branch of the facial nerve can be damaged. The Lynch external ethmoidectomy approach, the extended lateral canthotomy approach, and the bicoronal scalp-flap approach were also described in the literature [20, 21].

5.4.1 Reconstruction Materials

In cases of extensive destruction of the floor of orbit then reconstruction of the floor must be resorted to using implants. When deciding which material to use in order to reconstruct the orbital floor, we need to ask ourselves what would be the ideal material to use for the purpose? The answer to this question would be a material that is easy to adapt to the complex 3D anatomy of the orbital floor, that will provide an adequate "gliding" surface for the orbital tissues, and that will be less prone to infections due to the probable exposure of the material to respiratory mucosa. Another important feature of this material would be an ability to remove it easily in case of a complication. **These materials include autologous bone grafts, usually the** iliac crest bone, high-density porous polyethylene, **and titanium plates/meshes.**

The autografts might be suitable in cases with large defects. The chances for infection are low since it is an autogenous graft. The disadvantage of it is a need for a secondary surgical sight and the additional morbidity as well as cases with a significant resorption of the graft. The synthetic alloplasts are commonly used since they are usually easily placed within the orbital cavity and no additional surgical site is needed. Their disadvantage would be a higher risk for infection and the fibrous reaction they cause, which can lead to their removal. Titanium is the material commonly used as an inert material which causes minimal tissue irritation and good integration. It is also the least prone to infections. Titanium is an easily molded material which can be fitted to the anatomic structure of the orbit and thus preserving the 3D structure of the orbital cavity. **The reconstruction** materials containing titanium mesh have good tissue compatibility with minimal postoperative reactions such as infection and/or rejection. The material is easy to shape, and communication through micropores firmly bonds bone tissue of the orbit so that the surrounding tissue can grow effectively with good blood supply.

The pre-bent titanium mesh (MatrixORBITAL, Synthes GmbH, Switzerland; MEDPOR®, Stryker, USA, or similar, see further on Figs. 5.11a and 5.16) can be 1.5, 2.0, or 2.5 mm thick. The most frequently used is 1.5 mm thick. These implants may be contoured with surgical scissors in the sterile field to fit the individual orbital problem of a patient. In fact, these reconstruction materials can be manufactured by 3D technologies as patient-specific implants (PSI). It permits achieving a perfect adaption to the orbital structure and reducing operative time. The implants with embedded titanium mesh provide strength, shape retention when bent, and flexibility for various orbital trauma surgical procedures. Interconnected, omni-directional pore structure of the mesh promotes native tissue in-growth for enhanced biocompatibility. The implants usually require a titanium screw fixation.

5.4.2 The Minimally Invasive Revolution

The conventional approaches involving the transfacial incisions, blepharoplasty, or transconjunctival incisions further complicate the dilemma. As aforementioned, these surgeries can be considered as esthetic surgeries and when weighing the potential complications of the standard techniques as entropion and ectropion and conjunctival scaring we may be exchanging one esthetic problem with another esthetic defect. When considering the option of orbital floor reconstruction without skin incision and outside the orbital cavity, the decision to operate or not may be much easier. The transantral technique involves only intraoral incisions and thus all related complications are eliminated without any hardware inside the orbit. This enables us to perform an anatomic reduction with minimal potential complications.

The endoscopic surgical approach to the orbital blowout fractures was previously described in general and specifically for the endonasal reduction of blowout fractures of the orbital floor [22–24]. We present the new technique in detail as practiced at our department resulting in minimal morbidity and a very low rate of complications.

5.5 The Endoscopic Reconstruction of Orbital Floor Fractures

Access to the facial skeleton is very variable and the facial trauma with multiple facial lacerations has its own considerations. While less extensive trauma cases may require only esthetic considerations, there is a great deal of concern regarding the esthetic result following transfacial incisions.

By closely reading descriptions of different endoscopic techniques applicable to the orbital trauma, a great variability in the technique is apparent among them. Walter [25] first described surgical repair of blowout fractures of the orbital floor using the transantral approach but without a direct view obtained using an endoscope. Ducic and Verret described their endoscopic transantral approach to the repair of orbital floor fractures. In their series, the authors used the bony window on the lateral wall or a medpor inside the orbital cavity [26]. Strong et al. described an endoscopic transmaxillary technique for the repair of orbital blowout fractures [27]. This study was conducted on cadaver heads and ten clinical cases. The technique of these authors consisted of removing all prolapsed fragments of bone and reconstruction with a medpor inside the orbital cavity. This technique is not based on an anatomic consideration. Persons and Wong described a trans-antral endoscopic orbital floor repair using resorbable plate [28]. These authors also used an intraorbital placement of the reconstruction plate and described the remaining, medial posterior and lateral bony shelves as a rest for the material. This technique can be very hard to perform in cases where the bony shelves are not stable or missing. Finally, Fernandes et al. described his technique of reconstructing the orbital floor fracture through a transmaxillary approach and placed a resorbable medpor inside the orbital cavity [29]. This technique is also dependent from an intact posterior shelf to stabilize the medpor.

In short, our approach consists of only transoral incisions; a vestibular incision is made in order to gain access to the lateral astral wall. Next, an osteotomy is performed using piezosurgery or a bur, and the bone window is preserved in saline for further readaptment. After the access has been achieved, the orbital floor is inspected with a 30° endoscope and the muscle entrapment is released. If there is a prolapse of the orbital content, then the tissue is retrieved back to the orbital cavity. In order to reconstruct the anatomy of the orbital floor, we use a titanium mesh that is being molded to the anatomy of the sinus roof and fixated outside of the sinus on the access window performed. Usually, there is no need for further stabilization. This reconstruction type is an anatomic reduction and uses the prolapsed bony fragments as a scaffold for the reconstruction of the orbital floor.

In 2007, Farwell et al. analyzed the endoscopic repair of orbital blowout fractures [30]. The authors concluded then that while these fractures can be approached endoscopically, the technique is not perfected yet. Specifically, the authors indicated that endoscopic repair became very difficult and often not possible when a large amount of soft tissue was herniated through the floor defect and when dissection medially onto the lamina papyracea and lateral to the infraorbital nerve was required for implant placement [30]. It was our aim to overcome these limitations.

5.5.1 The Operative Technique

Step by step the endoscopic reconstruction of orbital floor fractures is performed by the following ways:

1. Forced duction test should be performed to determine whether the absence of movement of the eyeball is of neurological origin or a mechanical restriction is present. The anesthetized conjunctiva is grasped with forceps, and the eyeball is gently moved in the direction where the movement is restricted. If an orbital trauma caused a mechanical restriction, it will not be possible to induce a passive movement of the eyeball.
2. It follows with the sublabial, subperiosteal incision of the oral mucosa in the premolar-molar teeth area.
3. Osteotomy is usually performed with a piezosurgery (Mecatron) as a lateral antrostomy 2–1.5 cm.
4. Insertion of the endoscope is performed through the orifice.
5. Following the visualization and exploration of the fracture site, the reduction with a blunt, curved periosteal elevator and an indwelling balloon is performed.

6. Forced duction and "pulse" tests should be repeated (the direct view of the prolapsed content of the orbital cavity into the maxillary sinus while moving the globe).
7. At this point, an identification of the infraorbital nerve and inferior rectus muscle is needed followed by the retrieval of prolapsed fatty tissue back into the orbit and removal of sharp bony fragments.
8. The next step consists of adaptation of the titanium mesh to the orbital floor, insertion of an indwelling balloon, molding, and fixation with screws to stable bony structures.
9. Forced duction test should be repeated again; the endoscopic inspection through the sinus is necessary at this point.
10. Reattachment of the osteotomized lateral wall is performed.
11. Postoperative CT scan is obligatory to ensure adequate floor position.

To expand the suggested treatment protocol in more details, after the patient is under general anesthesia, a forced duction test is performed to depict the exact degree of globe motion, and then a sublabial, subperiosteal flap is raised to reach the lateral sinus wall. The infraorbital nerve should be identified and retracted. An osteotomy 2–1.5 cm is performed with extreme care taken to avoid damaging the teeth roots. The osteotomy should be performed with a piezosurgery device in order to prevent infraorbital nerve damage. The osteotomized bone is removed and maintained in saline solution during the procedure. The endoscope (DCI, 4 mm, 30°; Karl Storz, Tuttlingen, Germany) should be introduced to the maxillary sinus, and direct visualization of the fracture site can be obtained. A "pulse test" should be done so as to visualize the prolapsed periorbit through the bony defect from the antral view, and the periorbit is retrieved back into the orbit with a blunt curved periosteal elevator. If sharp bone fragments are encountered in the periorbit, they may be removed through the same approach. The inferior rectus muscle and the infraorbital nerve are identified with the aid of the forced duction test, and decompression of the muscle should be performed if necessary.

The titanium mesh (1.5 mm, A-O; Synthes, Solothurn, Switzerland) is inserted and placed in the antral roof, molded according to the curvature of the posterior border, and fixed to the anterior and lateral surfaces with 2–4 screws. It is important that one screw is fixed to the buttress area and one screw is fixed to the pyriform fossa to provide optimum stabilization.

An indwelling balloon should be placed in the maxillary sinus while the plate is fixed with the screws; once fixation is complete, the balloon is withdrawn. The osteotomized bone is then fixed back to the lateral wall. The procedure is completed with a forced duction test.

5.5.2 Specific Approaches to Various Cases

5.5.2.1 Illustrative Case 1

A 22-year-old patient presented with an injury of his right orbit after being involved in a fist fight. He arrived 3 h after his injury. His main complaint was diplopia in an upward gaze, local pain, and infraorbital paresthesia (Fig. 5.4). The oph-

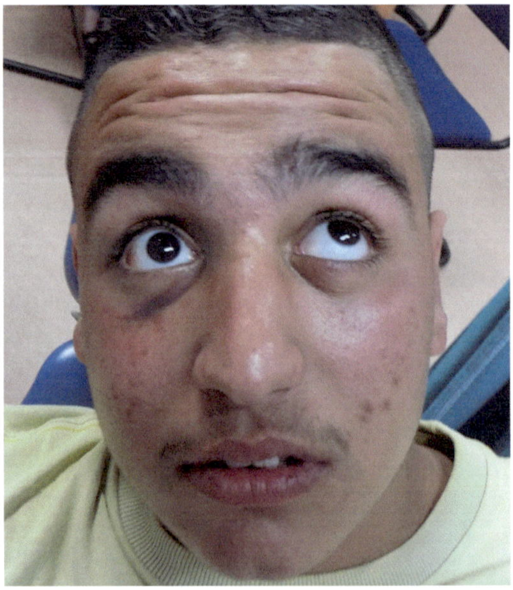

Fig. 5.4 A patient with an injury of the right orbit with diplopia in an upward gaze, local pain, and infraorbital paresthesia. The visual equity was not disturbed. (The patient's permission was obtained)

thalmologic evaluation demonstrated restricted eye movement and diplopia <30° in an upward gaze. The visual equity was not disturbed. The radiologic findings revealed orbital blowout fracture with prolapse of orbital content and inferior rectus entrapment. The inferior rectus as presented in the CT scan is elongated and the oval regular is not seen (Fig. 5.5a, b).

The patient was taken to the operating room, where a lateral antrostomy was performed under general anesthesia. Endoscopy demonstrated a trap door deformity and prolapsed orbital fat through the bony fragments (Fig. 5.6). The orbital contents were retrieved and pushed into the orbit with curved periostal elevators. The titanium mesh plate was molded to the orbital floor with the aid of curved periostal elevators and a Foley catheter balloon (Fig. 5.7a, b) and then fixed to the lateral surface with screws (Fig. 5.8). The osteotomized bone was brought and fixed back to the lateral walls. An obvious esthetic improvement with patient satisfaction was obtained with resolution of the diplopia noted after 48 h (Fig. 5.9). Postoperative CT scan demonstrated excellent bony reduction (Fig. 5.10). The complete **reconstruction of the floor of the orbit was achieved with** the titanium mesh plate (Fig. 5.11).

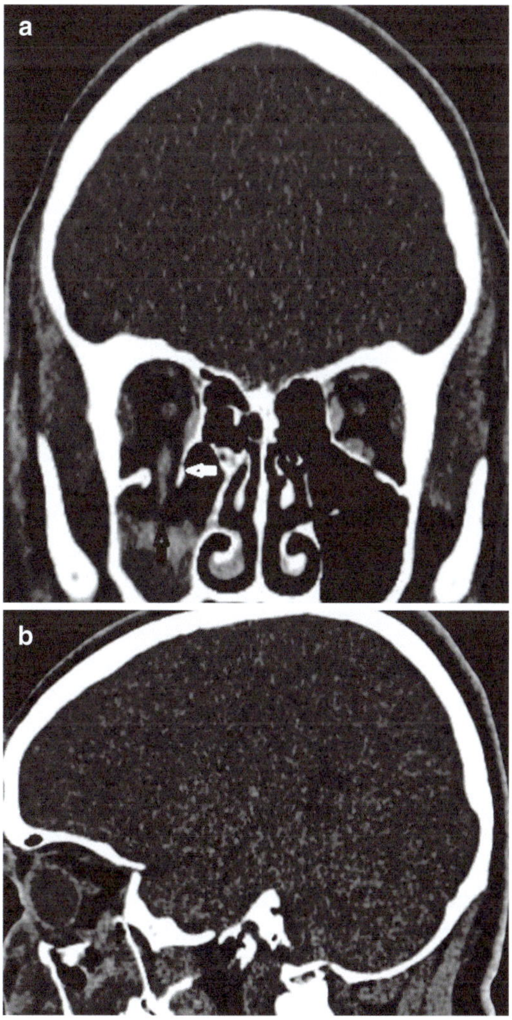

Fig. 5.5 The same patient with an injury of the right orbit. (**a**) The radiologic findings revealed orbital blowout fracture with prolapse of orbital content and inferior rectus entrapment. (**b**) The inferior rectus as presented in the CT scan is elongated and the oval regular is not seen

5.5.2.2 Illustrative Case 2

This unique in its clinical presentation and radiologic appearance case represents the clinical dilemma we confront in many of the cases regarding the time of the intervention and the dilemma weather to wait for spontaneous resolution and risk the loose of the time window for surgical intervention.

The 28-year-old patient was admitted to the emergency room after an assault to his left eye. An ophthalmologic assessment revealed diplopia with a severe restriction in an upward gaze (Fig. 5.12). The CT scan image presented a very

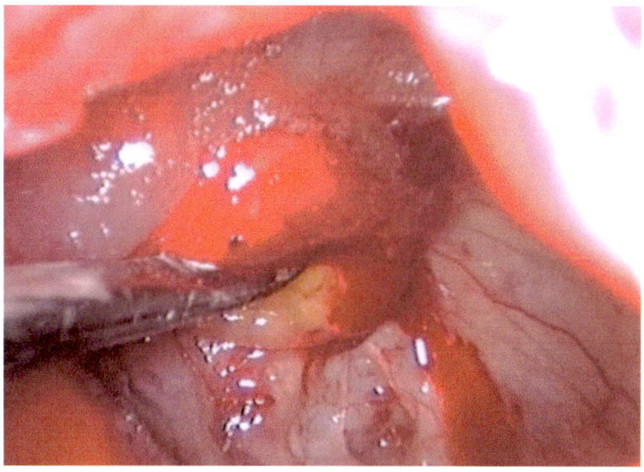

Fig. 5.6 The same patient with an injury of the right orbit during the surgery. Endoscopy demonstrated a trap door deformity and prolapsed orbital fat through the bony fragments

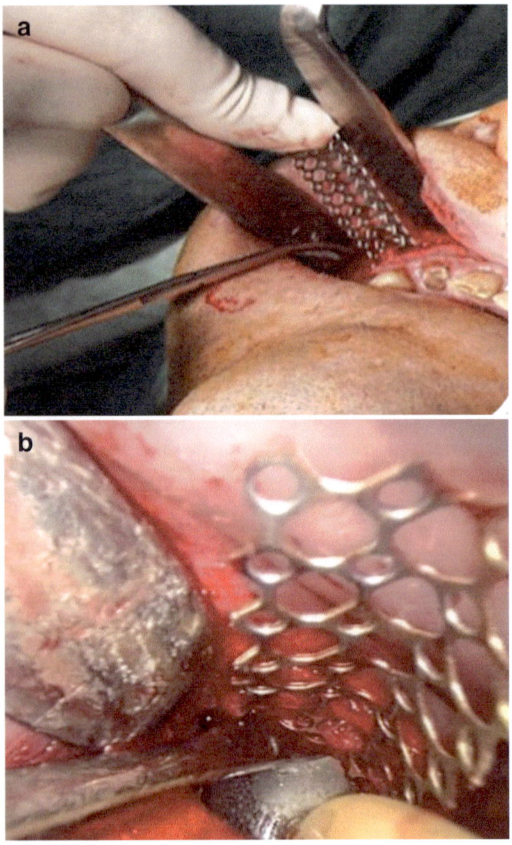

Fig. 5.7 (**a**, **b**) The same patient with an injury of the right orbit: continuation of the surgery. Titanium mesh plate was molded to the orbital floor with the aid of curved periostal elevators and a Foley catheter balloon

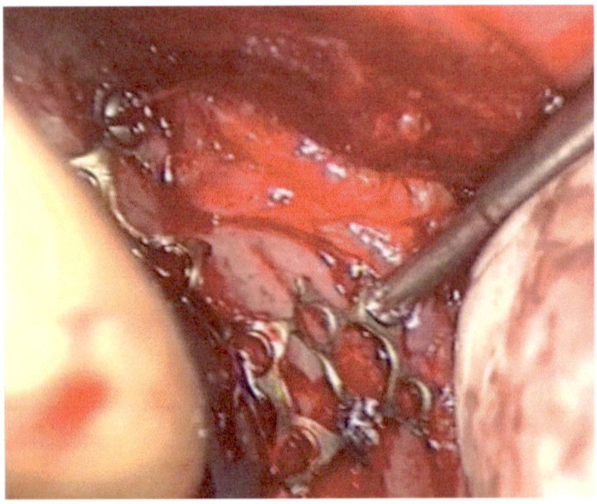

Fig. 5.8 The titanium mesh plate is fixed to the lateral surface of the orbit with screws

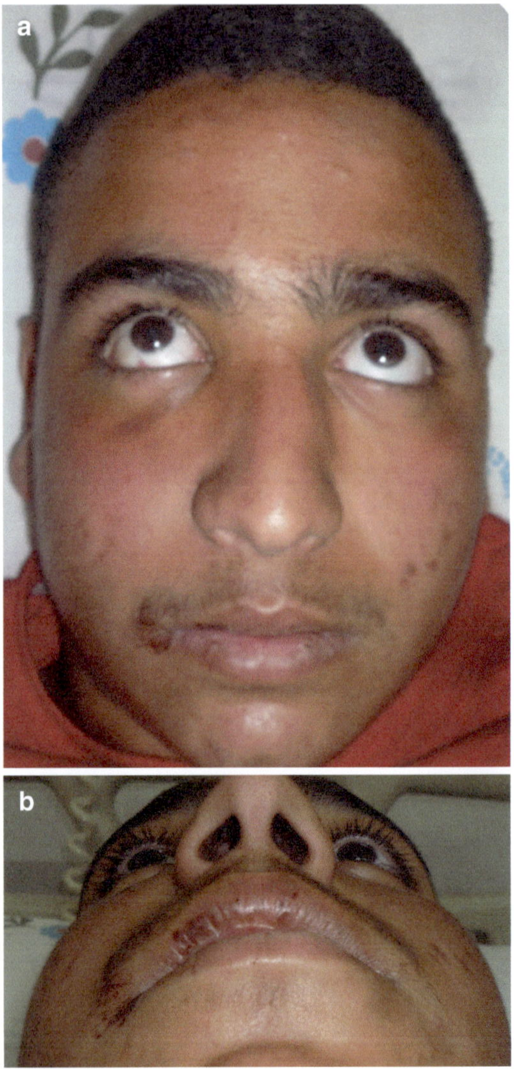

Fig. 5.9 (**a**, **b**) The same patient after the surgery. An obvious esthetic improvement with patient satisfaction was obtained. (The patient's permission was obtained)

mild displacement if any (Fig. 5.13). The involvement was in the posterior medial part of the floor of the orbit. As it was mentioned previously, it is very hard to reach this area that is located very close to the orbital apex. This case was very challenging since there was a discrepancy between the clinical (more severe) and radiological (less severe) findings. We decided to start with a conservative approach and wait for spontaneous res-

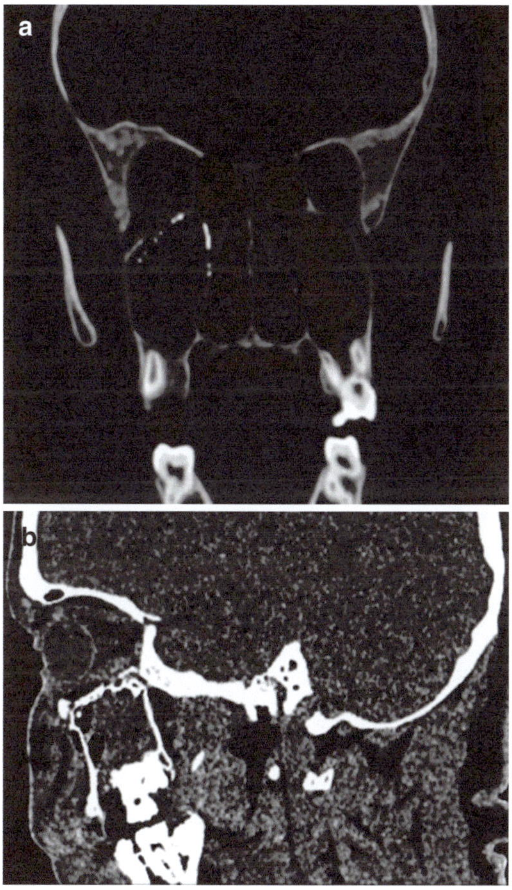

Fig. 5.10 (**a**, **b**) The same patient after the surgery. Postoperative CT scan demonstrated excellent bony reduction. Compare B with Fig. 5.5b

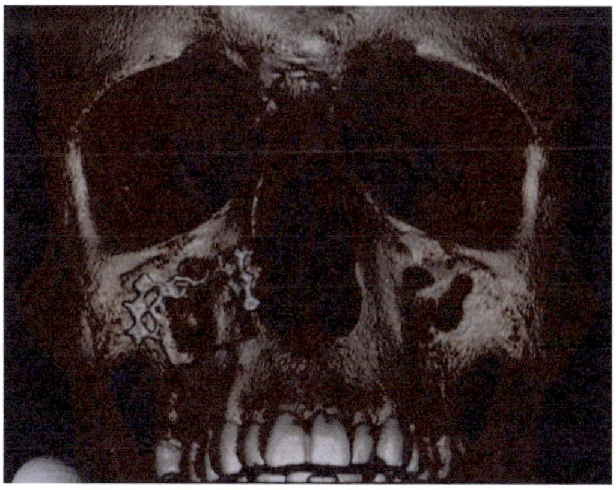

Fig. 5.11 The same patient after the surgery. Postoperative 3D CT scan images demonstrated the complete **reconstruction of the floor of the orbit with** the titanium mesh plate

olution of the condition. We initiated a protocol of dexamethasone 20 mg 3 h after the patient's arrival and continued downward scale by reducing 2 mg each subsequent day. The eyeball physiotherapy was also prescribed. Having 5 days of no improvement we decided to go to the operating theater.

We assessed that this case would be very challenging if using conventional transcutaneous methods and the above-described transantral endoscopic approach was selected. During the exploration of the orbital floor, a clear entrapment of the inferior rectus muscle was present with a minimal involvement of the orbital content (Fig. 5.14). The muscle was released and the titanium mesh (1.5 mm) was embedded. The procedure was uneventful, an intraoperative forced duction test was performed showing a release of the entrapped muscle and direct visualization of the movement of the inferior rectus muscle. The postoperative CT scan images demonstrated the adaptation of the mesh to the orbital floor outline (Fig. 5.15a–c) and the 3D CT reconstruction indicated the repositioning of the lateral antrostomy bony window (Fig. 5.16).

The postoperative follow-up a week after surgery showed no improvement of eye upward gaze (Fig. 5.17). The awake forced duction test was performed showing a release of the entrapment compared to the pre-surgical status (Fig. 5.18). This case is a classic case of a trap door fracture that needed an immediate intervention. The follow-up was continued for 3 weeks with an improvement of diplopia. The patient did not show for further follow-ups.

Traumas of the orbit are common and challenging to manage assuming the necessity of restoring the orbital anatomy, the eyeball physiology, and appreciation of good esthetic results. Such fractures can have an impact on the orbital globe, eye movement and esthetic consequences because of the change of the orbital volume. The minimally invasive approach to the orbital fracture site depends upon the type of injury, surgeon experience, and available equipment. After excluding any visual acuity disturbances, we

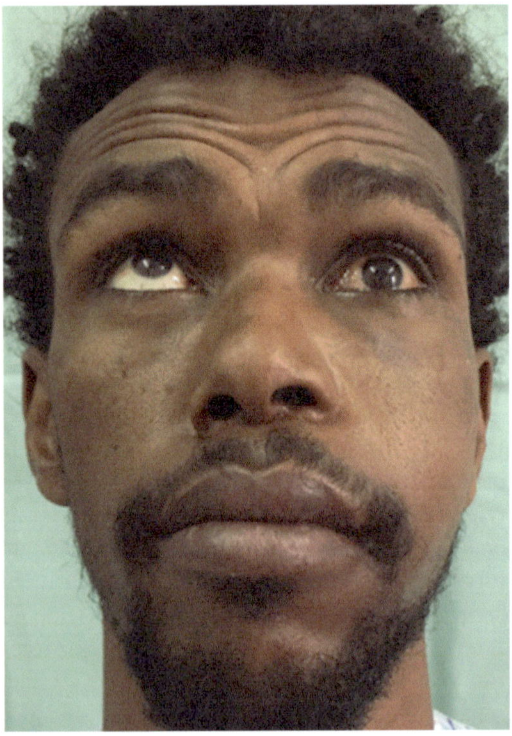

Fig. 5.12 Illustrative case 2. A patient with an injury of the left orbit with diplopia and a severe restriction in an upward gaze. (The patient's permission was obtained)

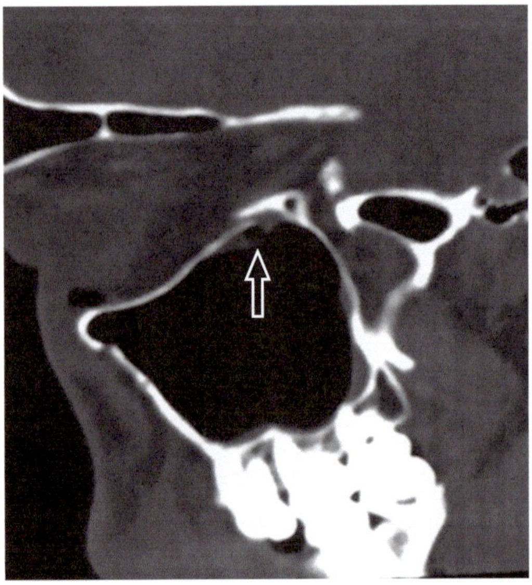

Fig. 5.13 Illustrative case 2. The CT scan image presented a very mild displacement if any

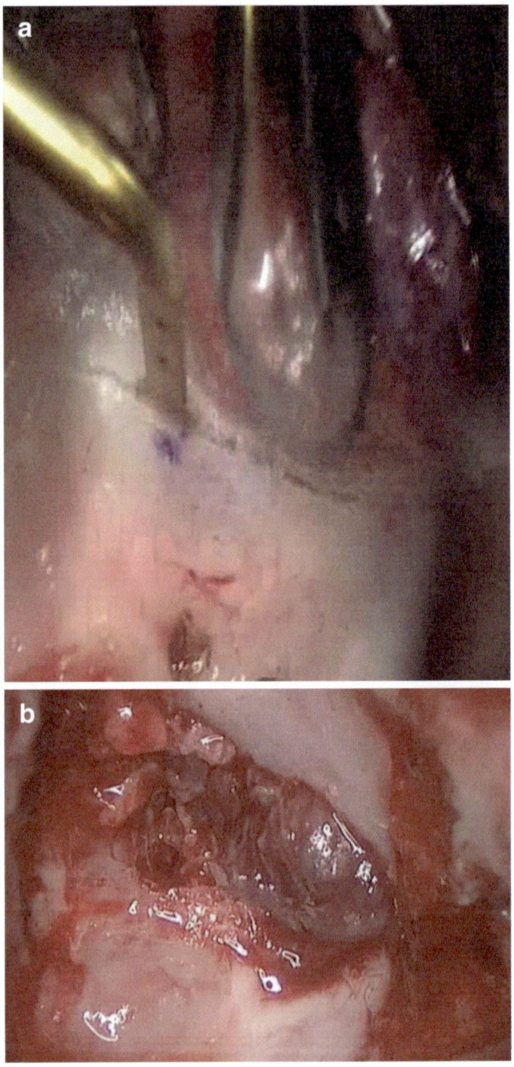

Fig. 5.14 Illustrative case 2. During the endoscopic exploration of the orbital floor, a clear entrapment of the inferior rectus muscle was present (**a**) with a minimal involvement of the orbital content (**b**)

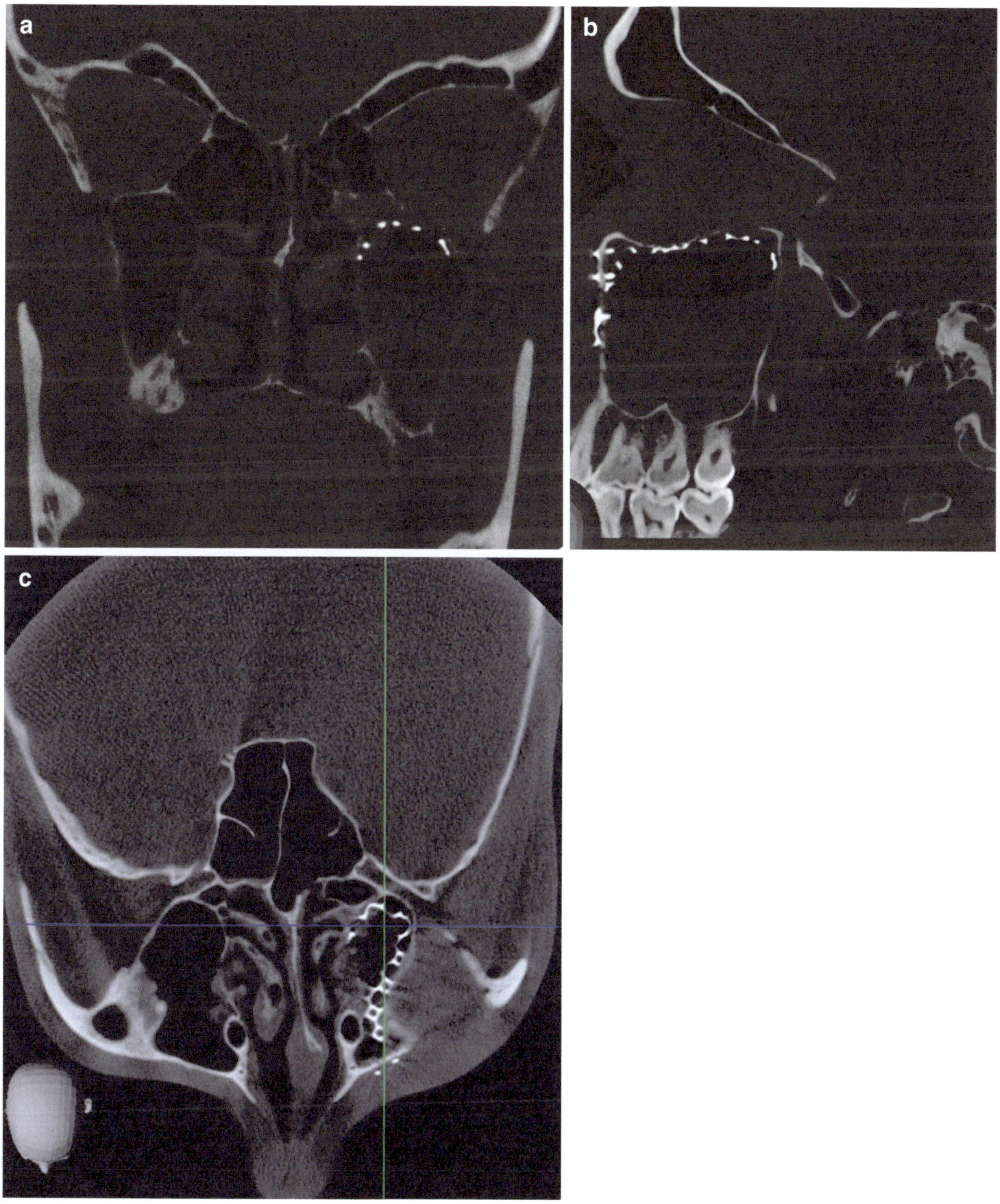

Fig. 5.15 Illustrative case 2. (**a–c**). The postoperative CT scan images demonstrated the adaptation of the mesh to the orbital floor outline

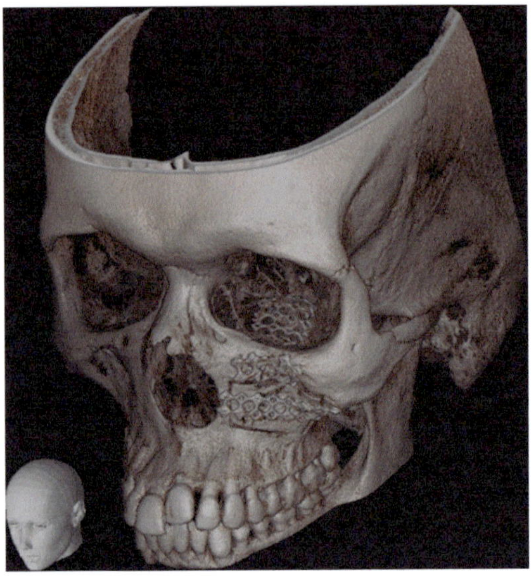

Fig. 5.16 Illustrative case 2. The 3D CT reconstruction indicated the repositioning of the lateral antrostomy bony window

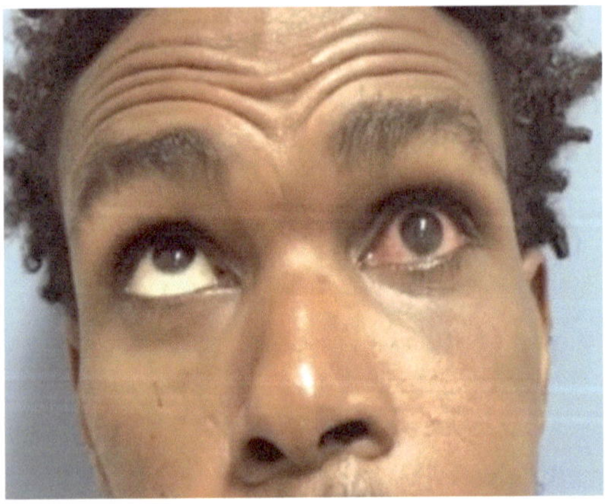

Fig. 5.17 Illustrative case 2. The postoperative follow-up a week after surgery showed no improvement of eye upward gaze

must decide on the need of intervention because of eye movement restriction or because of an anticipated enophthalmos. When deciding on the need of a surgical intervention, we must take into consideration the aesthetic result and the consequences of the facial incisions scaring and possible ectropion. The described endoscopic approach

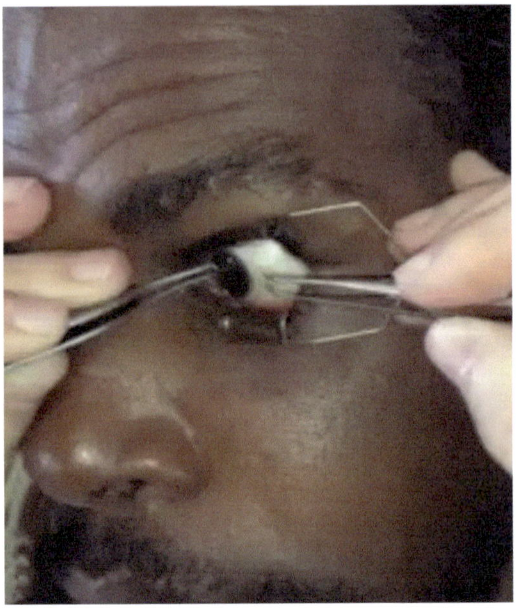

Fig. 5.18 Illustrative case 2. The awake forced duction test was performed showing a release of the entrapment compared to the pre-surgical status

to the floor and medial wall helps to avoid eyelid complications and improve visualization of the orbital walls. When there is no functional impairment, the surgeon faces a dilemma of trading one esthetic deformity with another and thus the minimal invasive intervention described in this chapter makes the decision process easy. Such approach is the only way we can achieve an anatomical reduction of the orbital floor using the bone fragments as a scaffold for the floor reconstruction. The described procedure enables the surgeon to perform a safer intervention in the posterior part of the orbital cavity near the orbital apex. Another advantage of this procedure is the ability to perform surgery in cases of muscle entrapment and globe involvement as in cases with increased intraocular pressure, a situation which can delay surgery. The disadvantage of this technique would be the slow learning curve as in all minimal invasive techniques. We believe that the above-described surgical technique may help in numerous cases of the blowout orbital trauma.

References

1. Smith B, Regan WF. Blow-out fracture of the orbit: mechanism and correction of internal orbital fracture. Am J Ophthalmol. 1957;44(6):733–9.
2. Crikelair GF, Rein JM, Potter GU, Cosman B. A critical look at the "blowout" fracture. Plast Reconstr Surg. 1972;49(4):374–9.
3. Putterman AM, Stevens T, Urist MJ. Nonsurgical management of blow-out fractures of the orbital floor. Am J Ophthalmol. 1974;77(2):232–9.
4. Dulley B, Fells P. Orbital blow-out fractures: to operate or not to operate, that is the question. Br Orthopt J. 1974;31:47–54.
5. Liss J, Stefko ST, Chung WL. Orbital surgery: state of the art. Oral Maxillofac Surg Clin North Am. 2010;22(1):59–71.
6. Dortzbach RK, Elner VM. Which orbital floor blowout fractures need surgery? Adv Ophthalmic Plast Reconstr Surg. 1987;6:287.
7. Kim YS, Kim JH, Hwang K. The frequency of decreased visual acuity in orbital fractures. J Craniofac Surg. 2015;26(5):1581–3. https://doi.org/10.1097/SCS.0000000000001860.
8. Joshi S, Kassira W, Thaller SR. Overview of pediatric orbital fractures. J Craniofac Surg. 2011;22(4):1330–2. https://doi.org/10.1097/SCS.0b013e31821c9365.
9. Perry M. Maxillofacial trauma—developments, innovations and controversies. Injury. 2009;40(12):1252–9. https://doi.org/10.1016/j.injury.2008.12.015.
10. Fraioli RE, Branstetter BF IV, Deleyiannis FW. Facial fractures: beyond Le Fort. Otolaryngol Clin N Am. 2008;41(1):51–76, vi. https://doi.org/10.1016/j.otc.2007.10.003.
11. Ducasse A. Surgical orbital anatomy. In: Guthoff RF, Katowitz JA, editors. Oculoplastics and orbit. New York: Springer; 2007. p. 73–95.
12. Laxenaire A, Levy J, Blanchard P, Lerondeau JC, Tesnier F, Scheffer P. Silastic implants and reconstruction of the orbital floor: review of twenty years' experience. Ann Chir Plast Esthet. 1996;41(6):631–8.
13. Chen CT, Chen YR. Update on orbital reconstruction. Curr Opin Otolaryngol Head Neck Surg. 2010;18(4):311–6. https://doi.org/10.1097/MOO.0b013e32833aafd2.
14. Dubois L, Steenen SA, Gooris PJ, Mourits MP, Becking AG. Controversies in orbital reconstruction—I. Defect-driven orbital reconstruction: a systematic review. Int J Oral Maxillofac Surg. 2015;44(3):308–15. https://doi.org/10.1016/j.ijom.2014.12.002.
15. Koornneef L. Orbital septa: anatomy and function. Ophthalmology. 1979;86(5):876–80.
16. Harris GJ, Garcia GH, Logani SC, Murphy ML. Correlation of preoperative computed tomography and postoperative ocular motility in orbital blowout fractures. Ophthal Plast Reconstr Surg. 2000;16(3):179–87.
17. Harris GJ. Orbital blow-out fractures: surgical timing and technique. Eye (Lond). 2006;20(10):1207–12.
18. Tenzel RR, Miller GR. Orbital blow-out fracture repair, conjunctival approach. Am J Ophthalmol. 1971;71:1141–2.
19. Mullins JB, Holds JB, Branham GH, Thomas JR. Complications of the transconjunctival approach. A review of 400 cases. Arch Otolaryngol Head Neck Surg. 1997;123(4):385–8.
20. Humphrey CD, Kriet JD. Sugical approaches to the orbit. Otolaryngology. 2008;19:132–9.
21. Collin R, Rose G, editors. Plastic and orbital surgery. London: BMJ Books; 2001.
22. Cheung K, Voineskos SH, Avram R, Sommer DD. A systematic review of the endoscopic management of orbital floor fractures. JAMA Facial Plast Surg. 2013;15(2):126–30.
23. Jin H-R, Yeon J-Y, Shin S-O, Choi Y-S, Lee D-W. Endoscopic versus external repair of orbital blowout fractures. Otolaryngol Head Neck Surg. 2007;136(1):38–44.
24. Hinohira Y, Yumoto E, Shimamura I. Endoscopic endonasal reduction of blowout fractures of the orbital floor. Otolaryngol Head Neck Surg. 2005;133(5):741–7.
25. Walter W. Early surgical repair of blowout fracture of the orbital floor by using the transantral approach. South Med J. 1972;65(10):1229.
26. Ducic Y, Verret DJ. Endoscopic transantral repair of orbital floor fractures. Otolaryngol Head Neck Surg. 2009;140(6):849–54.
27. Strong EB, Kim KK, Diaz RC. Endoscopic approach to orbital blowout fracture repair. Otolaryngol Head Neck Surg. 2004;131(5):683–95.
28. Persons BL, Wong GB. Transantral endoscopic orbital floor repair using resorbable plate. J Craniofac Surg [Internet]. 2002;13(3):483–9.
29. Fernandes R, Fattahi T, Steinberg B, Schare H. Endoscopic repair of isolated orbital floor fracture with implant placement. J Oral Maxillofac Surg. 2007;65(8):1449–53.
30. Farwell DG, Sires BS, Kriet JD, Stanley RB. Endoscopic repair of orbital blowout fractures: use or misuse of a new approach? Arch Facial Plast Surg. 2007;9(6):427–33.

Applications of Distraction Osteogenesis in Oral and Maxillofacial Surgery

6

Adi Rachmiel and Dekel Shilo

Abstract

Distraction osteogenesis (DO) of facial bones provides an excellent system of membranous bone formation. The bone is generated by stretching a callus that develops following corticotomy or an osteotomy of the facial bones. The use of DO in oral and maxillofacial surgery (OMS) has increased enormously in the last two decades especially for severe bone deficiency. DO is used in the hypoplastic retruded maxilla and midface, such as in cleft palate or Crouzon patients and in the mandible for the treatment of facial asymmetries or in patients with a hypoplastic mandible which may cause airway obstruction associated with obstructive sleep apnea (OSA). In addition, alveolar distraction osteogenesis (ADO) is used for augmentation in patients with severe deficient alveolar bone, prior to dental implantation. The aim of this chapter is to review the current application of distraction osteogenesis in oral and maxillofacial surgery upon the authors experience and based on the literature.

6.1 Introduction

The use of distraction osteogenesis (DO) in oral and maxillofacial surgery (OMS) has increased from the beginning of the 1990s, following the clinical application of the method by McCarthy for mandibular elongation in syndromatic children [1] associated with severe cases of hypoplastic mandible and facial asymmetry. DO is a method of generating new bone following a corticotomy or an osteotomy and gradual distraction. The method is based on the tension-stress principle described by Ilizarov. Ilizarov also stressed the influence of blood supply and loading

A. Rachmiel, DMD, PhD (✉)
Department of Oral and Maxillofacial Surgery, Rambam Medical Center, Haifa, Israel

Faculty of Medicine, Technion-Israel Institute of Technology, Haifa, Israel
e-mail: adi_rach@netvision.net.il

D. Shilo, DMD, PhD
Department of Oral and Maxillofacial Surgery, Rambam Medical Center, Haifa, Israel

O. Nahlieli (ed.), *Minimally Invasive Oral and Maxillofacial Surgery*,
http://doi.org/10.1007/978-3-662-54592-8_6

on the shape of bones and joints. He also pointed out the distraction device should be stable and not rigid, and there should be full control on the vector of lengthening [2, 3]. In this technique, gradual bone distraction stimulates molecular responses which promote bone formation. This process includes differentiation of stem cells, promotion of angiogenesis, osteogenesis, and bone mineralization [4–7].

Distraction osteogenesis includes four stages:

1. Corticotomy or osteotomy and placement of a distraction device.
2. Latency period of several days for primary callous organization.
3. Gradual distraction in a rate of 0.5–1 mm/day.
4. Retention/consolidation period of several months for callous maturation and mineralization.

In facial bones, the method was proved to be predictable in animal studies [4, 5] with generation of new bone as well as in clinical practice for elongation of the mandible, maxilla, and midface [1, 8–13]. In this chapter, we will review the current application of distraction osteogenesis in oral and maxillofacial surgery upon the authors experience and based on the literature. We will describe the use of distraction osteogenesis in the mandible for facial asymmetry and obstructive sleep apnea (OSA), in the maxilla for cleft palate patients, midface distraction by Le Fort III in syndromatic patients and in the deficient alveolar bone.

6.2 Mandibular Distraction

In the mandible, DO is used for the treatment of maxillofacial asymmetry as seen in hemifacial microsomia or in pediatric OSA due to severely hypoplastic mandible resulting in decreased pharyngeal airway as seen in Pierre Robin or Treacher Collins syndromes [1, 13–16]. The first distraction devices used for mandibular distraction were external distraction devices which were based on external pins introduced to the bones and connected to an external device [1, 13, 15]. Later, smaller internal devices applied directly on the bone were developed [16, 17]. Main advantages of internal distraction devices include a more predictable and precise rate of lengthening due to a direct contact of the device to the bony segments. Internal devices are invisible to the patients and to others around them, they are not vulnerable to external trauma and allow for nearly complete jaw function and they do not result in two visible buccal scars as seen when using external devices, but in a submandibular less visible scar. Internal devices are more comfortable to young patients compared to external devices. External devices allow for greater distraction length and are easily removed with no need for a second operation. Advantages and disadvantages of the two devices are described in Table 6.1 adopted from Rachmiel et al. [18].

Distraction devices are classified according to the required vector of distraction—(a) unidirectional, (b) bidirectional, and (c) multidirectional. Unidirectional devices are used for lengthening in a single vector a part of the mandible. Bidirectional devices are used for concomitant elongation of the ascending ramus and the body of the mandible. Multidirectional devices may offer an addition of transverse horizontal correction, mainly for the gonial angle [19].

In recent years, intraoral curvilinear distraction devices were introduced due to the difficulty of controlling the vector of distraction. These devices allow for a better forward control of the vector of lengthening [20, 21].

The severely hypoplastic mandible in pediatric patients can compromise the airway and is a serious life-threatening condition which can occur commonly in individuals with craniofacial anomalies associated with micrognathia [22]. The reduced size of the mandible and the retruded position observed in these cases can cause a posterior collapse of the tongue which may lead to upper airway obstruction [23, 24]. Severe cases of OSA in syndromatic children are frequently treated by tracheostomy. Permanent tracheostomy is associated with frequent morbidity which includes cannula tube dislodgment and tube obstruction secondary to mucus plugs or blood clots [25, 26].

Table 6.1 Summary of advantages and disadvantages of external and internal distraction devices in mandibular lengthening for correction of OSA

	External	Internal
Approach	Intraoral, two external pin insertion, simpler, shorter operation	Extraoral submandibular, with soft tissue dissection to the mandible
Osteotomy	Easier to perform and place the pins in various anatomic structures, more "freedom of osteotomy design"	According to local anatomy and device dimension
Placement	Easy to place in limited space as in micrognathic children	Limited by subperiosteal space for the distractor or difficulty in screw fixation
Distraction length	Permits longer distraction	Limited by subperiosteal space
Comfort	Uncomfortable, may be damaged by accidental external forces	Comfortable, safer
Vector of distraction	Less predictable	More predictable, pre-fixed by the device
Precision of lengthening	Less precise	More precise
Change of device	Possible	Need additional operation
Device stability	Possible pin loosening may compromise retention period	Stable for longer retention period and better ossification
Relapse after 1 year	Greater relapse	Decreased relapse
Facial nerve damage	Less risk	Greater risk
Infection	More pin tract infection	Less pin tract infection
Device removal	Simple, by unscrewing the pins	Need second operation under general anesthesia
Skin scars	Two buccal—Visible	One submandibular—Less visible

Adopted from Rachmiel et al. [18]

One of the main challenges during the distraction process is controlling the direction of the newly formed bone [27]. In cases of mandible elongation as a treatment for OSA, the vector of lengthening should be forwarded in order to advance the mandible and hyoid bone, thus enlarging the airway and inspiratory airflow. For this reason, there is great emphasis on controlling the forward vector of distraction osteogenesis, this can be accomplished by using orthodontic appliances, such as temporary anchorage devices (TADs). Mandibular distraction may be used for unilateral or bilateral mandibular deficiencies. Unilateral mandibular distraction is used for unilateral deficiency as in hemifacial microsomia (HFM).

The goal of the treatment in hemifacial microsomia is to elongate the hypoplastic mandible (mainly the ramus) and to prevent secondary restriction of maxillary vertical growth and canting of the occlusion. The vector of elongation should be mainly vertically downward, with slight anterior protrusion of the hypoplastic mandible [14, 16]. Some authors advocate an increased relapse in treatment during early age of childhood [28].

Mandibular osteotomies are usually performed in three anatomical sites (Fig. 6.1a):

1. Ramus osteotomy for vertical ramus elongation, as is needed in the treatment of HFM for example.
2. Mandibular angle oblique osteotomy in which a downward and forward vector of elongation of the ramus and mandibular body is required. A common application in facial asymmetries in which a concomitant vertical ramus and body deficiency exists.
3. Mandibular body osteotomy directly anterior to the ramus. For forward elongation of the mandible, as needed in OSA.

Mandibular distraction procedure includes exposure of the mandible according to the planned osteotomy. An osteotomy is performed in the required site and distraction devices are mounted across the osteotomy on both sides, one

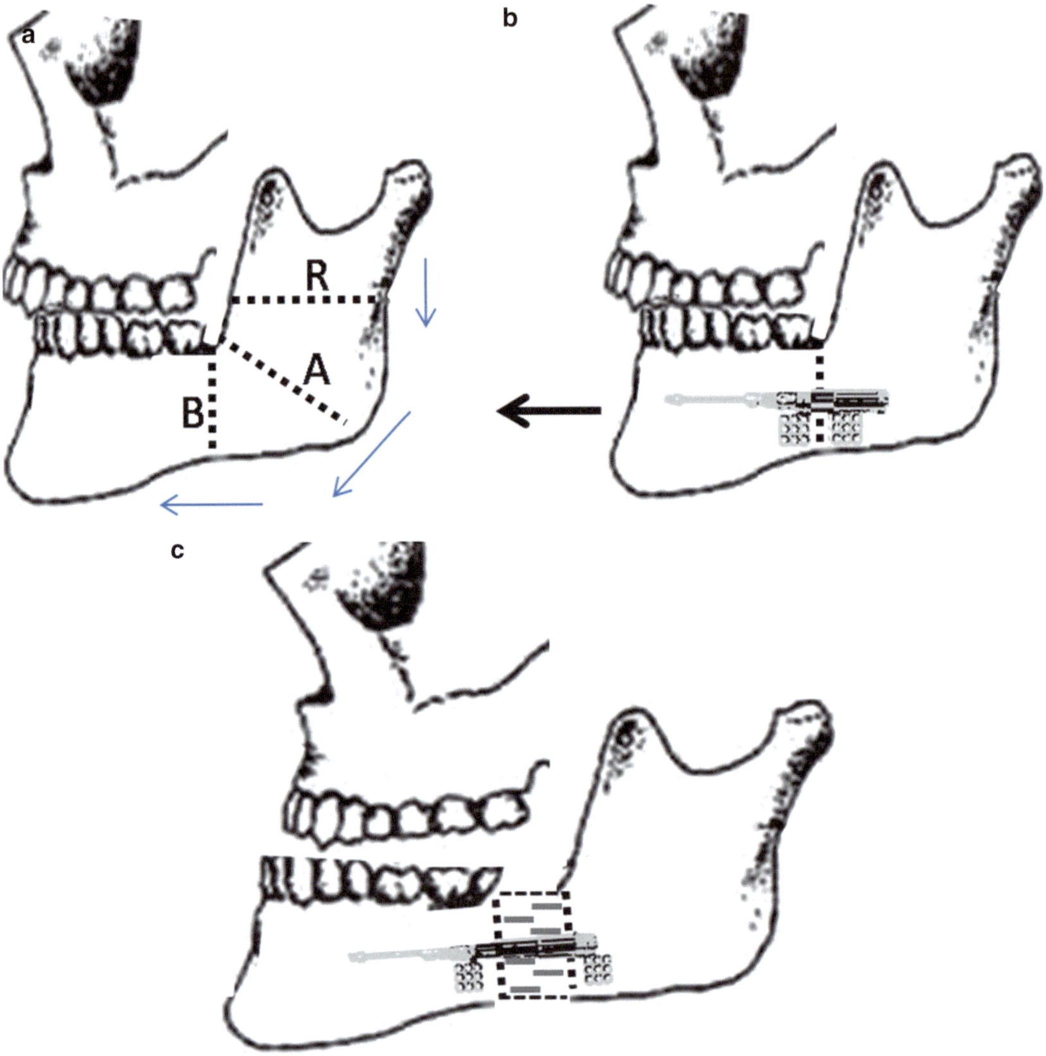

Fig. 6.1 An illustration of a mandible distractor used for different mandibular lengthening. (**a**) An osteotomy is performed as demonstrated by the dashed line. R—ramus osteotomy. A—mandibular angle oblique osteotomy. B—Mandibular body osteotomy. (**b**) An example of a mandibular body osteotomy, the distractor is fitted on both fragments. (**c**) Bone elongation of the mandibular body is performed gradually, dashed square demonstrates the newly formed bone

on each side of the mandible in case of bilateral distraction (Fig. 6.1b). After a latency period of 4 days for primary callus organization, gradual lengthening of the mandible is performed bilateral by activation of the distraction devices at a rate of 1 mm/day (Fig. 6.1c). In order to enable bone mineralization with minimal load bearing and thus minimize relapse, the devices are left for 3–4 additional months before removal after active distraction is finished—consolidation period.

An additional application of distraction osteogenesis is transport distraction in which a segment of osteotomized bone is transported using distraction osteogenesis to bridge a mandibular body bony gap (Fig. 6.2). This is performed following tumor resection or post-traumatic avulsion of a mandibular segment. Condyle transport is performed mainly following subcondylar avulsion or post-ankylotic temporomandibular joint (TMJ) resection [29–31].

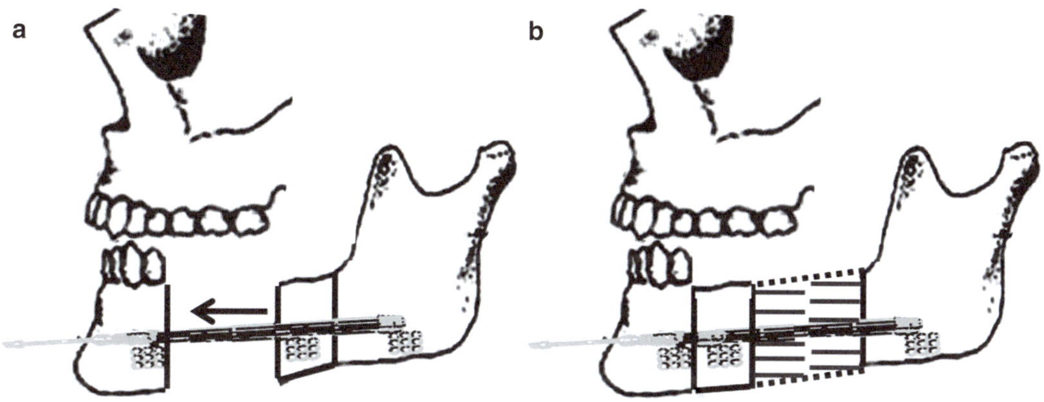

Fig. 6.2 An illustration of a reconstruction of mandibular body gap by the use of mandibular transport segmental distraction. (**a**) An mandibular transport segmental distractor is fixed across the segmental gap. (**b**) Forward gradual transport of the segment to bridge the gap. The dotted line illustrates the newly formed bone

6.3 Maxilla and Midface Distraction

In the maxilla and midface, the main use of distraction osteogenesis is in the treatment of hypoplastic cleft maxilla using external or internal maxillary distraction devices [11, 12], midface distraction by Le Fort III, as in Crouzon and Apert patients [32, 33] and frontofacial monobloc advancement (FFMA) in patients with faciocraniosynostosis [34]. Cleft patients usually undergo several surgical interventions throughout infancy, childhood, and adolescence to correct the upper lip when cleft lip exists, cleft palate closure, velopharyngeal insufficiency, and the alveolar cleft augmentation. These improve the facial appearance, speech, and deglutition, yet the scars formed from those operations cause impairment in maxillary growth in vertical and horizontal directions thus resulting in a hypoplastic maxilla [35]. Correction of the hypoplastic maxilla in cleft patients is a great challenge due to the difficulty in mobilizing the hypoplastic maxilla caused by scarring from previous operations in the soft and hard palate or after the lip closure. Moreover, following conventional orthognathic surgery of Le Fort I advancement, the hypoplastic maxilla in cleft lip and palate patients has a great tendency to relapse after major movements of over 10 mm [36–38]. Maxillary advancement by orthognathic surgery and miniplates fixation can be useful only in mild deficiencies in adult patients [39, 40].

The surgical procedure includes—different osteotomies are performed according to the maxillary deficiency and the correction needed. Osteotomies may be horizontal for forward distraction of the maxilla, oblique for forward and downward distraction of the maxilla or step osteotomy when the canine and premolar roots or buds are unerupted in a higher position in the maxilla [41]. An osteotomy at Le Fort I level and a downfracture are performed. In case of intraoral devices, two intraoral maxillary distractors are inserted and fixed (Fig. 6.3), one on each side with anchorage to the zygomatic buttresses where the bone is thickest. In case of extra-oral devices, the RED system (Polley/RED II System, Rigid External Distraction, KLS Martin, Tuttlingen, Germany) (Fig. 6.4) can be used. A halo is anchored to the skull by special fixation screws. An external adjustable distraction system is attached to the halo. The distraction device is connected to the maxilla by miniplates or by a circum dental metal arch connected to the teeth by wires.

Following 4 days of latency period, bone elongation is initiated by turning the distraction rods at a rate of 1 mm a day as desired. Following a 3–4-month period of retention, the devices are removed, in case of external devices by simple unscrewing of the device screws and in case of

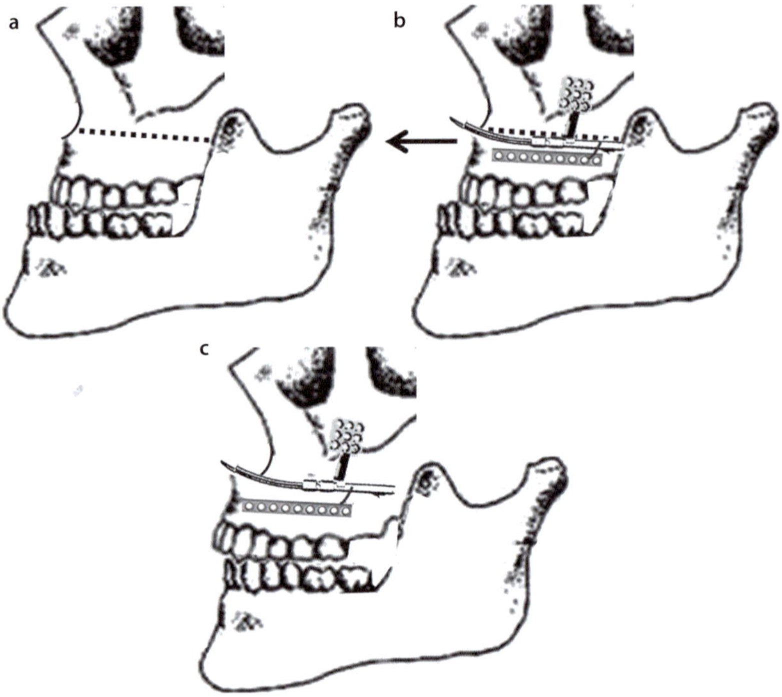

Fig. 6.3 An illustration of a maxillary distractor used for maxillary advancement. (**a**) An osteotomy at the level of Le Fort I is performed as demonstrated by the dashed line. (**b**) The distractor is fitted on both fragments. (**c**) Bone elongation is performed gradually

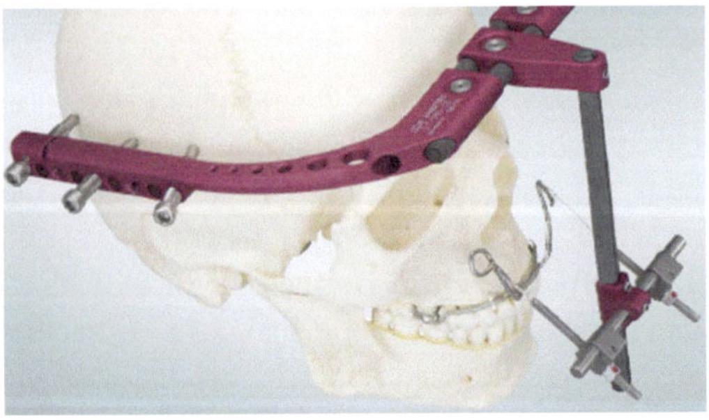

Fig. 6.4 The Rigid External Distractor (RED II System, KLS Martin, Tuttlingen, Germany) is anchored by pins to the parietal bone for midface and maxillary distraction

internal devices by an additional operation under general anesthesia.

The external device RED system is uncomfortable to the child to wear for long periods is exposed to external trauma forces during that period, and there is a risk of parietal bone penetration. The RED system offers greater distraction length, permits to perform the osteotomy in a hypoplastic deficient bone, offers a control over the vector of lengthening, and is easily removed by unscrewing the pins. Internal distraction devices are fixated directly to the bone. They are safer to wear for long periods, do not create social discomfort, and therefore permit longer retention periods which may contribute to better stability than external devices. Their major disadvantage is the need for a second operation under general anesthesia for device removal [11].

The hypoplastic maxilla in cleft patients is usually associated with moderate to severe retrusion and is better treated by distraction osteogenesis than by conventional orthognathic surgery as are moderate to severe cases of midface deficiency. Maxillary orthognatic surgery has the major advantage of a single, one stage operation and is indicated in mild adult maxillary or midface deficiency when craniofacial growth has ceased. However, in moderate or severe hypoplasia or in growing patients, distraction osteogenesis has a great advantage over conventional orthognatic surgery.

Distraction osteogenesis as a treatment modality in craniofacial surgery revolutionized the treatment of midface hypoplasia characteristic of craniofacial synostotic syndromes such as Apert and Crouzon. New bone is generated in the osteotomy sites as elongation is applied.

As in mandibular distraction osteogenesis, the gradual elongation and newly bone formation minimizes the resistance observed in extreme advancement and the relapse prevalence encountered in orthognatic advancement techniques. One of the main objectives of the distraction osteogenesis advancement in these patients is to establish normal size and position of the bony orbits. Timing of midface advancement is debatable, yet previous observations [32] revealed orbit growth forward between ages 8.5 and 15.5 was <4 mm thus making this procedure feasible already in childhood.

The surgical procedure includes the following steps. A coronal flap is elevated. An Osteotomy at the Le Fort III level is created and the distal fragment is downfractured. Both external and internal devices can be used. The internal distraction devices are fitted to the zygoma bilateral and then fixated. The activating pin is passed through a percutaneous cannula. After a latency period, elongation is initiated at a rate of 1 mm/day. After achieving the desired elongation, the cannula and activating pin are detached and the distraction device is left for a consolidation period. The device is then removed, in case of internal devices by a second operation [32].

6.4 Deficient Alveolar Bone

Another indication for DO is the bone augmentation of deficient alveolar ridge prior to dental implant placement [42–45]. Many patients lacking adequate bone height and width desire nowadays rehabilitation using endosseous implants. Bone deficiency may be a result of maxillofacial trauma, periodontal disease, or post-resection of aggressive large jaw cysts or tumors. These conditions require bone augmentation for insertion of endosseous implants. In cases of moderate to severe bone deficiency, alveolar distraction osteogenesis (ADO) is a very useful technique [43–45].

Possible methods for bone reconstruction in cases of mild-to-moderate alveolar bone loss up to 6 mm include onlay block bone graft or a sandwich osteotomy combined with an interpositional autogenous graft [46, 47]. In these methods, donor site morbidity is unavoidable and some resorption of the autogenous grafted bone occurs.

In the anterior region, ADO is most frequently applied in the maxilla [48] though in the anterior mandible it might be applied in order to allow inter-foraminal implant placement for an overdenture [49, 50]. In the posterior region, ADO is applied more frequently to the mandible to improve crown-implant ratio [51].

The alveolar distraction can be divided into:

(a) Unidirectional
(b) Bidirectional
(c) Horizontal

In unidirectional distraction when facing large alveolar segments of over 3 cm, the use of two distraction devices on both sides of the osteotomy may be needed in order to control the sagittal plane on both sides of the vector of elongation.

Bidirectional distraction is used for concomitant vertical and buccal vector control of elongation [52].

Horizontal expansion is recommended in cases of bucco-lingual or bucco-palatal deficiency which does not permit an insertion of a dental implant [53, 54].

The ADO devices can also be divided into:

(a) Extraosseous devices which are the most prevalent (e.g., the Track devices by KLS Martin, Tuttlingen, Germany) [44]
(b) Intraosseous devices which include central application devices (e.g., the LEAD System, Stryker CMF, Portage, MI, USA) [43]
(c) Distraction by implants (e.g., 3i Implant Distractors, Implant Innovations, West Palm Beach, Florida, USA) [48].

Advantages of ADO include simultaneous expansion of both bone and soft tissue, bone at the alveolar crest remains as cortical and mature bone, no donor site morbidity as opposed to autogenous block bone grafts and greater bone lengthening than other methods [45].

The ADO procedure includes paracrestal mucoperiosteal incision on the buccal side and is performed leaving the crestal attached mucosa intact. Two vertical and one horizontal osteotomies are to be performed creating a trapezoidal osteotomy that forms the transported segment (Fig. 6.5). Bone elongation is initiated after a latency period of several days in a rate of 0.5 mm/day and continues as necessary and according to the length of the distraction device. Following bone elongation, a consolidation period of 3–4 month is required. Subsequently, the devices are removed and endosseous implants can be placed followed by prosthetic restoration.

In patients with severe atrophy or after bone resection or bone loss due to trauma, two stages of jaw reconstruction can be performed: bone graft as the first stage followed by distraction osteogenesis as a second stage. It is important to be aware of the vector of distraction, the stability of the bone, the final alveolar height and the timing of placement of dental implants.

Alveolar distraction osteogenesis is a procedure in which a segment of mature bone is transported in order to lengthen the alveolar crest for better implant anchorage, either for esthetic purposes or functional prosthetic or occlusal requirements. The procedure offers an alternative method for bone reconstruction without donor site morbidity and sufficient stability of the final result.

Conclusions

Gradual bone lengthening using distraction osteogenesis principles is a useful method for treatment of moderate to severe deficient facial bones. The method is well established both in the mandible, maxilla, and midface. The development of new miniature distraction devices allowed for the advancements in alveolar distraction osteogenesis prior to dental implants. Distraction osteogenesis exhibits good results with long-term stability. The internal distraction devices are more comfortable to the patients and permit greater retention periods which contribute to long-term stability. Better understanding of the biomolecular mechanisms that mediate distraction osteogenesis may allow for the improvement of bone regeneration using different molecular mediators, growth factors, or stem cells. Shortening of the consolidation period is one of the main goals of future research. Development of biodegradable devices may spare the need for a second surgery to remove the distraction devices. Another important issue is the control of the vector of distraction osteogenesis, better control will improve clinical and functional results significantly. 3D imaging and custom devices designed specifically for each patient will allow for better prediction of bone and soft tissue formation.

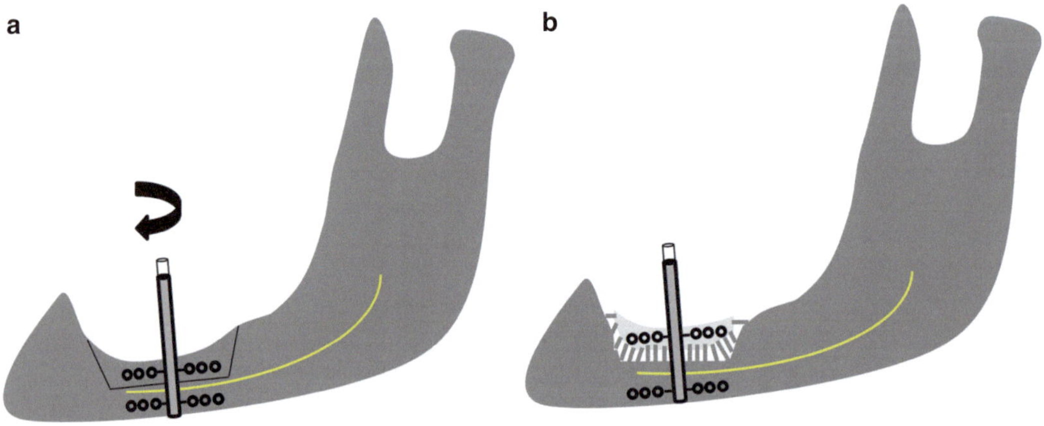

Fig. 6.5 Vertical augmentation of alveolar bone using an extraosseous device. (**a**) Trapezoid osteotomy is performed. The distractor is composed of an activator pin and two plates which are fixated to the basal segment and the alveolar transport segment. (**b**) Following gradual elevation, new bone is formed between the transport segment and the basal segment. Adopted from Shilo et al. [55]

In this chapter, we reviewed the use of distraction osteogenesis in facial bones for different indications ranging from treatment of life-threatening conditions to ridge augmentation prior to dental implants placement.

References

1. McCarthy J, Schreiber J, Karp N, Thorne C, Grayson B. Lengthening the human mandible by gradual distraction. Plast Reconstr Surg. 1992;89(1):1–10.
2. Ilizarov G. The tension-stress effect on the genesis and growth of tissues. Part I. The influence of stability of fixation and soft-tissue preservation. Clin Orthop Relat Res. 1989;238:249–81.
3. Ilizarov G. The tension-stress effect on the genesis and growth of tissues: part II. The influence of the rate and frequency of distraction. Clin Orthop Relat Res. 1989;239:263–85.
4. Rachmiel A, Jackson I, Potparic Z, Laufer D. Midface advancement in sheep by gradual distraction: a 1-year follow-up study. J Oral Maxillofac Surg. 1995;53:525–9.
5. Rachmiel A, Laufer D, Jackson I, Lewinson D. Midface membranous bone lengthening: a one-year histological and morphological follow-up of distraction osteogenesis. Calcif Tissue Int. 1998;62(4):370–6.
6. Rachmiel A, Leiser Y. The molecular and cellular events that take place during craniofacial distraction osteogenesis. Plast Reconstr Surg Glob Open. 2014;2(1):e98.
7. Rachmiel A, Rozen N, Peled M, Lewinson D. Characterization of midface maxillary membranous bone formation during distraction osteogenesis. Plast Reconstr Surg. 2002;109:1611–20.
8. Marchac D, Arnaud E. Midface surgery from Tessier to distraction. Childs Nerv Syst. 1999;15(11–12):681–94.
9. Polley J, Figueroa A. Distraction osteogenesis: its application in severe mandibular deformities in hemifacial microsomia. J Craniofac Surg. 1997;8(5):422–30.
10. Polley J, Figueroa A. Management of severe maxillary deficiency in childhood and adolescence through distraction osteogenesis with an external, adjustable, rigid distraction device. J Craniofac Surg. 1997;8(3):181–6.
11. Rachmiel A, Aizenbud D, Peled M. Long-term results in maxillary deficiency using intraoral devices. Int J Oral Maxillofac Surg. 2005;34(5):473–9.
12. Rachmiel A, Aizenbud D, Peled M. Distraction osteogenesis in maxillary deficiency using a rigid external distraction device. Plast Reconstr Surg. 2006;117:2399–406.
13. Rachmiel A, Levy M, Laufer D. Lengthening of the mandible by distraction osteogenesis: report of cases. J Oral Maxillofac Surg. 1995;53(7):838–46.
14. Rachmiel A, Aizenbud D, Eleftheriou S, Peled M, Laufer D. Extraoral vs. intraoral distraction osteogenesis in the treatment of hemifacial microsomia. Ann Plast Surg. 2000;45(4):386–94.
15. Rachmiel A, Aizenbud D, Pillar G, Srouji S, Peled M. Bilateral mandibular distraction for patients with compromised airway analyzed by three-dimensional CT. Int J Oral Maxillofac Surg. 2005;34:9–18.
16. Rachmiel A, Manor R, Peled M, Laufer D. Intraoral distraction osteogenesis of the mandible in hemifacial microsomia. J Oral Maxillofac Surg. 2001;59(7):728–33.
17. Rachmiel A, Emodi O, Aizenbud D. Management of obstructive sleep apnea in pediatric craniofacial anomalies. Ann Maxillofac Surg. 2012;2(2):111–5.
18. Rachmiel A, Nseir S, Emodi O, Aizenbud D. External versus internal distraction devices in treatment of obstructive sleep apnea in craniofacial anomalies. Plast Reconstr Surg Glob Open. 2014;2(7):e188.
19. McCarthy J, Williams J, Grayson B, Crombie J. Controlled multiplanar distraction of the mandible: device development and clinical application. J Craniofac Surg. 1998;9(4):322–9.
20. Kaban L, Seldin E, Kikinis R, Yeshwant K, Padwa B, Troulis M. Clinical application of curvilinear distraction osteogenesis for correction of mandibular deformities. J Oral Maxillofac Surg. 2009;67:996–1008.
21. Schendel S, Linck D. Mandibular distraction osteogenesis by sagittal split osteotomy and intraoral curvilinear distraction. J Craniofac Surg. 2004;15:631–5.
22. Cosman B, Crikelair G. Mandibular hypoplasia and the late development of glossopharyngeal airway obstruction. Plast Reconstr Surg. 1972;50:573–9.
23. Cohen S, Simms C, Burstein F. Mandibular distraction osteogenesis in the treatment of upper airway obstruction in children with craniofacial deformities. Plast Reconstr Surg. 1998;101:312–8.
24. Williams J, Maull D, Grayson B, Longker M, McCarthy J. Early decannulation with bilateral mandibular distraction for tracheostomy-dependent patients. Plast Reconstr Surg. 1999;103:48–57.
25. Cohen S, Simms C, Burstein F, Thomsen J. Alternatives to tracheostomy in infants and children with obstructive sleep apnea. J Pediatr Surg. 1999;34:182–6.
26. Guilleminault C. Obstructive sleep apnea syndrome and its treatment in children: areas of agreement and controversy. Pediatr Pulmonol. 1987;3:429–36.
27. Vendittelli B, Dec W, Warren S, Garfinkle J, Grayson B, McCarthy J. The importance of vector selection in preoperative planning of bilateral mandibular distraction. Plast Reconstr Surg. 2008;122(4):1144–53.
28. Meazzini M, Mazzoleni F, Bozzetti A, Brusati R. Comparison of mandibular vertical growth in hemifacial microsomia patients treated with early distraction or not treated: follow up till the completion of growth. J Craniomaxillofac Surg. 2012;40(2):105–11.
29. Bansal V, Singh S, Garg N, Dubey P. Transport distraction osteogenesis as a method of reconstruction of the temporomandibular joint following gap arthroplasty for post-traumatic ankylosis in children: a clinical and radiological prospective assessment of outcome. Int J Oral Maxillofac Surg. 2014;43(2):227–36.

30. Schwartz H. Transport distraction osteogenesis for reconstruction of the ramus-condyle unit of the temporomandibular joint: surgical technique. J Oral Maxillofac Surg. 2009;67(10):2197–200.
31. Stucki-McCormick S, Fox R, Mizrahi R. Transport distraction: mandibular reconstruction. Atlas Oral Maxillofac Surg Clin North Am. 1999;7(1):65–83.
32. Chin M, Toth B. Le Fort III advancement with gradual distraction using internal devices. Plast Reconstr Surg. 1997;100(4):819–30.
33. Jensen J, McCarthy J, Grayson B, Nusbaum A, Eski M. Bone deposition/generation with LeFort III (midface) distraction. Plast Reconstr Surg. 2007;119(1):298–307.
34. Arnaud E, Marchac D, Renier D. Quadruple internal distraction with early frontal-facial advancement for faciocraniodysostosis. Rev Stomatol Chir Maxillofac. 2004;105(1):13–8.
35. Ross R. Treatment variables affecting facial growth in complete unilateral cleft lip and palate: an overview of treatment and facial growth. Cleft Palate Craniofac J. 1987;24:5–77.
36. Adlam D, Banks P. A retrospective study of the stability of midface osteotomies in cleft lip and palate patients. Br J Oral Maxillofac Surg. 1989;27:265–76.
37. Drommer R, Luhr H. The stabilization of osteotomised maxillary segment with Luhr miniplates in secondary cleft surgery. J Maxillofac Surg. 1981;9:166–9.
38. Houston W, James D, Jones E, Kavvadia S. Le Fort I maxillary osteotomies in cleft palate cases: surgical changes and stability. J Maxillofac Surg. 1989;17:9–15.
39. Cheung L, Chua H, Hägg M. Cleft maxillary distraction versus orthognathic surgery: clinical morbidities and surgical relapse. Plast Reconstr Surg. 2006;118(4):996–1008.
40. Rachmiel A, Even-Almos M, Aizenbud D. Treatment of maxillary cleft palate: distraction osteogenesis vs. orthognathic surgery. Ann Maxillofac Surg. 2012;2(2):127–30.
41. Rachmiel A, Aizenbud D, Ardekian L, Peled M, Laufer D. Surgically-assisted orthopedic protraction of the maxilla in cleft lip and palate patients. Int J Oral Maxillofac Surg. 1999;28:9–14.
42. Aizenbud D, Hazan-Molina H, Cohen M, Rachmiel A. Combined orthodontic temporary anchorage devices and surgical management of the alveolar ridge augmentation using distraction osteogenesis. J Oral Maxillofac Surg. 2012;70(8):1815–26.
43. Chin M, Toth B. Distraction osteogenesis in maxillofacial surgery using internal devices: review of five cases. J Oral Maxillofac Surg. 1996;54:45–53.
44. Hidding J, Lazar F, Zöller J. Initial outcome of vertical distraction osteogenesis of the atrophic alveolar ridge. Mund Kiefer Gesichtschir. 1999;3(1):S79–83.
45. Rachmiel A, Srouji S, Peled M. Alveolar ridge augmentation by distraction osteogenesis. Int J Oral Maxillofac Surg. 2001;30:510–7.
46. Jensen O. Alveolar segmental "sandwich" osteotomies for posterior edentulous mandibular sites for dental implants. J Oral Maxillofac Surg. 2006;64(3):471–5.
47. Jensen O, Kuhlke L, Bedard J, White D. Alveolar segmental sandwich osteotomy for anterior maxillary vertical augmentation prior to implant placement. J Oral Maxillofac Surg. 2006;64(2):290–6.
48. Jensen O, Cockrell R, Kuhike L, Reed C. Anterior maxillary alveolar distraction osteogenesis: a prospective 5-year clinical study. Int J Oral Maxillofac Implants. 2002;17:52–68.
49. Feichtinger M, Gaggl A, Schultes G, Karcher H. Evaluation of distraction implants for prosthetic treatment after vertical alveolar ridge distraction: a clinical investigation. Int J Prosthodont. 2003;16:19–24.
50. Krenkel C, Grunert I. The endo-distractor for preimplant mandibular regeneration. Rev Stomatol Chir Maxillofac. 2009;110(1):17–26.
51. Garcia-Garcia A, Somoza-Martin M, Gandara-Vila P, Saulacic N, Gandara-Rey J. Alveolar distraction before insertion of dental implants in the posterior mandible. Br J Oral Maxillofac Surg. 2003;41:376–9.
52. Jensen O, Ueda M, Laster Z, Mommaerts M, Rachmiel A. Alveolar distraction osteogenesis. SROMS. 2002;10(4):1–48.
53. Laster Z, Rachmiel A, Jensen O. Alveolar width distraction osteogenesis for early implant placement. J Oral Maxillofac Surg. 2005;63(12):1724–30.
54. Laster Z, Reem Y, Nagler R. Horizontal alveolar ridge distraction in an edentulous patient. J Oral Maxillofac Surg. 2011;69(2):502–6.
55. Shilo D, Emodi O, Aizenbud D, Rachmiel A. Distraction osteogenesis of deficient alveolar bone prior to dental rehabilitation. Refuat Hapeh Vehashinayim (1993). 2015;32(3):38–42, 69.

Minimally Invasive Orthognathic Surgery

7

Nardi Casap and Heli Rushinek

Abstract

Recent advances in imaging, instrumentation, and fiberoptic technology have allowed surgeons to develop and refine new minimally invasive orthognathic procedures. In this chapter, minimally invasive Le Fort I osteotomy is outlined with emphasis on the reduction of complications. In addition, navigation-assisted Le Fort I osteotomy is detailed to illustrate its advantages in minimally invasive procedures.

7.1 Introduction

Orthognathic surgery for correction of dentofacial deformities is a well-established, safe, and reliable treatment. The improvement of surgical techniques, the progress in anesthesia, and the introduction of rigid internal fixation have made orthognathic surgery more predictable, and decreased its morbidity. During the last four decades, only moderate modifications have been made to this long-familiar procedure [1]. Yet, recent advances in imaging, instrumentation, and fiberoptic technology have allowed surgeons to develop and refine new minimally invasive orthognathic procedures.

Minimally invasive surgery aims to minimize morbidity and complications that are usually associated with traditional procedures by reducing tissue trauma and the resultant bleeding, edema, and injury, and so maximize the rate and quality of healing, thus to result in faster patient recovery. In orthognathic surgery, minimally invasive approaches include reduction of the incision length, endoscope-assisted procedures, and distraction osteogenesis [2]. Nonetheless, we consider distraction osteogenesis not to be a minimally invasive procedure because it requires two surgeries, and the incisions for the application of the distractors are often not minimal, and the distractor must be opened daily, slowing the patient's recovery.

The first to describe minimally invasive orthognathic surgery was Kostecka in 1931, who described his technique of horizontal osteotomy of the ramus, and also condylar osteotomy as a

N. Casap, MD, DMD
Department of Oral and Maxillofacial Surgery, Hadassah Medical Center, Jerusalem, Israel

H. Rushinek, DMD (✉)
Department of Oral and Maxillofacial Surgery, School of Dental Medicine, Hebrew University, Hadassah Medical Center, Jerusalem, Israel
e-mail: heliru@walla.com

O. Nahlieli (ed.), *Minimally Invasive Oral and Maxillofacial Surgery*,
http://doi.org/10.1007/978-3-662-54592-8_7

"blind procedure" that is carried out with a Gigli saw through a stab incision [1]. Later, the reported cases of endoscopically assisted orthognathic procedures failed to allow full mobilization of the maxilla or mandible but enabled the application of facial bone distractors [3–5].

The development of virtual surgical planning and real-time navigation systems has provided very detailed analysis of anatomic deformities and aided the surgeon to accurately plan operative corrections of dentofacial deformities. These technologies have enabled minimally invasive surgery and precise surgical performance [6].

In 2013, Alfaro and Guijarro-Martínez described a minimally invasive approach to the Le Fort I osteotomy where the size of mucoperiosteal flap was reduced to only the anterior maxilla. This modified approach has minimized the risk of ischemic events by preservation of most of the bone's vascular supply through the buccal corridors. The author considered that decreasing the incision length represented technical progress from the classic approach but not a primary objective for the inexperienced orthognathic surgeon [7].

The overall complication rate of Le Fort I osteotomies varies between 6% and 9%, mostly represented by hemorrhage, infection, and maxillary necrosis [8]. Hemorrhage was considered a major complication in the first 48 postoperative hours, requiring blood transfusion in 1% to 1.1% of cases. Ischemic complications reported to occur in approximately 1% of cases, including aseptic necrosis of the alveolar process [9, 10].

The sequelae of insufficient vascularity can vary from tooth devitalization, periodontal defects, tooth loss, loss of major segments of alveolar bone to the slough of the entire maxilla. In 1975, Bell documented that the vascular supply to the downfractured, completely mobilized maxilla is preserved via the buccal and palatal soft tissues, and that the descending palatine vessels can be sacrificed without vascular compromise to the surgically repositioned maxilla [11]. The traditional large gingivobuccal exposure leaves the maxilloalveolar segment dependent on the ascending palatine branch of the facial artery and the anterior branch of the ascending pharyngeal artery. Although these vessels are sufficient to support this method, improvements in vascular protection could decrease healing times, lower infection rates, and reduce the risk of bone necrosis [11]. Tunneling technique used to access the anterior maxillary bone was found to be superior in maintaining the blood supply to the anterior maxillary labial pedicle technique, especially with minimally invasive technique [12].

The incidence of pterygoid plate fracture following Le Fort I osteotomy, as identified on postoperative computed tomography (CT) scanning, can range from 58% to 75%. Lanigan and Guest, working on cadavers [9], concluded that it is "probably impossible to totally prevent untoward fractures from occurring during pterygomaxillary dysjunction and downfracture," despite their suggestion of using a micro-oscillating saw or a straight osteotome to facilitate "separation" through the maxillary tuberosity [9]. Alfaro focused on the twist technique for pterygomaxillary disjunction, with a frontal approach to the pterygomaxillary junction, as opposed to the classic lateral approach, and emphasized that a pterygoid plate fracture should not be considered a complication because it is not necessarily the cause of hemorrhage or nerve injury [7].

In this chapter, we describe the use of minimally invasive Le Fort I osteotomies and use of computer-assisted surgery for their planning and execution.

7.2 Minimally Invasive Orthognathic Surgery

Through a minimally invasive incision from lateral incisor to lateral incisor, the nasal spine is osteotomized from the maxilla with a sharp 6 mm osteotome.

After this osteotomy, the nasal mucosa is detached from the nasal floor with periosteal elevators. Subsequently, subperiosteal tunneling is performed from the pyriform fossa to the maxillary buttress (Fig. 7.1). Le Fort I horizontal osteotomies are made with a reciprocating saw using small retractors as not to extend the original small mucosal incision (Fig. 7.2). To visual-

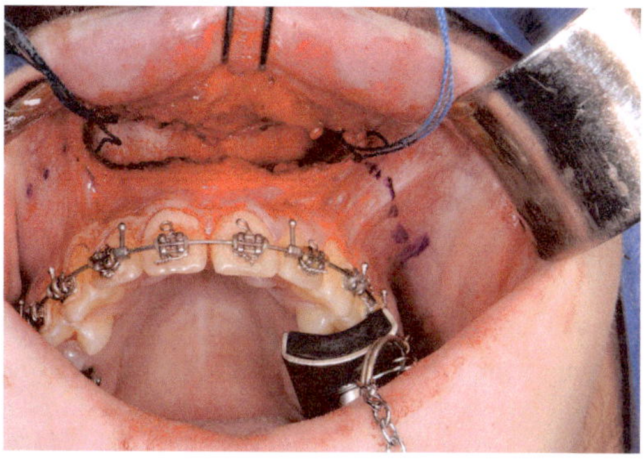

Fig. 7.1 Mucosal incision between the laterals

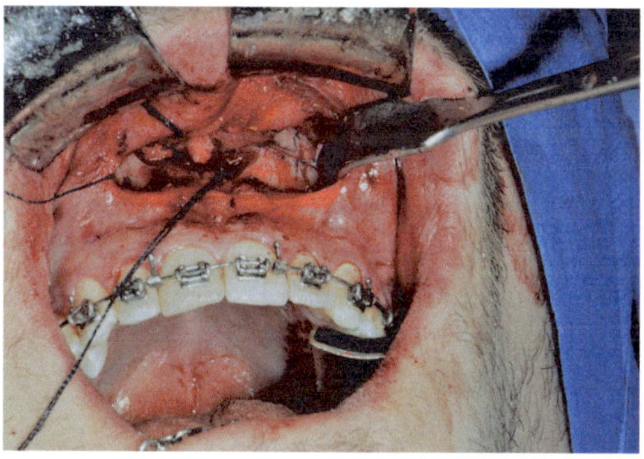

Fig. 7.2 Use of retractors for Le Fort I horizontal osteotomy. Demonstrating the minimal incision

ize the posterior completion of the osteotomy, an endoscope can be used posteriorly (Fig. 7.3). The classic pterygomaxillary disjunction with a lateral approach (i.e., driving a curved osteotome at the pterygomaxillary fissure) is not performed; instead, a straight osteotome is driven through the horizontal osteotomy from the pyriform fossa back to the junction of the posterior wall of the maxillary sinus to the pterygoid plates (Fig. 7.4). Subsequently, once the osteotome is fixed at the pterygomaxillary junction and underneath the zygomatic buttress, it is rotated inwardly, thus provoking downfracture of the maxilla. Separation of maxilla from cranial base can be verified under direct vision. Sufficient maxillary fixation is performed only in the anterior pyriform buttress (Fig. 7.5). If posterior fixation due to inadequate bone contact is required, an extension of the incision to the first premolar will be needed.

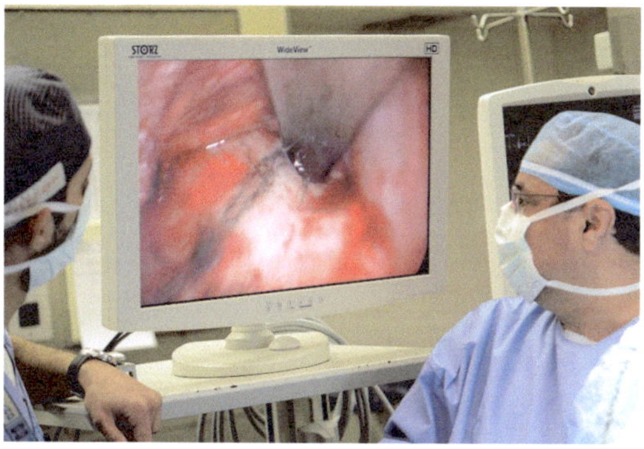

Fig. 7.3 Endoscopic visualization of the osteotomy

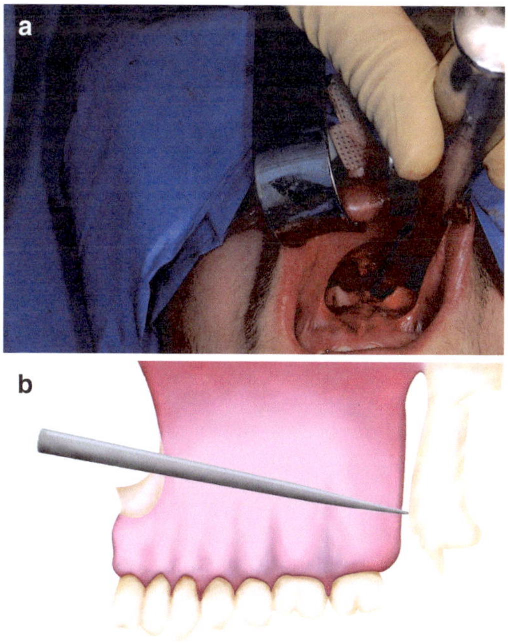

Fig. 7.4 A straight osteotome is driven through the horizontal osteotomy: (**a**) the image and (**b**) the schema

7.3 Navigation-Assisted Le Fort I Osteotomy

Advances in 3D imaging technology have resulted in a series of projects that have provided new computerized tools for use in preoperative planning and for the manufacture of surgical splints [13]. In maxillofacial surgery, computer-aided surgery can assist in preoperative planning or be used in the intraoperative navigation.

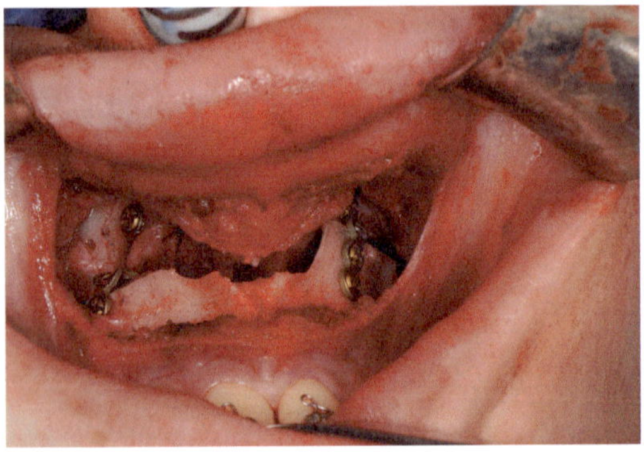

Fig. 7.5 Maxillary fixation in the anterior pyriform buttresses

Computer planning systems have been developed for use in the craniofacial skeleton, and they provide for 3D manipulation of CT data, which can further be combined with intraoperative navigation to facilitate accurate implementation of a virtual plan [14]. Virtual bone-based surgery planning can be performed through mirror imaging of the opposite "healthy" side, by segmentation of the desired bone or it can be combined with a printed stereolithographic model, to simulate osteotomies, to pre-bend reconstruction plates, or to construct custom guide stents and splints.

Currently, standard software is used for virtual surgical simulation in orthognathic surgery. These programs provide multiple functions, such as image segmentation, identification, and delineation of specified anatomic structures in CT images, simulation of common osteotomy procedures, relocation of bony segments according to planned surgical movement, and prediction of soft tissue changes. The surgical plan can then be transferred back to the navigation software by using DICOM or STL formatted files.

A real-time navigation system can be applied to definitely determine the final bone position in the absence of positioning guides as an additional instrument for guiding the osteotomies and checking the movement of bone [6].

Commercially available navigation systems employ predominantly optical tracking technologies for the determining the position of the patient and the surgical tools. Typically, an infrared stereoscopic camera system measures the positions of infrared light emitting or reflecting tracking elements that are rigidly attached to the patient and the surgical tools [15] (Fig. 7.6). When using a real-time navigation system, a reference star (tracker) is fixed to patient's skull to mark the location of the patient in the navigation system (Fig. 7.7). Then, the patient is registered in the navigation system, using marker-based or surface matching registration modalities, to establish the mathematical relationship that links the patient's CT imaging space coordinates to the physical space coordinates of a patient [6]. Either bony or skin surface landmarks can be used, and for bony landmarks we use three temporary anchorage devices (TADs) between maxillary teeth and three anatomical landmarks on the face (Fig. 7.8).

The application of computerized navigation is more complicated in surgery of the lower jaw due to the mobile nature of the mandible. Generally, three approaches can be applied to enable navigation in relation to the lower jaw. The first approach relies on maxillomandibular fixation that immobilizes the jaw. However, this approach limits considerably the access to the surgical site, and in most cases makes surgery impossible. The more commonly used approach is based on the positioning of the mandible in a reproducible position that allows its synchronization. Such positioning may be accomplished by juxtapositioning the mandible to the maxilla in a reproducible posture, based on the centric occlusion of the teeth or with the use of special templates. However, this strategy is highly sensitive to the relative movements of the mandible, which can greatly undermine the accuracy of the navigation. The third possible approach is to mount a special sensor frame onto the mandible, thereby allowing surgeons to optically track the mandible's

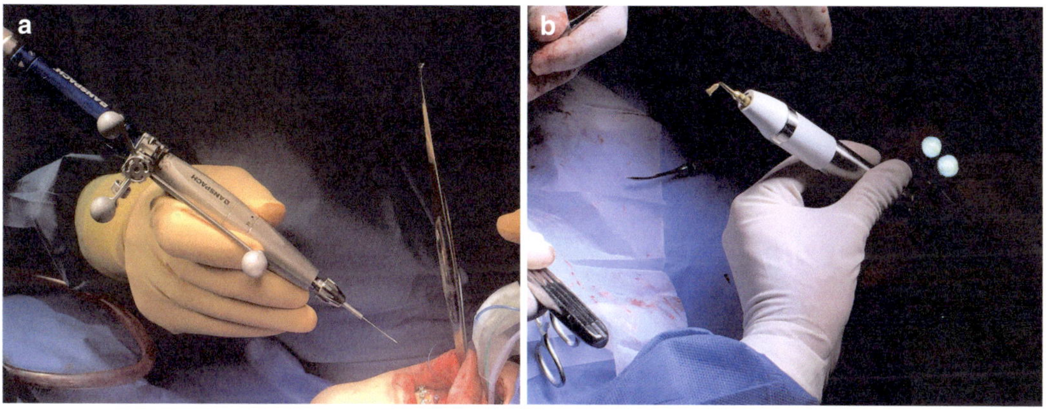

Fig. 7.6 The surgical tools for maxillary osteotomy with reflecting tracking elements: (**a**) oscillating saw and (**b**) piezoelectric oscillating device (Brainlab AG, Germany)

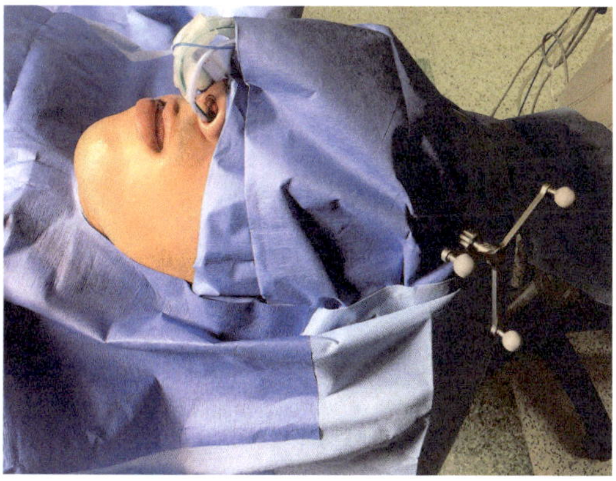

Fig. 7.7 Tracker fixed to the patient's skull (Brainlab AG, Germany)

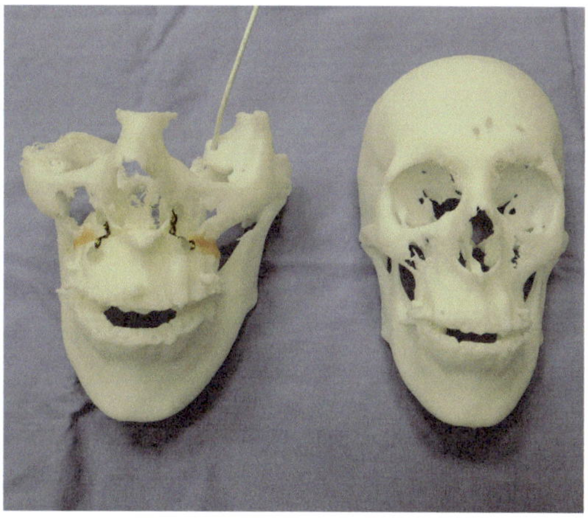

Fig. 7.9 Stereolithographic model printed for simulation of surgery

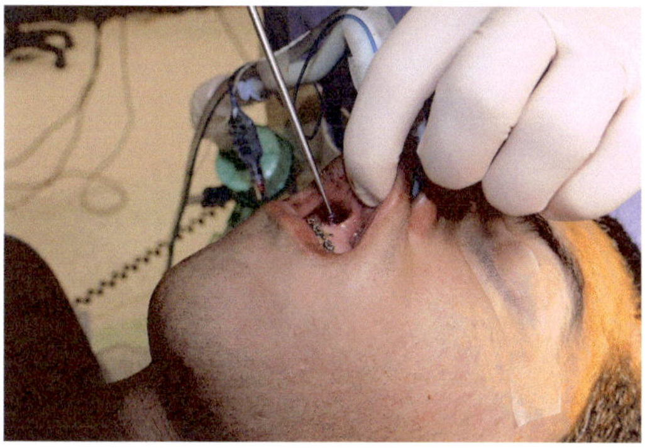

Fig. 7.8 Use of temporary anchorage device as registration marker

position and to compensate for its continuous movement during surgery. In this strategy, the position of the mandible is monitored directly, rather than by its position relative to other cranial structures, and so improves the accuracy of navigation [16].

Another method to be used with navigation systems is a stereolithographic model printed for the simulation of the surgery (Fig. 7.9). Miniplates are bent to fit the new position of the maxilla on the stereolithographic model. The "operated"

a b

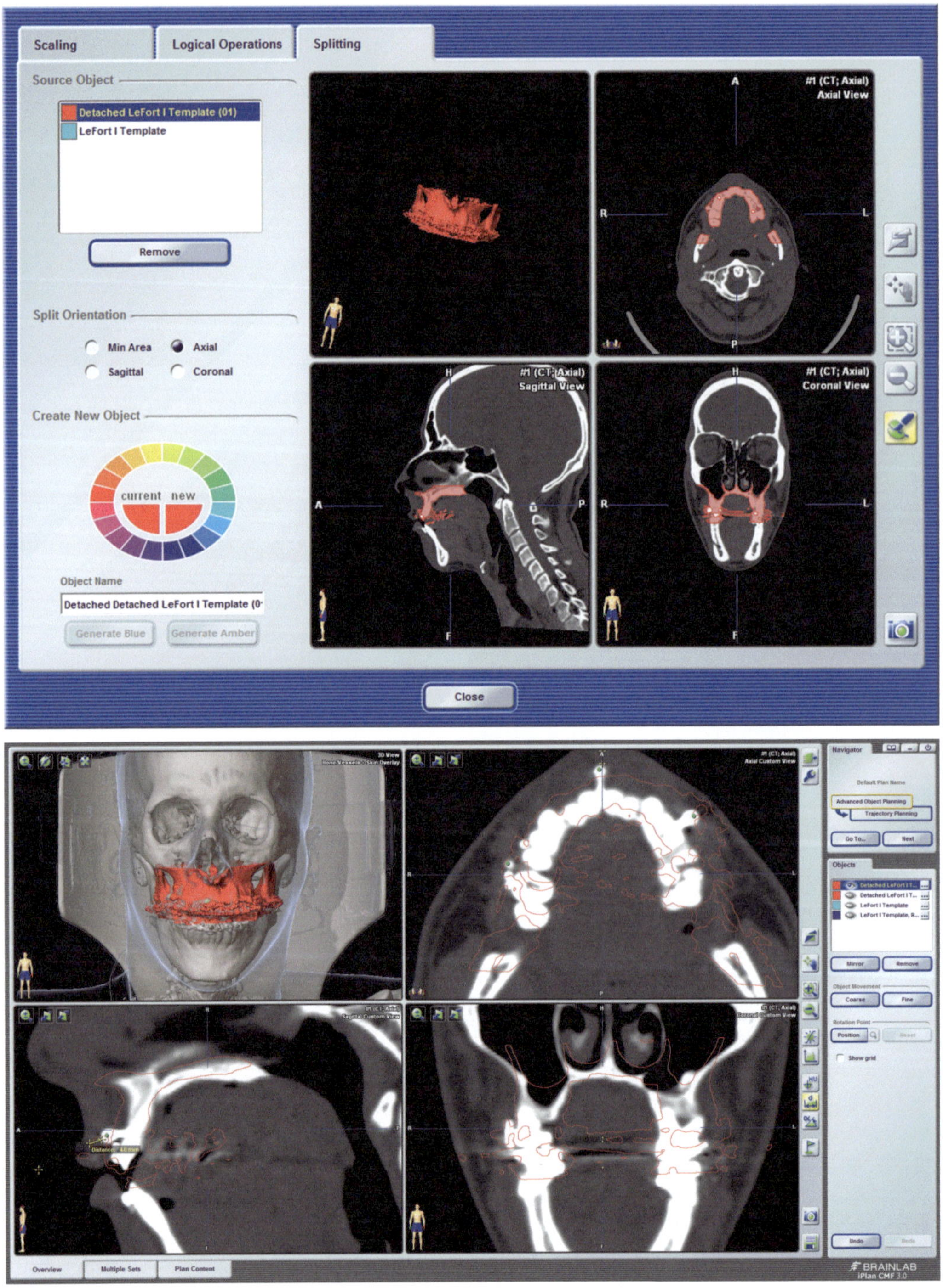

Fig. 7.10 Transferring the surgical plan. (**a**) The osteotomized maxilla displayed on the navigation system monitor to guide Le Fort I osteotomy, (**b**) advancement of 4 mm is demonstrated (iPlan CMF Brainlab AG, Germany)

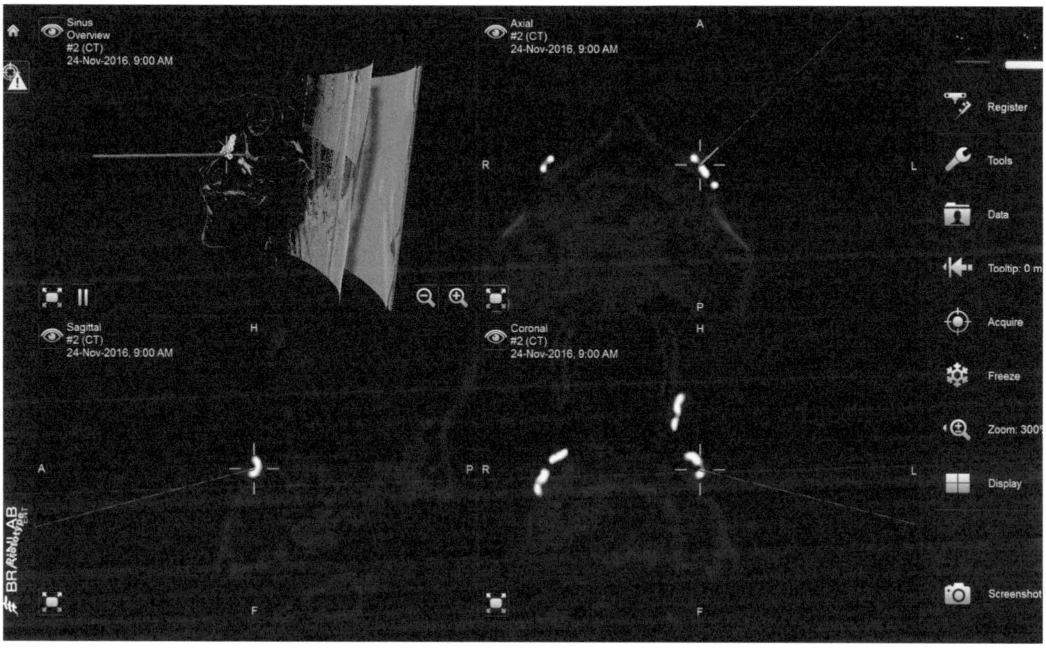

Fig. 7.11 Verification of maxillary positioning after Le Fort I osteotomy and fixation (Brainlab AG, Germany)

model is CT scanned, and the STL file can be merged to the patient's CT scan on the navigation system software.

In the operating room, the osteotomized maxilla is displayed on the navigation system's monitor to guide its repositioning as planned (Fig. 7.10). When the optimal position is achieved, the maxilla is fixed using the titanium plates that had been pre-bent. Finally, the position of the maxilla after the Le Fort I osteotomy and rigid fixation can be verified with the navigation system (Fig. 7.11).

This minimally invasive approach maxillary orthognathic surgery enables using a substantially smaller soft tissue incision than the classic "molar-to-molar" exposure, and the postoperative swelling is considerably reduced when compared to the classic approach, enabling faster patient recovery. The computer planning and navigation systems assist in making this procedure more accurate.

References

1. Steinhäuser EW. Historical development of orthognathic surgery. J Craniomaxillofac Surg. 1996;24:195–204.
2. Resnick CM, Kaban LB, Troulis MJ. Minimally invasive orthognathic surgery. Facial Plast Surg. 2009;25:49–62. https://doi.org/10.1055/s-0028-1112232.
3. Troulis MJ, Perrott DH, Kaban LB. Endoscopic mandibular osteotomy, and placement and activation of a semiburied distractor. J Oral Maxillofac Surg. 1999;57:1110–3.
4. Wiltfang J, Kessler P. Endoscopically assisted Le Fort I osteotomy to correct transverse and sagittal discrepancies of the maxilla. J Oral Maxillofac Surg. 2002;60:1142–5.
5. Taylor JA, Maercks RA, Runyan CM, Jones DC, Gordon CB. Endoscopically assisted Le Fort III osteotomy using an ultrasonic scalpel: a feasibility study in cadavers. J Craniofac Surg. 2009;20:2211–4. https://doi.org/10.1097/SCS.0b013e3181bf84a7.
6. Lin HH, Lo LL. Three-dimensional computer-assisted surgical simulation and intraoperative navigation in orthognathic surgery: a literature review. J Formos Med Assoc. 2015;114:300–7.

7. Hernández-Alfaro F, Guijarro-Martínez R. "Twist technique" for pterygomaxillary dysjunction in minimally invasive Le Fort I osteotomy. J Oral Maxillofac Surg. 2013;71:389–92. https://doi.org/10.1016/j.joms.2012.04.032.
8. Rohner D, Yeow V, Hammer B. Endoscopically assisted Le Fort I osteotomy. J Craniomaxillofac Surg. 2001;29:360–5. https://doi.org/10.1054/jcms.2001.0248.
9. Lanigan DT, Guest P. Alternative approaches to pterygomaxillary separation. Int J Oral Maxillofac Surg. 1993;22:131–8.
10. Pereira FL, Yaedú RYF, Sant'Ana AP, Sant'Ana A. Maxillary aseptic necrosis after Le Fort I osteotomy: a case report and literature review. J Oral Maxillofac Surg. 2010;68:1402–7.
11. Bell WH, Fonseca RJ, Kenneky JW, Levy BM. Bone healing and revascularization after total maxillary osteotomy. J Oral Surg. 1975;33:253–60.
12. Brusati R, Bottoli V. Maxillary anterior segmentary osteotomy: experimental research on vascular supply of osteotomised segment. Fortschr Kiefer Gesichtschir. 1974;18:90–3.
13. Aboul-Hosn CS, Hernández-Alfaro F. 3D planning in orthognathic surgery: CAD/CAM surgical splints and prediction of the soft and hard tissues results - our experience in 16 cases. J Craniomaxillofac Surg. 2012;40:162–8.
14. Bell BR. Computer planning and intraoperative navigation in Orthognathic surgery. J Oral Maxillofac Surg. 2011;69:592–605.
15. Seeberger B, Kane G, Hoffmann J, Eggers G. Accuracy assessment for navigated maxillo-facial surgery using an electromagnetic tracking device. J Craniomaxillofac Surg. 2011;40:156–61.
16. Casap N, Wexler A, Eliashar R. Computerized navigation for surgery of the lower jaw: comparison of 2 navigation systems. J Oral Maxillofac Surg. 2008;66:1467–75.

Salivary Gland Endoscopy and Minimally Invasive Surgery

8

Oded Nahlieli

Abstract

In the 1990s and the beginning of the 2000s, the problem analyzed and discussed in articles on salivary gland surgery could reasonably be labeled: "minimally invasive surgery versus gland excision.". In the 2010s, the discussion has shifted to the question of which minimally invasive method to choose. At the same time, there is no clear borderline between radical and minimally invasive surgery of the salivary glands. Currently, both surgical approaches partially overlap and in some cases endoscopically assisted traditional surgery is applied. Minimally invasive approach, or "less aggressive surgery," for traditional parotidectomy suggests selective deep lobe parotidectomy instead of total excision of the gland in benign cases only involving the deep lobe. Combinations of various minimally invasive techniques are also possible. This chapter describes several modern techniques to choose from: the direct sialoendoscopic removal of the stones via the salivary ducts, the endoscopy-assisted intraoral surgery, the extracorporeal shock-wave lithotripsy (ESWL), a combination of the ESWL with the sialoendoscopic approach in order to remove stone fragments, and the ductal stretching.

8.1 Introduction

The rapid developments in technology in the XXI century especially optical miniaturization, lithotripsy equipment and micro-instruments, the influence from other surgical fields, and general knowledge about the regeneration potential of the salivary glands directed maxillofacial surgeons to develop new methods of treatment by means of noninvasive, minimally invasive, and less invasive interventions. In this chapter, we review the modern methods developed for salivary gland sialolithiasis and some other diseases of the salivary glands.

O. Nahlieli, DMD
Department of Oral and Maxillofacial Surgery, The Barzilai Medical Center, Ashkelon, Israel

The Faculty of Medicine, Ben Gurion University of the Negev, Beer Sheva, Israel

Department of Oral and Maxillofacial Surgery, Eastman Institute for Oral Health University of Rochester, Rochester, NY, USA

Department of Oral and Maxillofacial Surgery, University of Michigan Health System, Ann Arbor, Michigan, USA
e-mail: nahlieli@yahoo.com

O. Nahlieli (ed.), *Minimally Invasive Oral and Maxillofacial Surgery*,
http://doi.org/10.1007/978-3-662-54592-8_8

The methods, which we discussed on these pages, are the salivary gland endoscopic and endoscopic assistance techniques, extracorporeal shock-wave lithotripsy, the intracorporeal lithotripsy, the ductal stretching, and some other intraoral procedures.

8.1.1 Anatomical Considerations

The excretory ducts of the salivary glands are the gates for any minimally invasive interventions inside these glands when the duct is patent. The *submandibular gland* (Fig. 8.1) is located in the anterior cervical region in the submandibular triangle and its duct, the Wharton's duct, leaves the body of the gland between the mylohyoid, hyoglossus, and genioglossus muscles. The duct opens by a narrow orifice on the summit of a small papilla at the side of the frenulum of the tongue. When the tongue is elevated, these orifices are quite visible from both sides of the midline of the underside of the tongue (Fig. 8.2). From the orifice, the Wharton's duct runs into the gland via a gap between the above-mentioned muscles.

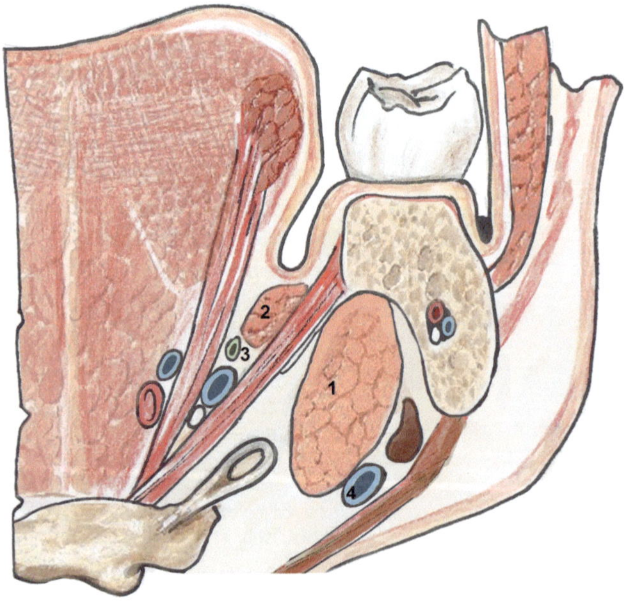

Fig. 8.1 The submandibular gland is located in the anterior cervical region in the submandibular triangle. *1*—the submandibular gland, *2*—the sublingual gland, *3*—the Wharton's duct, *4*—the facial vein

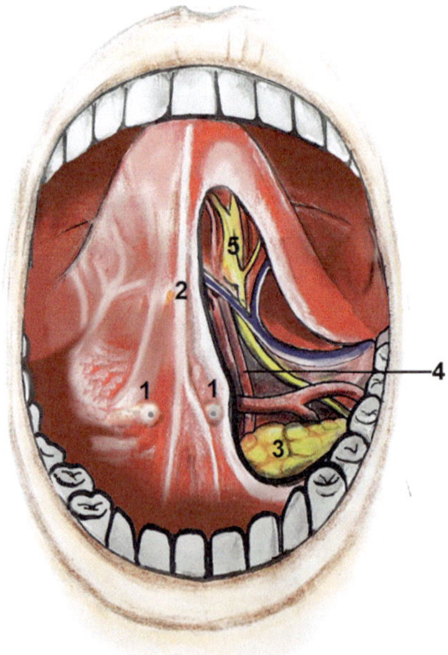

Fig. 8.2 The Wharton's duct opens by a narrow orifice on the summit of a small papilla (*1*) at the side of the frenulum of the tongue (*2*). *3*—the sublingual gland, *4*—deep lingual artery, *5*—the lingual nerve

Attention, surgeons: the lingual nerve and the lingual vein and sublingual gland travel along the path of the Wharton's duct (Fig. 8.3).

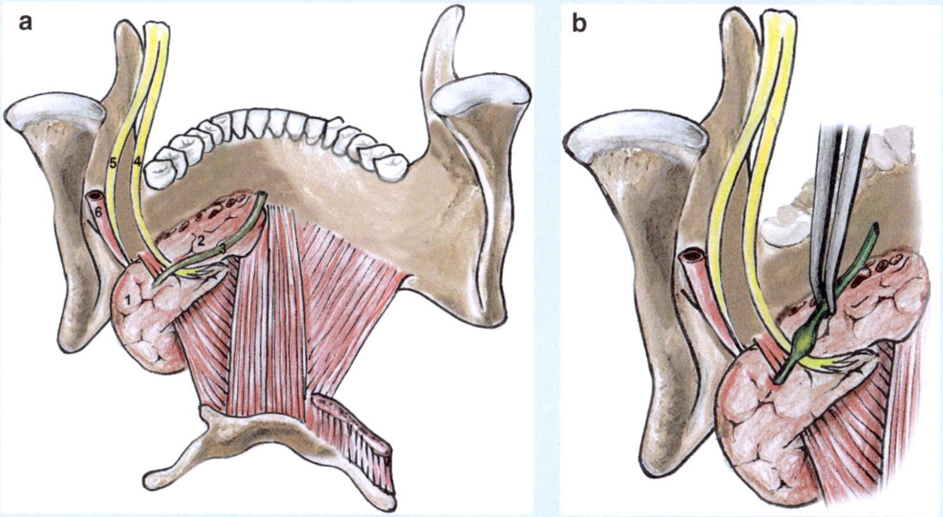

Fig. 8.3 (**a**) The Wharton's duct and the neighboring structures. *1*—the submandibular gland, *2*—the sublingual gland, *3*—the Wharton's duct, *4*—the lingual nerve, *5*—the inferior alveolar nerve, *6*—the inferior alveolar artery. (**b**) The stone is in the duct

The main part of the duct is surrounded by gland tissue from the submandibular and partly from the sublingual gland. From the orifice, the duct may run deep into the gland either almost horizontally backwards, or in a slightly curved semicircle, or obliquely downwards and backwards. As a rule, it curves around the mylohyoid muscle. That is why as it proceeds from its entrance in the oral cavity deeper it curves and the size of the angle of this curve varies between 24° and 178°. This fact is very important for minimally invasive endoscopic interventions because this angle is the most common site for stone formation and the formation of obstructing ductal kinks [1].

In adults, the Wharton's duct is 5 cm long. In 1998, Zenk et al. reported that its diameter ranges between 0.5 and 1.5 mm in various segments [2]. Ten years after that, Francis Marchal estimated the diameter of the Wharton's duct as 2–3 mm [3]. The narrowest duct diameter is identified at the ostium [2]. Inside the gland, the main duct is divided into the first, second, and third generation branches and finally the terminal branches. The practicality of these facts for the endoscopic intervention is obvious. For diagnostic and therapeutic purposes, sialoendoscopes with stone-extraction baskets or forceps and balloon catheters should conform as much as possible to physiological duct widths. While modern sialoendoscopes may be less than 1 mm in diameter, the diameter of 2.00 mm should be considered the upper limit for duct instruments. It is possible to introduce the exploration unit of 1.3, 1.6, and 2.00 mm through the natural orifice of the duct [3–5]. Yet, it is generally accepted that the best results can be achieved when the maximum size of a stone or a stone fragment does not exceed 1.2 mm. However, some investigators have suggested that a calculus 20% greater than the diameter of the duct should not be extracted via the duct itself [6].

The *parotid glands* are the largest salivary glands (Fig. 8.4). Each parotid gland lies behind the mandibular ramus and in front of the mastoid process of the temporal bone.

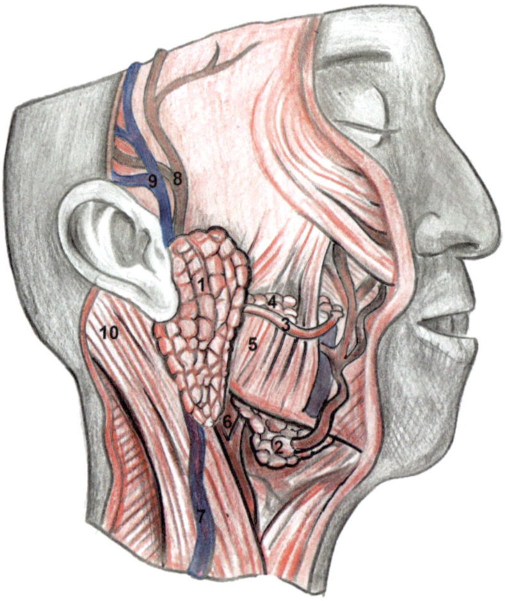

Fig. 8.4 The parotid glands are the largest salivary glands. Each parotid gland lies behind the mandibular ramus and in front of the mastoid process of the temporal bone. *1*—the parotid gland, *2*—the submandibular gland, *3*—the Stensen's duct, *4*—the accessory parotid gland, *5*—the masseter muscle, *6*—the external carotid artery, *7*—the external jugular vein, *8*—the superficial temporal artery, *9*—the superficial temporal vein, *10*—the starnocleidomastoid muscle

Attention, surgeons: A number of different structures pass through the parotid gland. From lateral to medial, these are: the facial nerve (Fig. 8.5), the retromandibular vein, the external carotid artery, the superficial temporal artery, several branches of the great auricular nerve, and the maxillary artery. Please revive your knowledge of the parotideomasseteric region and the buccal region (Fig. 8.6), the retromandibular region (Fig. 8.7), and the submandibular triangle (Fig. 8.8).

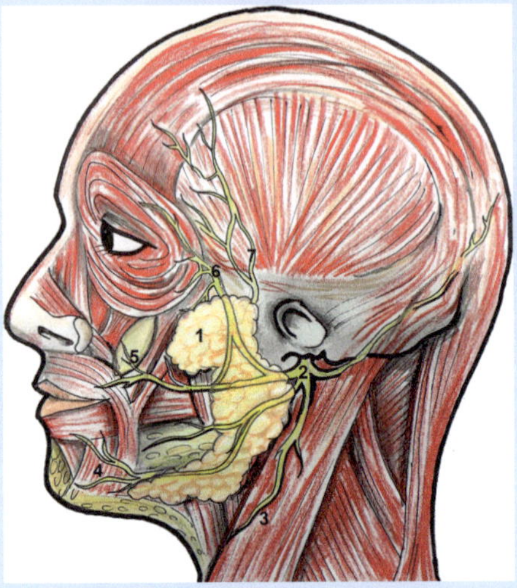

Fig. 8.5 The facial nerve passes through the parotid gland. *1*—the parotid gland, *2*—the facial nerve, *3*—the cervical branch of the facial nerve, *4*—the mandibular branches of the facial nerve, *5*—the buccal branches of the facial nerve, *6*—the zygomatic branches of the facial nerve, *7*—the temporal branches of the facial nerve

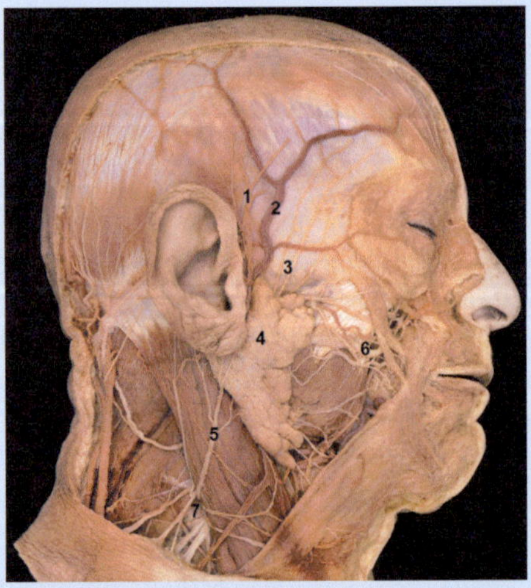

Fig. 8.6 The parotideomasseteric region and the buccal region (lateral view). *1*—N. auricotemporalis, *2*—*A. temporalis* superficialis, *3*—temporofacial branches of n. VII, *4*—the parotid gland, *5*—*N. auricularis* magnus, *6*—the parotid duct, *7*—Erb-point, where the cutaneous branches of cervical plexus appear to supply the skin of the neck and the scalp (by permission from Isradon Publishing House, Herzeliya, 2007)

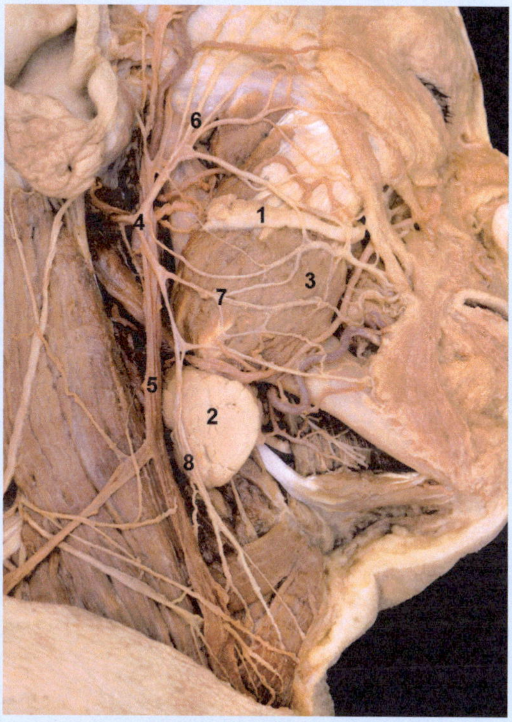

Fig. 8.7 The retromandibular region after removal of the parotid gland. *1*—the duct of the parotid, *2*—the submandibular gland, *3*—the masseter m., *4*—the facial nerve (VII), *5*—the retromandibular vein, *6*—temporofacial branches of the n. VII, *7*—zygomatic and buccal branches of the n. VII, *8*—the colli branch of the n. VII (by permission from Isradon Publishing House, Herzeliya, 2007)

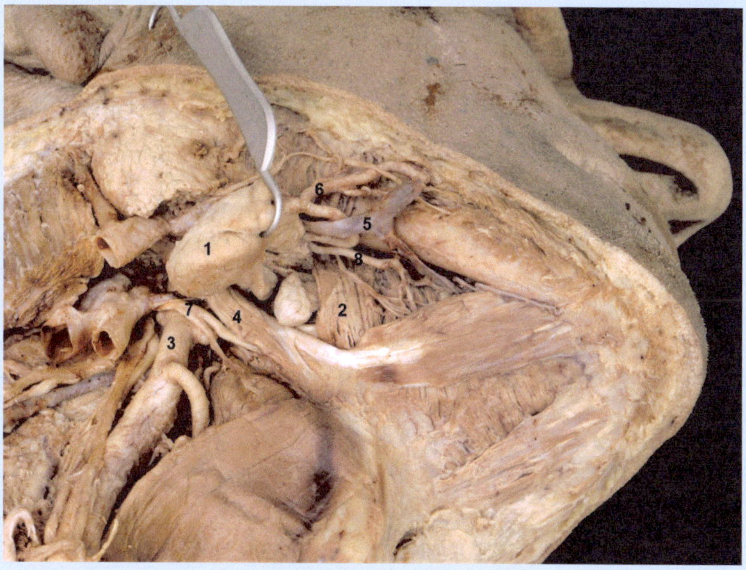

Fig. 8.8 The submandibular triangle, superficial dissection. *1*—the submandibular gland, *2*—the mylohyoid m., *3*—the external carotid a., *4*—the stylohyoid m., *5*—the facial vein, *6*—the facial a., *7*—N. hypoglossus (XII) followed by the lingual a., *8*—the submental a.

The parotid duct, the Stensen's duct, is formed from several large interlobular ducts inside the gland. Its orifice can be observed at the parotid papilla, which lies in the vestibule of the mouth between the cheek and the gums. The second superior molar tooth serves as the landmark.

Moving from the orifice to the gland, the duct passes through the buccinator muscle, takes a steep turn at the border of the masseter muscle and runs backward along the lateral side of the masseter muscle. In this course, the Stensen's duct is surrounded by the buccal fat pad.

The mean diameter of the Stensen's duct at four different segments along its length ranges between 0.5 and 1.4 mm [2]. As in the submandibular gland, the main duct is also divided into primary, secondary, tertiary, and terminal branches. Zenk et al. indicated a narrowing at the middle segment of the duct and found the minimum width of the secretory duct at the ostium [2]. Therefore, the diameter of 1.2–1.3 mm should be considered the upper limit for duct endoscopes in case of the Stensen's duct. According to Marchal however, the diameter of Stensen's duct can reach almost 2 mm that permits to use 1.6 mm endoscopes [3].

8.1.2 Salivary Gland Disorders for Minimally Invasive Surgery

Several disorders of the salivary glands welcome minimally invasive interventions. Of them, the obstructive sialadenitis, with or without sialolithiasis, represents the most common inflammatory disorder of the major salivary glands [7]. Sialolithiasis is one of the major causes of sialadenitis. Calculi in the salivary glands can be found in 1.2% of the general population [8]. Other common salivary gland pathologies (besides tumors) are sialadenitis, strictures and kinks, and rarely foreign bodies. The minimally invasive approach can be successfully tried for these disorders as well.

> Attention, surgeons: some tumors of the salivary glands can mimic sialadenitis and stones. Tumors mimicking sialadenitis and stones are the most serious rarities which can affect the prognosis of a patient and could delay an adequate treatment. Phleboliths mimic salivary stones.

Autoimmune diseases that might affect the salivary glands also can gain advantages by minimally invasive techniques. Such diseases are disorders in which the body's tissues are attacked by its own immune system, mostly by autoantibodies and T-cells. Of these diseases, the Sjögren's syndrome and systemic lupus erythematosus affect salivary glands. The salivary glands actually are the main target for the Sjögren's syndrome. This syndrome is a chronic inflammatory disease of the exocrine glands with a broad range of extraglandular manifestation. Symptoms of dry mouth, xerostomia, keratoconjunctivitis sicca, and dry eyes are common signs of the Sjögren's syndrome. Oral lesions such as desquamative gingivitis and marginal gingivitis or erosive mucosal lesions have been reported in up to 40% of these patients [9]. The systemic lupus erythematosus is a multi-system inflammatory disease of unknown cause, which affects the skin, joints, the kidneys, the lungs, the nervous system, serous membranes, and other organs of the body including the salivary glands [10, 11].

Strictures of the salivary ducts and an obstruction of the ductal system due to abnormal gelatin saliva are pathologies caused by the autoimmune sialadenitis. These pathologies can be managed by the sialoendoscopy as well.

8.1.3 The Tool #1: Sialoendoscope

Endoscopes designed for the salivary gland ducts, sialoendoscopes, are produced by various manufacturers (PloyDiagnost GmbH, Germany; Karl Storz, Germany) [5, 12, 13]. These sialoendoscopes are divided into diagnostic and therapeutic devices. The diagnostic endoscopes usually have the exterior diameter of 0.65–0.9 mm and are suitable for observation and irrigation. Semirigid optic specifications vary from 3000 to 30,000 pixels.

We believe that good sialoendoscope should contain a telescope with at least 6000 pixels illumination fibers and focal length of 2–15 mm and 70° field of view. However, the best results can be obtained with the 10,000 pixel optic with

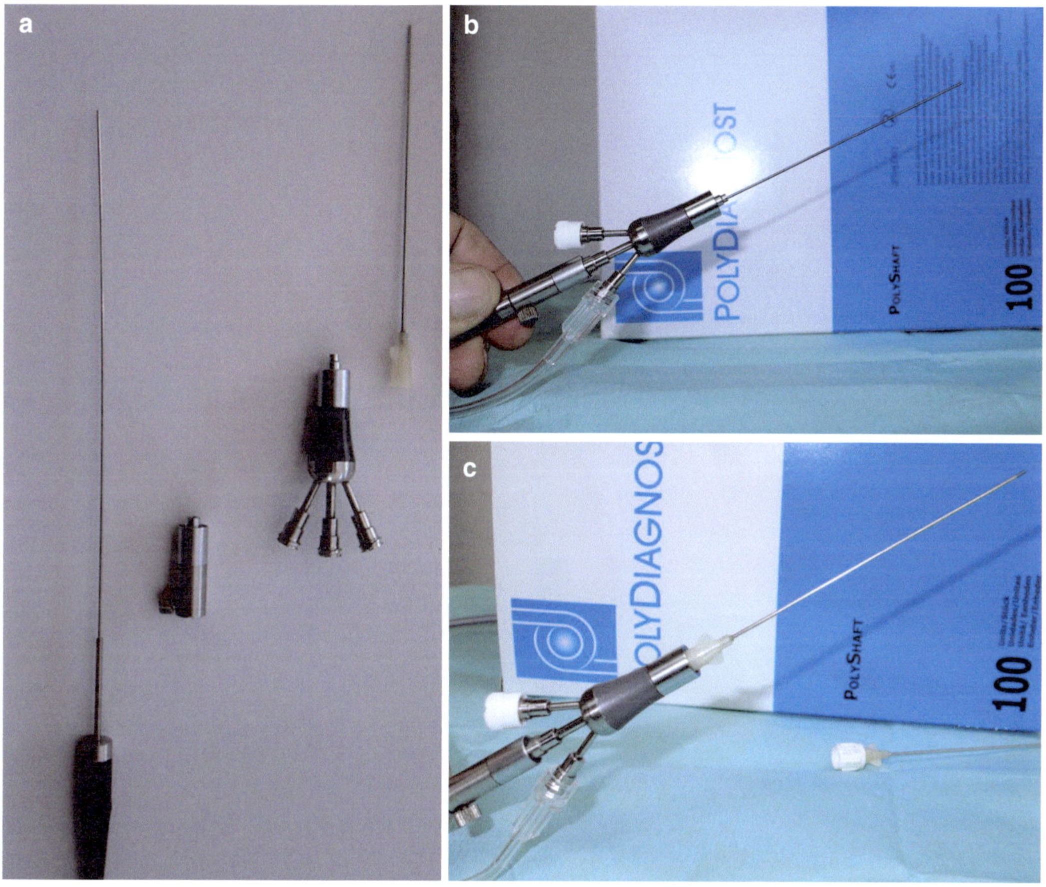

Fig. 8.9 (**a**) Modular sialoendoscope (Polydiagnost)—with reusable telescope, (**a**) handle and disposable cannula. (**b**) The modular sialoendoscope with the telescope inside, (**c**) the sialoendoscope with the disposable cannula covering the telescope

120° field of view. Such micro-endoscopes can change the view field from 0° to 70° and further to 120°. The diameter of the telescope is usually 0.5 mm. The endoscopes can be either designed with the fixed exterior diameter or have disposable sleeves of various diameters. For example, the Polydygnost Modular salivascope (POLYDIAGNOST GmbH, Hallbergmoos, Germany) has a reusable handle and four sets of disposable sleeves: 1.1, 1.3, 1.6, and 2.0 mm in diameter.

Therapeutic endoscopes start from 1.1 mm in diameter. The modular handle has three channels for the telescope, irrigation, and special channel for surgical instruments (Figs. 8.9 and 8.10).

All the sleeves are disposable. The optical part—the telescope—is autoclavable [5, 12, 13]. Other reliable endoscopes are the Karl Storz Erlangen—Sialoendoscope and the Marchal Sialoendoscope. Both these endoscopes represent the all-in-one type when the telescope and the working and irrigation channels are combined in one piece. The diameters of such devices are usually from 1.1 to 2 mm.

The instruments which are available today for use with the endoscopic system and that were used in our studies were: micro-baskets of 0.4–0.6 mm with three, four, or six wires suitable as stone extractors, miniforceps with double action jaws for foreign bodies, flexible minibiopsy forceps, high pressure balloons for dilatation, brushes for cytology, and micro-needles for injection. The forceps are autoclavable, the stone extractors are disposable.

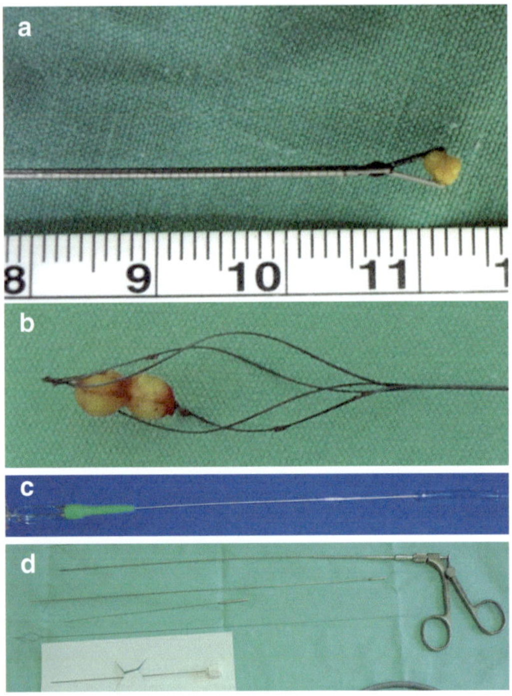

Fig. 8.10 Mini instruments for sialoendoscopy intervention: (**a**) miniforceps, (**b**) 4-wires mini baskets, (**c**) high pressure balloons, and (**d**) drills

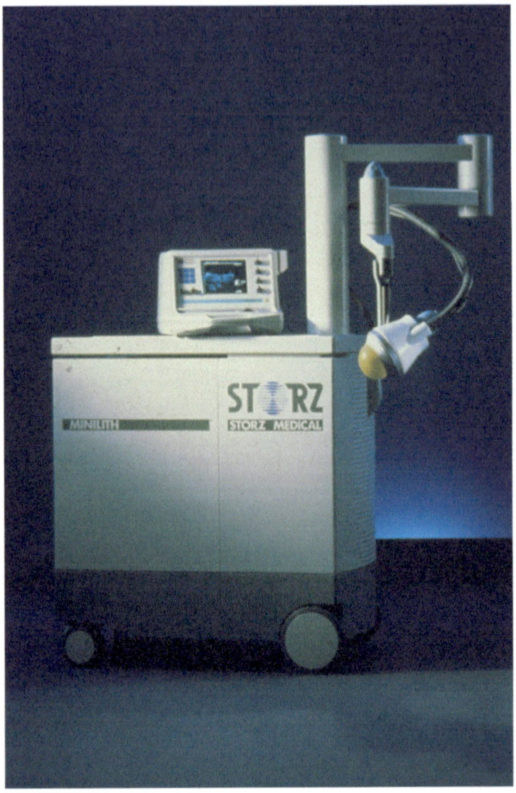

Fig. 8.11 The extracorporeal lithotripter (Storz Medical)

8.1.4 The Tool #2: Extracorporeal Shock-Wave Lithotripter

Extracorporeal shock-wave lithotripters are used against kidney stones since the 1970s and were introduced in orthopedics, pain medicine, and esthetic medicine since then. Specific modifications for the salivary gland calculi were developed mainly in the 1990s and the 2000s by several manufacturers (Medispec Ltd.—Israel; Storz Medical AG, Tägerwilen, Switzerland; Sialo Technology, Ashkelon, Israel). Of them, Minilith SL1 (Storz Medical) and Sialowave (Medispec) are most widely used (Figs. 8.11 and 8.12). The Shock Wave Unit of Sialowave consists of a reflector and a dry natural rubber membrane called contact membrane filled with water, an underwater electrode and a high voltage power supply. The energy of the shock wave can be adjusted between 10 and 24 kV. The shock wave applicator itself is a disposable part and needs to be replaced after 50,000 shocks (pulses). It is recommended to start the treatment at energy level of about 10 kV and to increase it progressively during the treatment according to the judgment of the physician and tolerance of the patient [14]. A local anesthetic may be spread on the area to be treated. While such lithotripters are usually quite heavy (up to 35 kg), the miniature External Lithotripter (Sialo Technology) was also designed. With electrohydraulic energy of 10–24 kV, it has a miniature generator and an applicator, focal point depth—15 × 15 × 25, large focus zone (focus at 50%)—35 mm, and penetration depth—120 mm. The diameter of the generator is not bigger than a computer box and the working head is reduced to fit the dimensions of the head and neck region.

Usually, extracorporeal shock-wave lithotripsy (ESWL) delivers 1000–1500 shock waves (pulses) per session. However, the intensity of the waves from 1300 to 7000 pulses was also reported [15]. The external lithotripsy is applied with low energy levels up to 130 atm. The lithotripter generates enough power to produce the cavitation

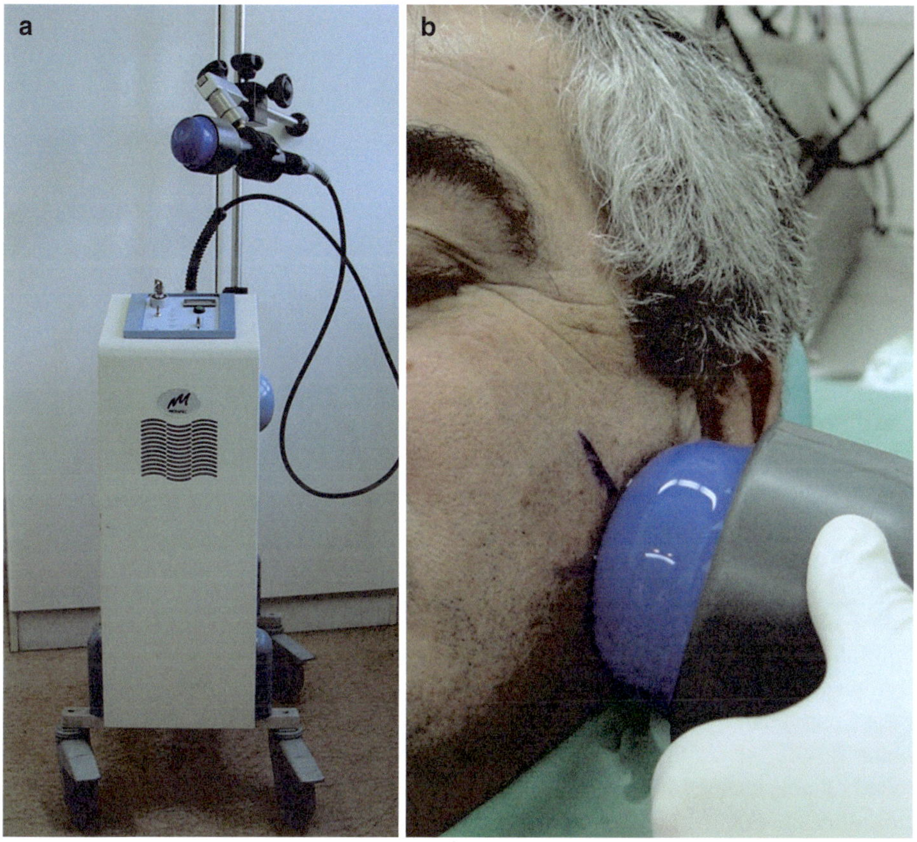

Fig. 8.12 (**a**) The extracorporeal lithotripter (Medispec), (**b**) the application of the lithotripter head to the stone location in the parotid gland

effect. The cavitation leads to reduction of the hydrodynamic pressure within the saliva, as by subjecting it to ultrasonic vibration. It helps the shock waves to disconnect the salivary stone from the ductal wall, reduce the volume of the stone, and can crush the stone. Due to the low energy levels of the shock waves, the procedure is not painful and do not require anesthesia.

The piezoelectric and electrohydraulic devices are also available.

8.2 The Types and the Technique of the Minimally Invasive Interventions

In the 1990s and the beginning of the 2000s, the problem analyzed and discussed in articles on salivary gland surgery could reasonably be labeled: "minimally invasive surgery versus gland excision." In the 2010s, the discussion has shifted to the question of which minimally invasive method to choose. At the same time, there is no clear borderline between radical and minimally invasive surgery of the salivary glands. Currently, both surgical approaches partially overlap and in some cases endoscopically assisted traditional surgery is applied. Minimally invasive approach, or "less aggressive surgery," for traditional parotidectomy suggests selective deep lobe parotidectomy instead of total excision of the gland in benign cases only involving the deep lobe. Combinations of various minimally invasive techniques are also possible.

There are several modern techniques to choose from: the direct sialoendoscopic removal of the stones via the salivary ducts, the endoscopy-assisted intraoral surgery, the ESWL, a combination of the ESWL with the sialoendoscopic approach in order to remove stone fragments, and the ductal stretching.

8.2.1 Sialoendoscopic Removal of the Stones

Since the 1990s, sialoendoscopy has added a significant new dimension to the surgeon's armamentarium for diagnosis and management of inflammatory salivary disease, specifically the obstructive sialadenitis, with or without sialolithiasis. The diagnostic purposes of sialoendoscopy were described separately [12, 13]. This chapter is dedicated to interventional sialoendoscopy. The only one absolute contraindication to this technique is acute sialadenitis.

In addition to a careful clinical evaluation, the proper imaging of the affected gland is of upmost importance. Assessing computed tomography (CT) imaging variations, the Cone Beam CT is the most reliable (Fig. 8.13). It gives an excellent resolution with minimum irradiation and with minimum interference from metals like a dental crown bridge and dental fillings. Another advantage of the Cone Beam CT (CBCT) is the option to combine it with the sialography (Fig. 8.14). The second reliable evaluation method is a high resolution ultrasonography. Due to introduction of these excellent methods into every day practice, we don't recommend the usage of plain X-rays (panorex, occlusal, occlusal oblique) for the salivary glands evaluation.

As it was mentioned in the anatomical introduction, diameters of the ducts vary. Therefore, the size of the duct should be measured by CBCT sialography and ultrasound imaging in order to determine the feasibility of entering the ductal lumen by use of sialoendoscopy. Sialography is used for mapping the ductal system for possible variations and assessment of its estimated dilatation capacity.

If the duct size and diameter offer a good entrance, we can proceed with endoscopy. There are four possible methods for introducing the endoscope into the ductal lumen:

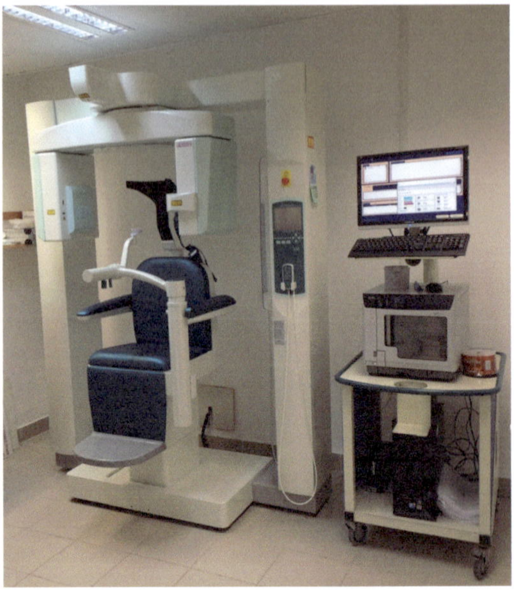

Fig. 8.13 The Cone Beam CT (Accuitomo Morita, Japan)

- Introducing the sialoendoscope (up to 1.3 mm) through the natural orifice of the duct. Sometimes there is a need for dilatation which can be done with lacrimal probes and ductal dilators.
- Introducing the endoscope through a papillotomy procedure. This is performed with an incision immediately posterior to the orifice of the duct, thus enlarging the opening.
- Introducing the sialoendoscope through ductal exploration ("ductal cutdown"), which involves surgical dissection and exposure of the anterior portion of the duct with a microsurgical technique. The duct is then incised longitudinally to allow the intraluminal insertion of the endoscope. If there are any difficulties in introducing the endoscope in the anterior part (e.g., stricture, too narrow ductal lumen), it may be necessary to expose the duct more posteriorly to arrive at a location where the diameter will accommodate the endoscope.
- Introducing the sialoendoscope through a sialolithotomy opening. The endoscope can be inserted through the same opening in the duct where the stone was extracted.

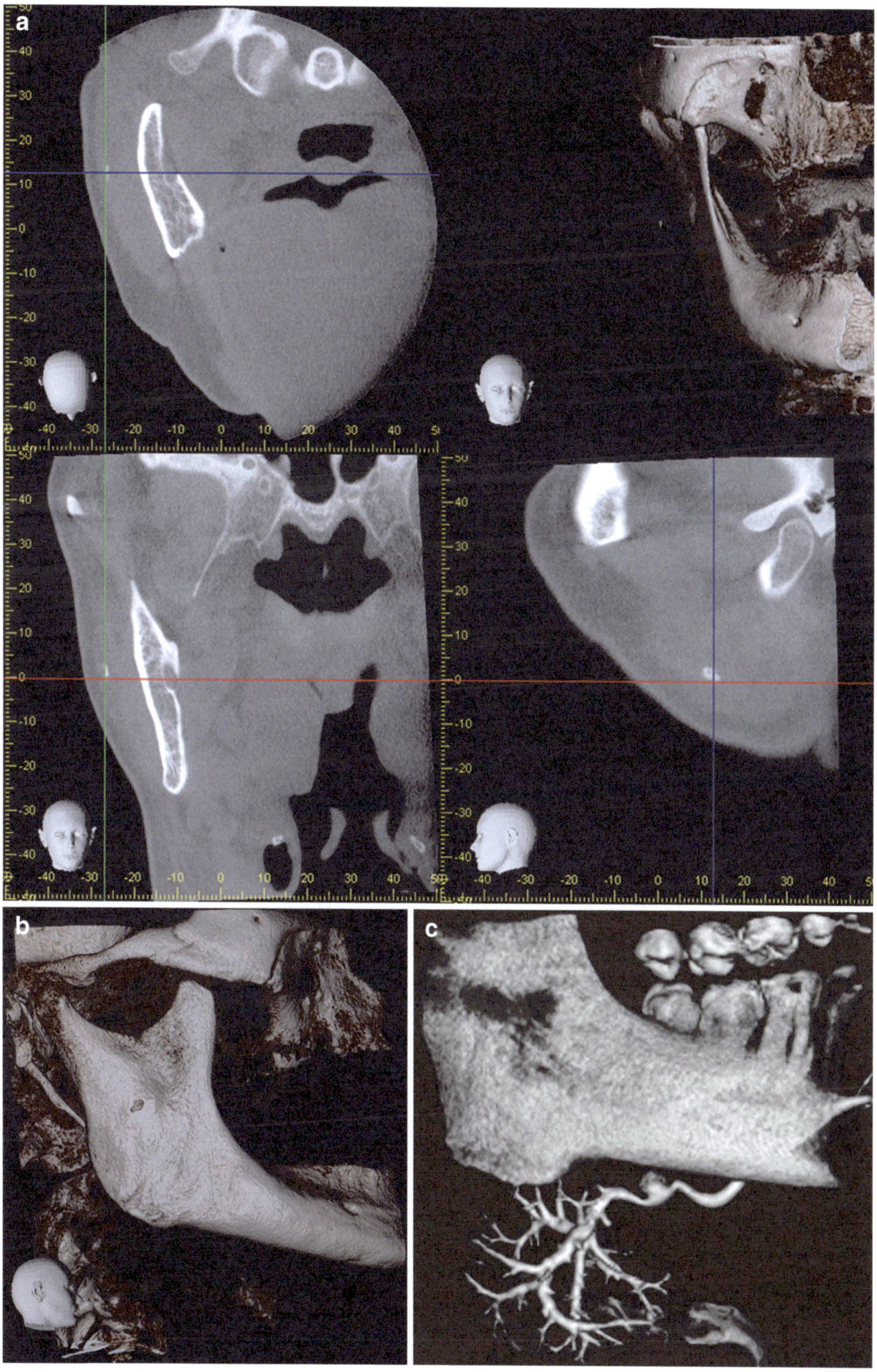

Fig. 8.14 The Cone Beam CT demonstrating 3 mm stone in the right parotid gland (**a**), (**b**) the 3D demonstration of stone in the parotid gland. (**c**, **d**) The Cone Beam 3D CT sialogram, coronal, and sagittal. The stone is near the hilum of the submandibular. Note that the stone location is extraductal

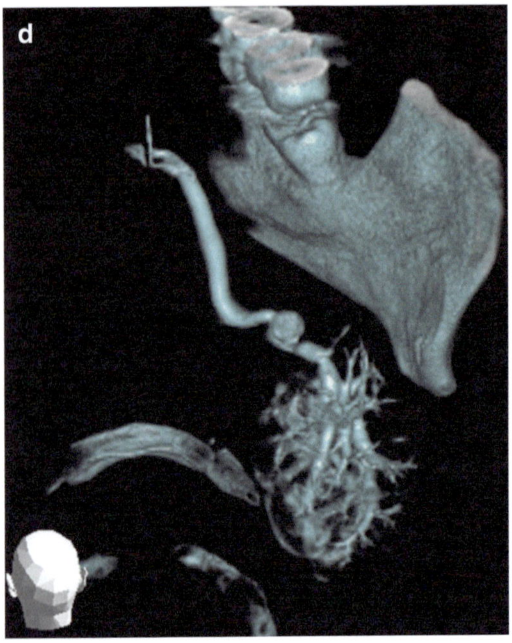

Fig. 8.14 (continued)

8.2.2 Irrigation During Sialoendoscopy

Irrigation is crucial for every endoscopic procedure. The cavity or the duct has to be filled with fluid to allow free movement of the instrument, and the area needs to be lavaged permitting good visualization. The isotonic saline is the fluid of choice. A 10–20 cm^3 syringe with luer lock containing isotonic saline is connected via extension tube to the irrigation port and the endoscope and moved forward being accompanied by a gentle flow of saline. Usually, 4 cm^3 of 2% lidocaine are also injected through this port, resulting in the anesthesia of the entire ductal system.

8.3 Techniques of Endoscopic Sialolithotomy

The following methods are available for removal of stones:

- Intraductal approach
- Extraductal approach

The intraductal approach is a pure endoscopic technique. The extraductal approach involves endoscopically assisted techniques. When a sialolith is encountered, its diameter is estimated and the method of choice for its removal is selected from two *intraductal sialolithotomy* possibilities:

- Removal of a stone in one piece with the help of grasping forceps, wire baskets, or hydrostatic pressure posterior to the stone (Fig. 8.15)
- Combined use of an ESWL and endoscopic removal

The primary goal is to remove the calculus in one piece. The following approaches are available in cases when the extraductal technique was chosen:

- Intraoral techniques. These techniques can be used for the submandibular, sublingual, and parotid stones.

- Extraoral technique. This technique is exclusively used for impacted parotid stones.

8.3.1 Endoscopy-Assisted Intraoral Surgery

Transoral/intraoral surgical approaches with or without endoscopic assistance are mainly used for removal of the salivary stones located in the ducts including giant sialoliths [16]. The main criterion for intraoral release is the presence of the palpable stone in the floor of mouth as otherwise the calculus lies within the gland where experience has shown it is difficult to identify at surgery. However, this technique can be applied for removal of hiloparenchymal submandibular calculi as well [17]. Since endoscopy became a commonly used minimally invasive technique, surgeons realized that endoscopic surgery is unable to overcome large posterior sialoliths that are connected to the ductal walls or located in the posterior part of the salivary ducts. Specific intraoral techniques were developed by Zenk [18] and McGurk [17] to reach the stones in various locations, mainly for the submandibular surgery. The Zenk's approach suggests the

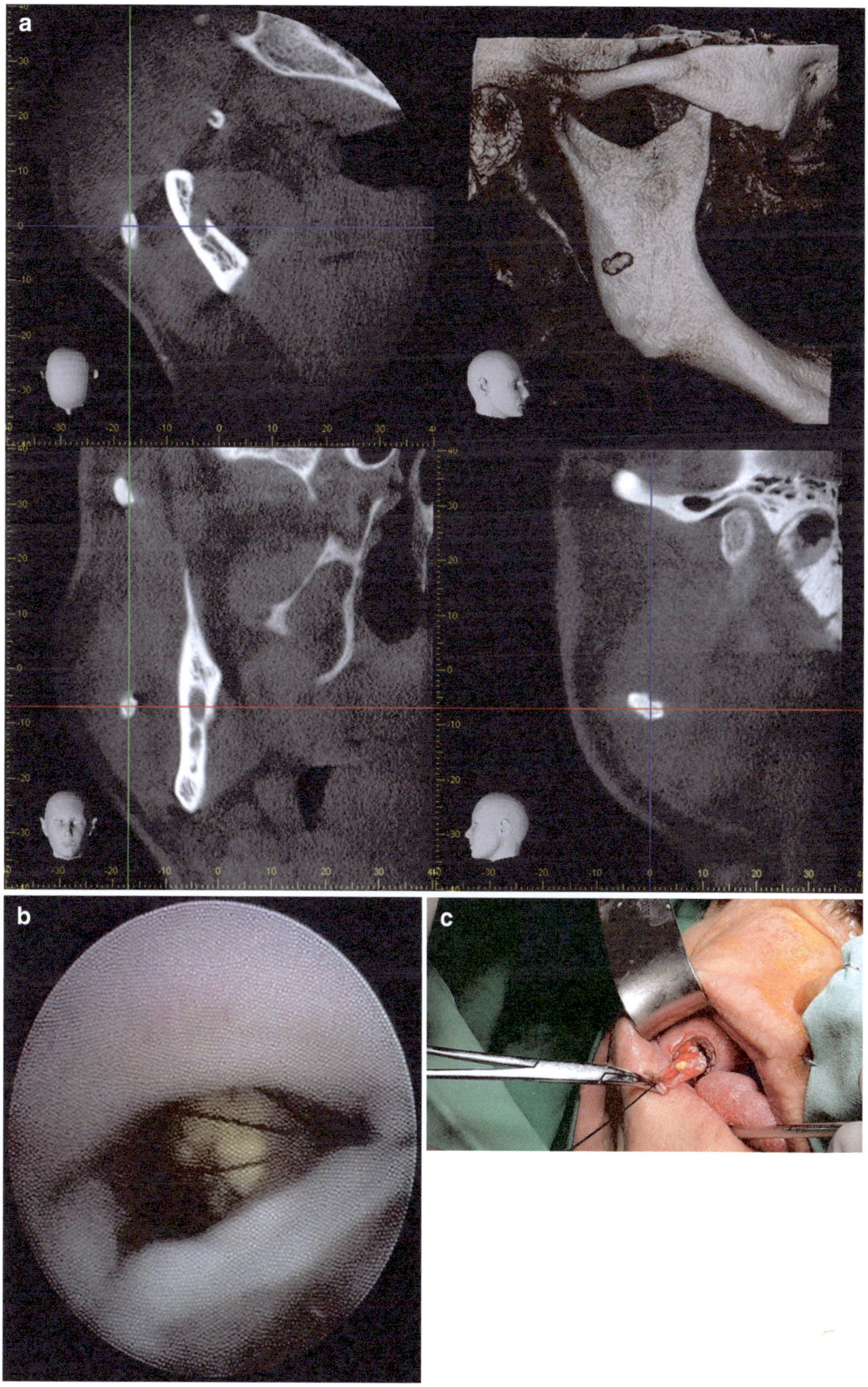

Fig. 8.15 The Cone Beam CT of 7 mm stone in the hilum of the right parotid gland (**a**). (**b**) Intraoperative endoscopic view of basket removal of the stone. (**c**) Removal of the stone via intraoral ductal excision. (**d**) Extraction of stone from the submandibular hilum with miniforceps

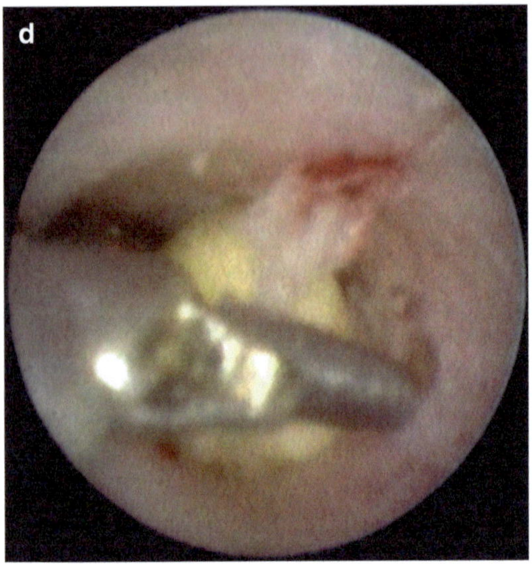

Fig. 8.15 (continued)

main duct should be exposed lengthwise by separating it from the surrounding tissues and sutured to the mouth floor after release of the calculus. Following McGurk, the duct should be exposed and opened specifically over the stone and then re-sutured. Therefore, an operating surgeon can chose either the dissection technique or the pinpoint technique. Nahlieli published his ductal stretching technique in 2007 dissecting the Wharton's duct for safe and easy exploration and removal of hilar submandibular stones [19] (Fig. 8.16).

8.3.2 Ductal Stretching

As it was mentioned before, there are large posterior sialoliths connected to the ductal walls, which intraductal endoscopic surgery cannot overcome. About 60% of such stones are located in the hilum, about 25% of stones are located in the posterior part of the duct, and in 15% patients have multiple stones in the hilum. The ductal stretching is a combined method for the removal of posterior and hilar stones. The procedure is mainly suitable for large and impacted submandibular calculi but occasionally can be implemented in the parotid surgery as well [20–24].

The ductal stretching technique helps to overcome sialoliths removal which cannot be solved with the pure endoscopic techniques. It is used also after failed attempt to extract the sialolith by pure endoscopic techniques.

The ductal stretching technique involves the following 12 steps:

1. Introduce the endoscope for exact location of the stone and lavage and disconnect the stone from the ductal wall.
2. Introduce a lacrimal probe into the duct and perform an incision above the duct with Erbium-laser, CO_2 laser, or electrosurgery.
3. Dissect and isolate the duct from the surrounding tissues up to the first molar (in submandibular cases) securing the safe zone above the nerve.
4. In submandibular cases, apply forwarding the gland towards the mouth with digital pressure from the submandibular region.
5. Stretch the duct with fine hemostat forward.
6. Perform ductal section above the calculus.
7. Perform sialolithotomy.
8. Apply endoscopic exploration for removal of additional calculi, the attachments of the stone to the duct, dilatation of strictures, and lavage for removal of mucous plaques and debris.
9. Perform an excision of the anterior 5 mm of the Wharton's duct suturing the duct to the orifice region with 4/0 vicryl, slitting the duct up to 5–7 mm from the ductal section.
10. Insert the Sialostent.
11. Suture the Sialostent (4/0 vicryl) to the floor of the mouth creating a new orifice.
12. Apply dexamethasone 12 mg injection into the surgical field and irrigation of the gland with hydrocortisone 100 mg via the stent and Hexcaprone (Tranexamic acid) 1 g.

During the follow-up, antibiotic treatment is usually administered over a period of 7 days; imaging of the affected gland, usually CBCT, CT, or US, should be performed on the same day of surgery. Hydration after the procedure includes drinking above 2 L a day without sialogoges or spicy food and massage of the affected gland.

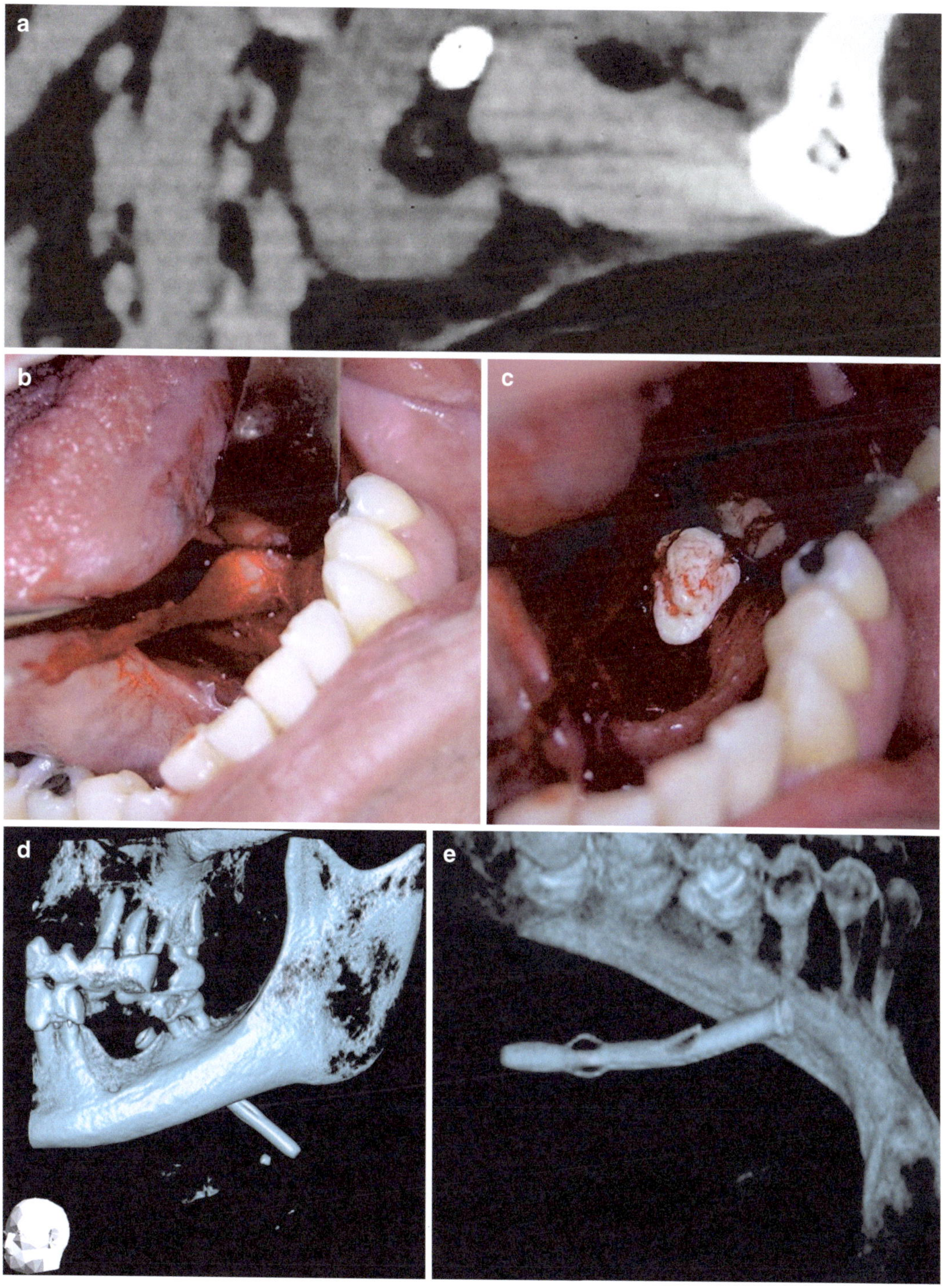

Fig. 8.16 (**a**) The CT of a sialolith in the hilum of submandibular gland, failure to remove with basket and mini-forceps; (**b**) stretching procedure, note the anterior location of the stone (S) after stretching the duct (D); (**c**) extraction of the stone; (**d**, **e**) the Cone Beam CT demonstrating the sialostent inside the submandibular duct; (**f**) a sialostent with flaps and the basket holding the sialostent in the duct; (**g**) insertion of the sialostent with the help of the sialoendoscope; (**h**) the sialostent is inside the submandibular duct

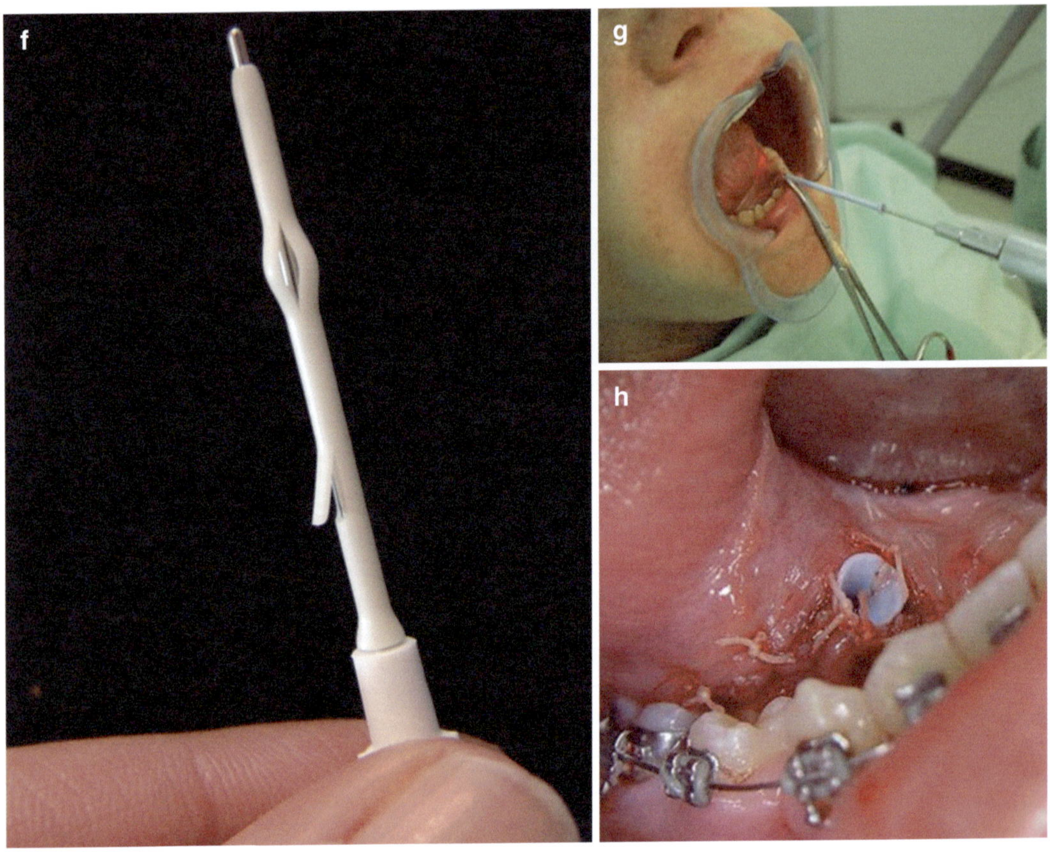

Fig. 8.16 (continued)

The leading arguments for endoscopy-assisted intraoral surgery are the size and the position of the calculus and/or the presence of a stricture associated with the calculus. Another important factor is the presence of multiple calculi and the diameter of the duct. Thus, the performing surgeons should choose their approach not because of advantages and disadvantages of the preferred technique but because of the dimensions and localization of the sialoliths. The dissection technique can be performed without endoscopy. The pinpoint technique also can be performed without endoscopy in cases when a large well-palpable sialolith is located in the main duct itself.

The surgeons however appreciate the endoscopy during surgery for the exact location of the stone and following the removal of the stone for direct visualization and assessment of pathologic changes in the salivary duct system (strictures) and the detection of additional stones.

Attention surgeons: this technique requires precise knowledge of the floor of the mouth and the lingual nerve anatomy.

8.3.3 Extraoral Approach to Parotid Stones

This approach is exclusively reserved for removal of parotid stones in the middle posterior and hilar part of the parotid duct which cannot be removed via intraductal approach and also for removal of intraparenchymal stones. Identification of the stones can be performed either by sialoendoscopic technique or by ultrasound technique. The endoscopic approach is indicated when there is a possibility to introduce the endoscope into the duct (Fig. 8.17).

Sialoendoscopic technique: The stone is located with the help of an insertion of the sialoendoscope into the Stensen's duct, identification of the stone on the endoscope monitor, and with the aid of the transillumination effect on the outer skin. The surgeon marks the exact location on the skin. The same technique is used during the surgery for final location of the stone.

Ultrasound technique: When insertion of the endoscope is impossible or in cases with intraparenchymal stones the only diagnostic method is to use high resolution ultrasound and to locate the stone with the aid of biopsy marker.

There are two options to explore and to remove the stone: Via face-lift approach and by direct incision. The author prefers the first option due to the better esthetic results. The second option can be used in older patients when there are prominent skin creases.

8.3.4 Endoscopic Sialolithotomy Face-Lift Approach

Endoscopic sialolithotomy face-lift approach is as follows (Fig. 8.18). After identification of the stone with the endoscope and marking the exact location of the stone on the skin, an incision along the preauricular line is performed. The dissection is directed towards the location of the transillumination from the light source of the endoscope. It is essential to dissect and to identify the parotid capsule and the Stensen's duct layer for the closure stage. When the surgeon reaches the area of the stone, a careful dissection is performed and an #11 blade is used to incise the duct. The stone is removed with the aid of dental excavators. The sialoendoscope is inserted via the duct incision to explore the gland for additional stones strictures dilatation and for secondary ducts irrigation.

The next step is to insert a stent via the ductal incision towards the duct oral orifice. We use parotid sialostent especially designed for this method. The duct and the parotid capsule closure is performed with 5/0 nylon suture. The stent fixation in the oral orifice is done with 5/0 silk suture. An irrigation of the duct via the oral orifice with saline after the final duct and capsule closure for leakage will prevent possible future sialocele and/or salivary fistule. Subcutaneous layer is closed with 4/0 vicryl suture, skin with 6/0 nylon suture.

After the subcutaneous and skin closure, it is essential to apply pressure for 48 h on the duct closure. This is done with external pressure by an elastic bandage. This is an essential step to prevent salivary fistule and sialocele formation. The stent should be removed after 2 weeks.

8.3.5 The Skin Incision Technique

The only difference of this technique from the face-lift approach is the location of the incision dictated by the stone location. The endoscopic transillumination directs the surgeon towards the exact location of the stone. The limitation of this technique is the location around the anterior part of the masseter (the curvature of the duct) where the damage of the buccal nerve is possible.

When the ultrasound technique is used, the biopsy marker is inserted touching the stone after the skin preparation. The same procedure (described for the endoscopic technique) is performed for the dissection. The identification of the stone with the aid of the biopsy marker is presented in Fig. 8.19. After the removal of the stone, the only change is to create a new salivary duct and oral orifice. The author prefers the technique with a small pediatric feeding tube (3 mm diameter) to be inserted towards the stone location in the duct. From this area, it can be directed towards the cheek near the correct anatomical area. All the other steps of the surgery are the same. Following the procedure, we irrigate the dissection area with tranexamic acid 1 g irrigation of the duct via the stent with hydrocortisone 100 mg and injection of dexamethasone 12 mg in the surgical field.

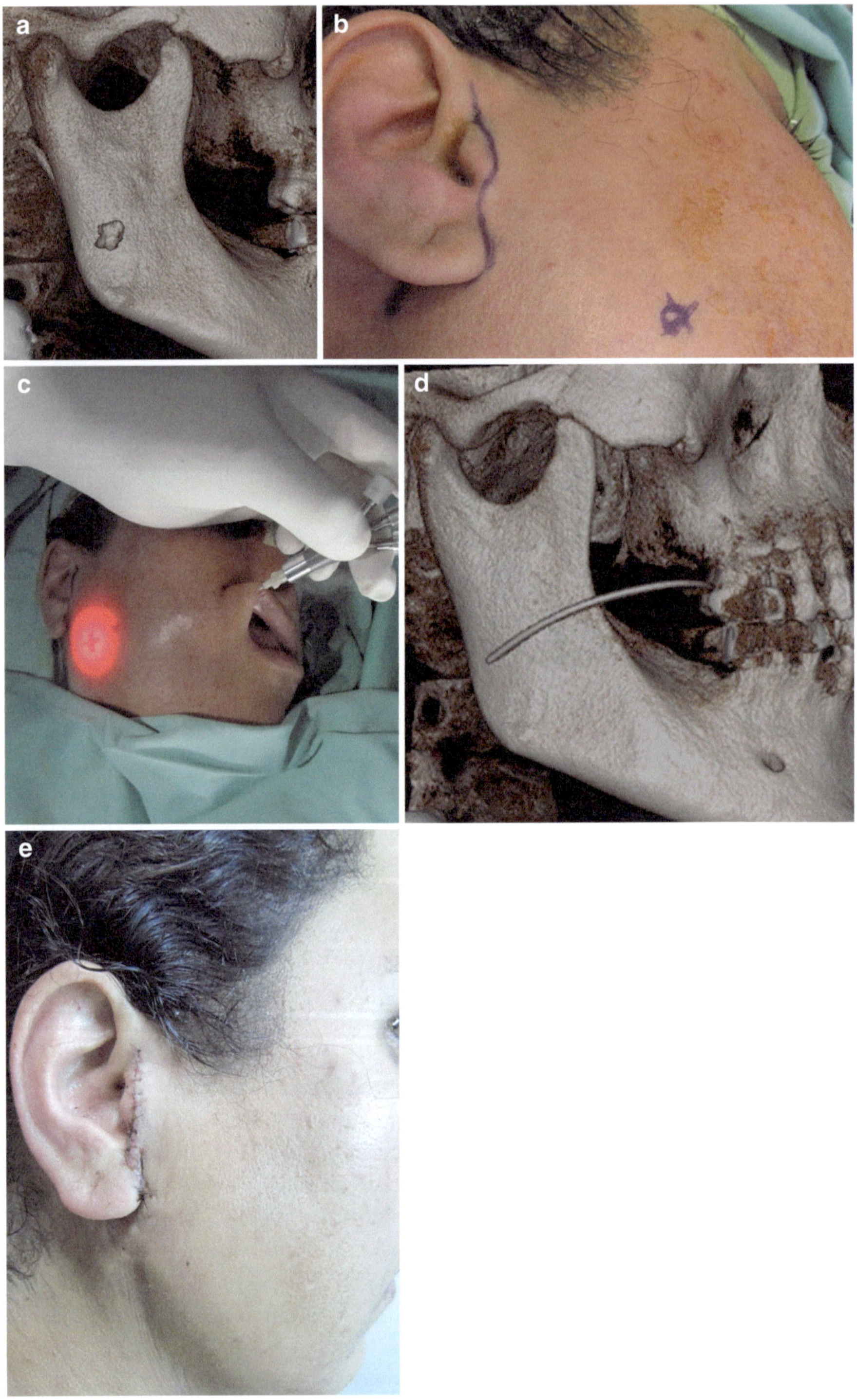

Fig. 8.17 (**a**) An external approach via face-lift technique for the 7 mm irregular stone (3D CBCT) in the hilum of the parotid gland; (**b**) the *blue mark* on the skin represents the location of the stone according to manual palpation; (**c**) an intraoperative view during the sialoendoscopy stage, note the actual location of the stone (X) and the location according to the manual palpation; (**d**) the CBCT demonstrates the stent location; (**e**) facial view one day after surgery

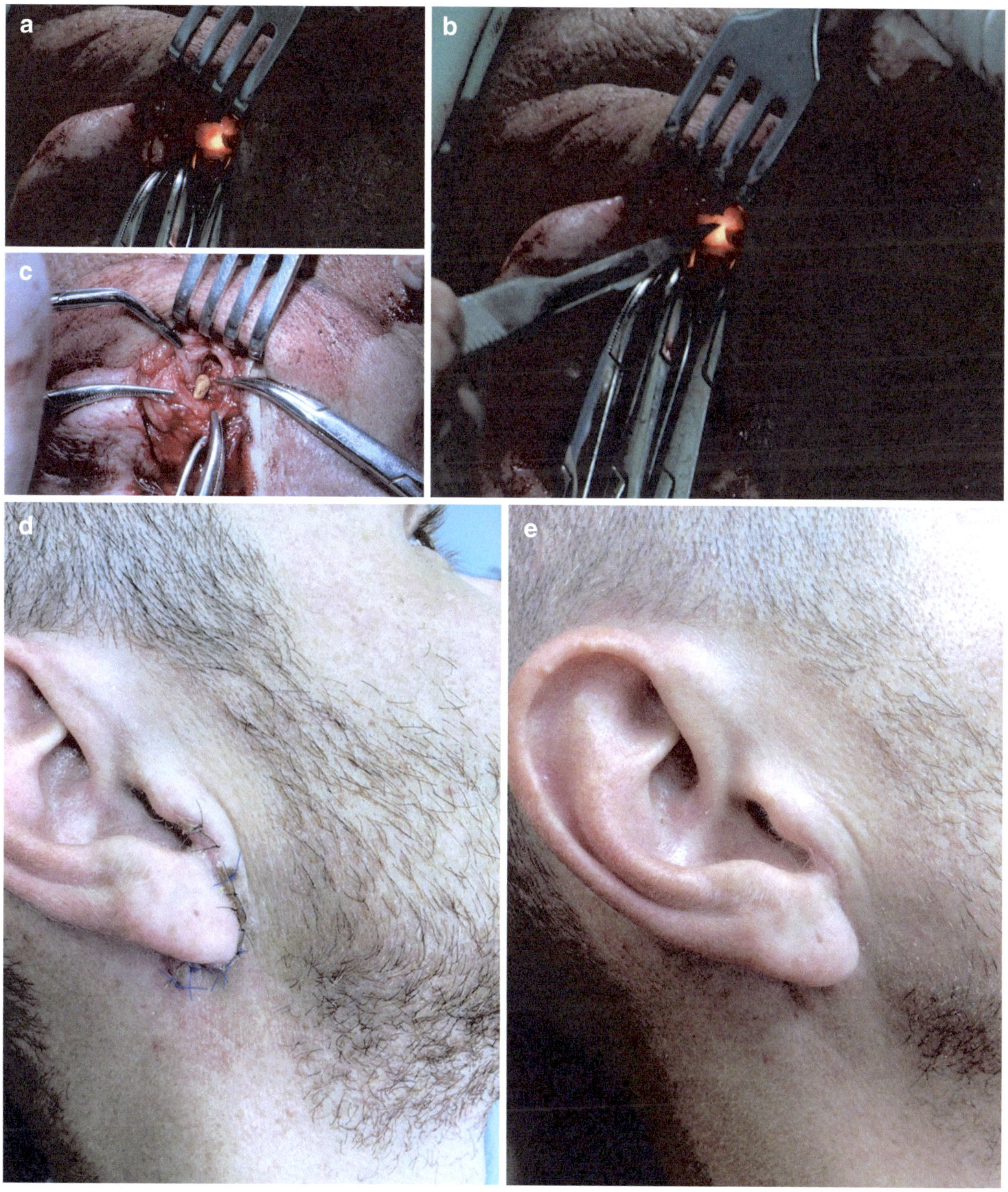

Fig. 8.18 An intraoperative view of the transillumination technique with face-lift approach. (**a**) Identification of the exact location of the stone according to the endoscopic transillumination effect; (**b**) an incision with #11 blade; (**c**) the stone removal from the parotid hilum; (**d**) the operated area 1 week after surgery; (**e**) the operated area 1 year after surgery

Antibiotic coverage for 7 days includes Augmentin 875 mg BID and dexamethasone 16 mg for the first day, 12 mg for the second day, 8 mg for the third day, 4 mg for the fourth day, and 2 mg for the fifth day after surgery. External bandage is essential for 48 h after surgery (Fig. 8.20).

Attention surgeons: this technique requires precise knowledge of the parotid anatomy, the facial nerve anatomy, and the Stensen's duct rout.

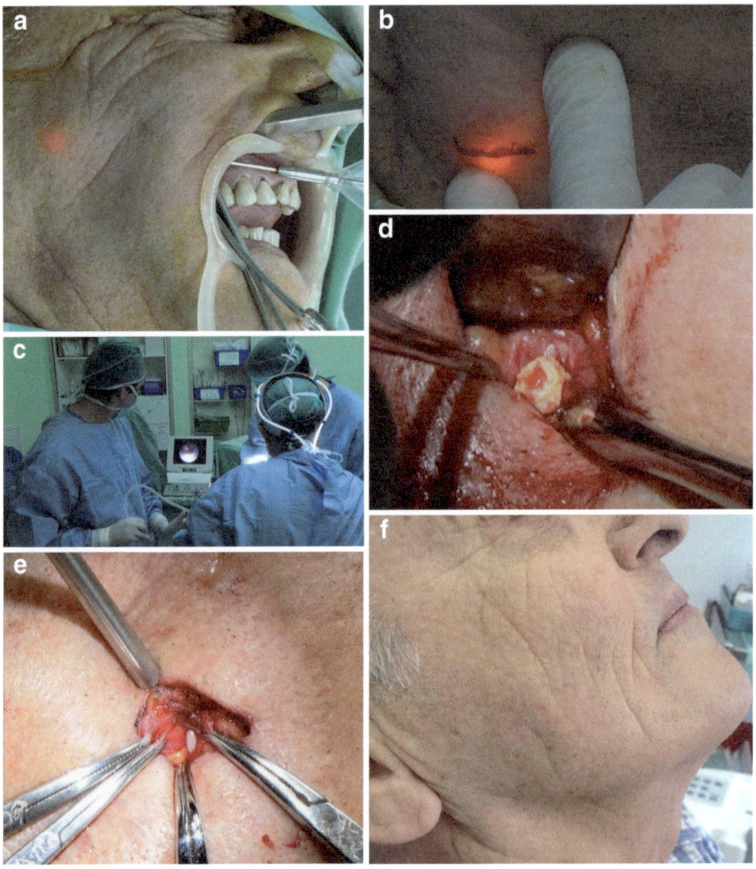

Fig. 8.19 An external approach for a parotid stone—the cheek approach. (**a**, **b**) The transillumination effect dictates the location of an incision; (**c**) ultrasound guided external approach with biopsy marker leading to the exact location of the stone; (**d**) intraoperative view—removal of the stone; (**e**) the stent is inside the duct after the removal of the stone; (**f**) final result 1 year after the stone removal via cheek approach

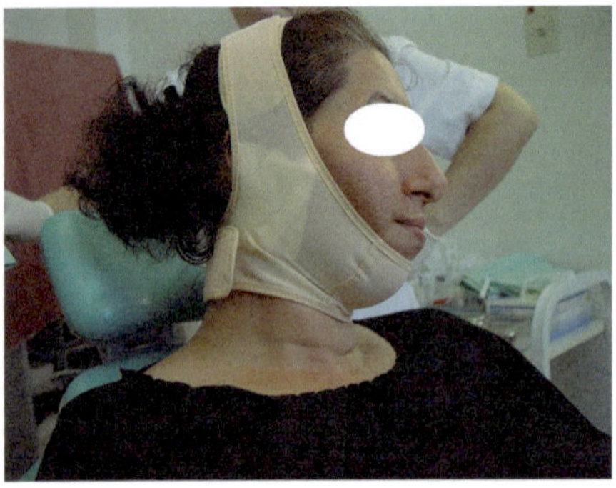

Fig. 8.20 Compression elastic bandage applied to the patient following external approach for removal of parotid stone

8.3.5.1 Extracorporeal Shock-Wave Lithotripsy

In general, the ESWL is a reliable, effective, and safe technique [25, 26]. An ultrasound assists in location of the stone. Three sessions of extracorporeal shock wave treatment per patient were administered with 1-month interval between each session. No sedation is needed. No specific ESWL-related side effects were detected [15, 25–30]. Disconnecting the outer cortex of the stone during/after lithotripsy and the positive effect on scar tissue provides a possibility for

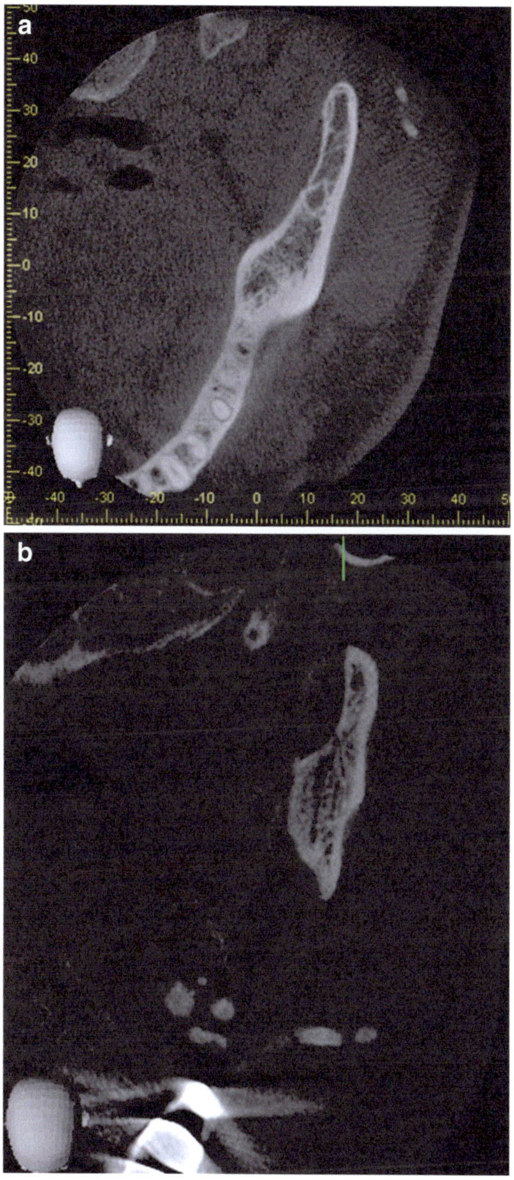

Fig. 8.21 (**a**) The Cone Beam CT image before treatment demonstrates two stones deep in the left parotid gland; (**b**) the Cone Beam CT image following three sessions of extracorporeal lithotripsy with Sialowave Lithotripter. Due to the treatment, the two stones moved to the anterior part of the duct

saliva leakage to the oral cavity bypassing the affected stone (Fig. 8.21).

ESWL however should be distinguished from laser lithotripsy of sialoliths. Subsequent fragmentation of salivary stones can be performed with a Ho:YAG laser or Er:YAG laser in a near-contact manner, but for this technique damage of salivary duct mucosa, ductal stenosis, and salivary fistula were reported as rare complications (less than 2%) [31–33]. A newly approved pneumatic lithotripter is still under investigation. An intraparenchymal repulsion of a residual fragment of a stone was reported as a complication so far [34].

The main problem with the ESWL is not the rate of specific complications but inability to fragment all the stones and to remove all the fragments from the ducts. Total elimination of the stone by lithotripsy alone can be achieved in 30–50% [19, 25–30]. The success of the technique is more impressive when the ESWL is combined with sialoendoscopic intervention [19].

8.3.6 Combination of ESWL and Sialoendoscopic Approach

The ESWL + the intraductal or extraductal endoscopic treatment of sialolithiasis is a highly effective surgical method of eliminating/removal of salivary stones, especially of deeply located stones and in advanced sialolithiasis cases. It has broader applications in comparison with pure ESWL but careful selection of patients is important for this technique to achieve sound results.

The selection of patients with the submandibular gland calculi is as follows:

1. A small (<5 mm) stone in secondary ducts or intraparenchymal stone
2. A small (<5 mm) fixed stone in the main duct or in the hilar region
3. A medium to large (>5 mm) hilar or intraglandular stone attached to the surrounding tissue—immobile or difficult to palpate

For the parotid duct and gland calculi, every stone located in the middle third part of the duct and posteriorly is considered as an advanced and complicated case. The combination of ESWL and sialoendoscopic approach is specifically indicated for such cases.

The treatment starts with an application of the ESWL (see above). Following the results of

ESWL being assessed by Cone Beam CT, CT, and ultrasonography variations for further management of a patient are possible.

Thus, three types of treatment can be performed following the ESWL:

- The ESWL as a solo treatment
- The ESWL + intraductal endoscopic approach (the pure endoscopy)
- The ESWL + endoscopic assisted extraductal approach

The third method is a stretching procedure for the submandibular stones or extraoral approach for the parotid stones [21, 35]. The second and the third methods can be used in cases when a salivary stone was not eliminated by the lithotripsy alone.

The endoscopic removal of the stones after the ESWL procedures is easier and less complicated due to disconnection of the stone from the surrounding ductal tissue that seems to be the major positive effect of the ESWL. We believe that this combined lithotripsy-endoscopy approach might help to overcome the various sizes and locations of the stones and most of the obstruction pathologies as it involves multiple techniques and technologies: the pure endoscopy, the endoscopic assistance technique, and the ESWL, which could be combined in a treatment of the same patient. The implementations of these three methods mainly rely not on the advantages of each method but rather on careful diagnostic evaluation of the size, location, and number of sialoliths. The ESWL + the intraductal or extraductal endoscopic treatment might lead to effective management of most of the obstruction and inflammatory conditions of the salivary glands.

8.4 The Author's Approaches to Various Cases

In this section, I will describe my way to treat sialolithiasis of the major salivary glands.

Approach #1. If the stones are located in the anterior third part of the Wharton's or Stensen's duct, the surgery includes

- Incision
- Extraction of a calculus
- Endoscopic exploration
- Sialostent insertion

Approach #2. If the stones are located in the middle third of the Wharton's duct, the surgery includes

- Ductal dissection and exploration
- Stone removal
- Endoscopic exploration
- Sialostent insertion

Approach #3. If mobile stone/stones are found in the hilum of the Wharton's duct, the approach depends of the stone diameter. The surgical procedure includes

- Endoscopic removal of the calculus

or

- Extraductal removal of the calculus via stretching procedure
- Endoscopic exploration
- Sialostent insertion

All advanced sialolithiasis cases should be treated according to the protocol of combined extracorporeal shock-wave lithotripsy with sialoendoscopic approach.

8.5 Non-calculus-Related Obstruction Pathology

There are three pathologies which can cause obstruction of the salivary ductal system without any stone involvement:

- Strictures
- Adhesions
- Changes in saliva viscosity

Most of such obstructions cases occur in the parotid glands. The diagnosis of a stricture is usually performed when swelling of the affected gland occurred without the presence of a stone being detected by imaging methods. Only the sialogram and MRI can demonstrate strictures. Ultrasonography can demonstrate the dilatation of the duct posteriorly to the stricture. The best way to diagnose the stricture is sialoendoscopy.

The *treatment* options are somewhat different for the submandibular and the parotid cases. Strictures of the submandibular glands are well treated with dilatation of the stricture with hydrostatic pressure, the high pressure balloon, or the mechanical dilatation. The selection of the approach depends from the diameter of a stricture. Following the dilatation, an irrigation with steroids is applied and we recommend stent insertion for 2–4 weeks.

The problem with parotid ductal strictures is the extreme sensitivity of the Stensen's duct. Any trauma to the ductal layer can cause total obstruction of the ductal lumen especially in the orifice leading to severe swellings and infections.

Due to these reasons, my philosophy of treatment is to treat strictures according to the initial results of the treatment and not according to the severance of the pathology. Sometimes, a single non-hazardously looking stricture can cause more problems that number of strictures accompanied by dilatations, a giant duct, and sialocele combined. In general, the approach is as follows.

Option #1. The first option is to overcome the strictures with an insertion of the sialoendoscope, thorough irrigation with pressure dilatation, and balloon dilatation if it is possible. Following this procedure, we recommend an irrigation with hydrocortisone 100 mg intraductally.

Option #2. If the Option #1 did not improve the situation, the injection of Botox can be performed under ultrasonographic control of the parenchyma of the affected gland.

Option #3. A stent insertion to the anterior part of the duct is possible for 4–6 weeks followed by injections of steroids around the orifice. Usually, hydrocortisone 100 mg can be injected every week for 4–6 weeks.

Option #4. The vein graft can be used to replace the problematic Stensen's duct.

Adhesions are easy treated with an endoscopic lavage. The same treatment is indicated for thick saliva viscosity like in cases of the Sjögren's syndrome.

8.6 Complications of Sialoendoscopy and How to Avoid Them

While endoscopic and endoscopy-assisted surgeries can have general postsurgical complications such as infection or hematoma [36], endoscopic interventions may produce several specific complications [37]. The emerging literature presents a general agreement that sialoendoscopy complications are minor [19, 38]. The endoscopy-related complications are of different origin in comparison with the traditional surgery complications. While most complications of the radical surgery are of neurological matter, these types of complications are minimal when sialoendoscopy is involved. The facial palsy/paralysis or the Frey's syndrome never occur [19, 23]. The lingual nerve paresthesia might occur if the submandibular gland is involved but the risk of complication is minimal (˂0.5%) [22, 39].

The major endoscopy-related complications are iatrogenic insults directly responsible for additional procedures [40, 41]. The minor complications are events leading to either failure of the procedure, a second surgical procedure, a change in the surgical plan, or deviation from the planned course of events as a result of the procedure itself. The major complications occur in only 2–3% of cases, and the minor complications occur in 19–23% [22–24, 36, 37, 39–43]. The avulsion of the salivary duct, postoperative strictures, the gland swelling, salivary fistulas and perforations (false rout), traumatic ranulas, and the lingual nerve paresthesia are the main endoscopy-related complications.

Avulsion of the duct occurs when an operating surgeon fixes a calculus in the wire basket and then tries to remove it out from the duct. If the traction is excessive, the avulsion can occur. This complication is rare, but it is possible if an operation is performed by inexperienced surgeon. *Postoperative strictures* of the salivary duct is the main complication following sialoendoscopic procedures [19, 22, 23, 44] (Fig. 8.22). The risk for such a complication remains after each operative endoscopic surgery at about 2–2.45% [19, 44, 45]. The strictures can be iden-

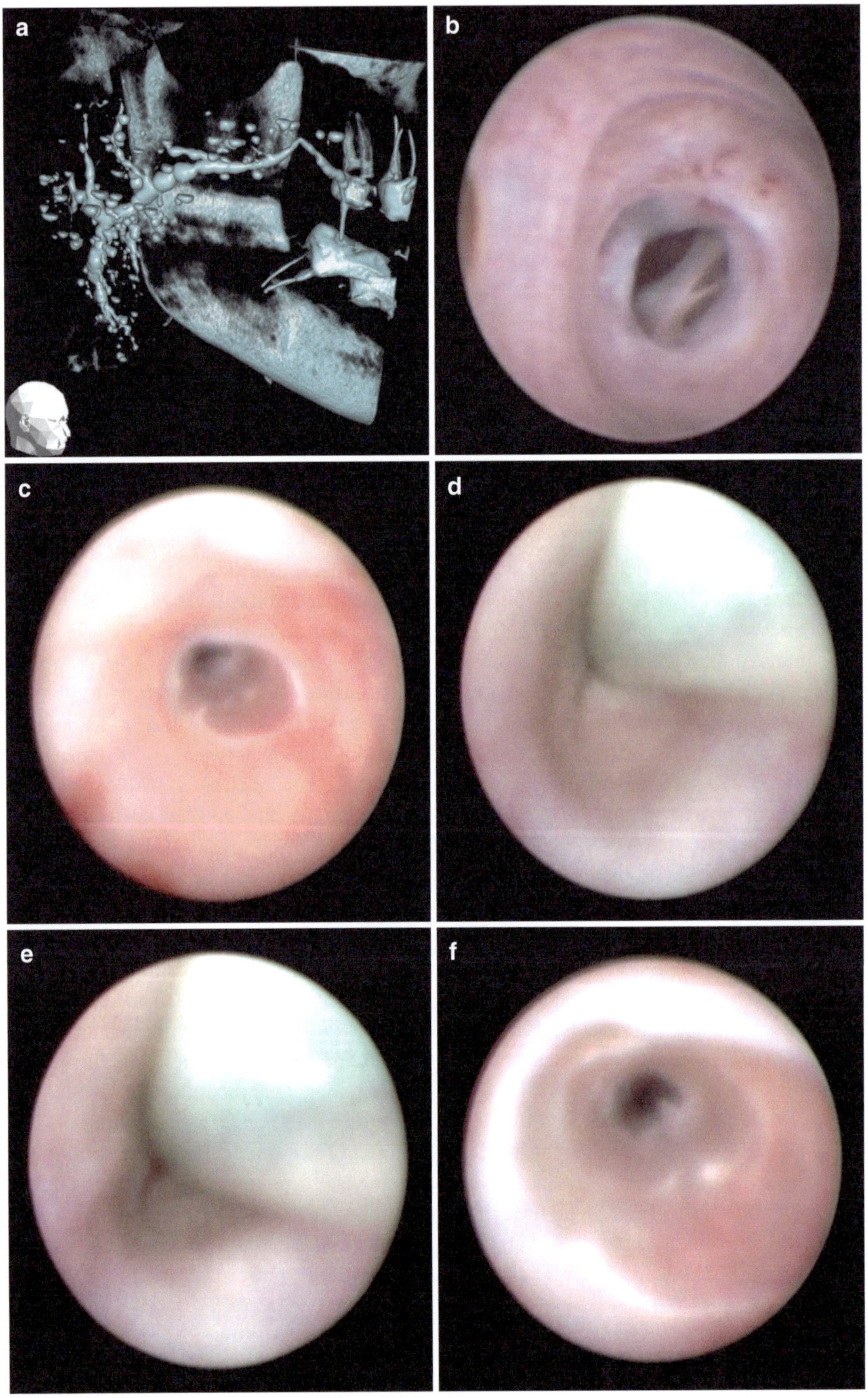

Fig. 8.22 (**a**) The Cone Beam CT image of multiple strictures in the parotid duct; (**b**) the endoscopic view of the same strictures; (**c**–**f**) the intraoperative endoscopic view of the steps for the stricture dilatation with high pressure balloon

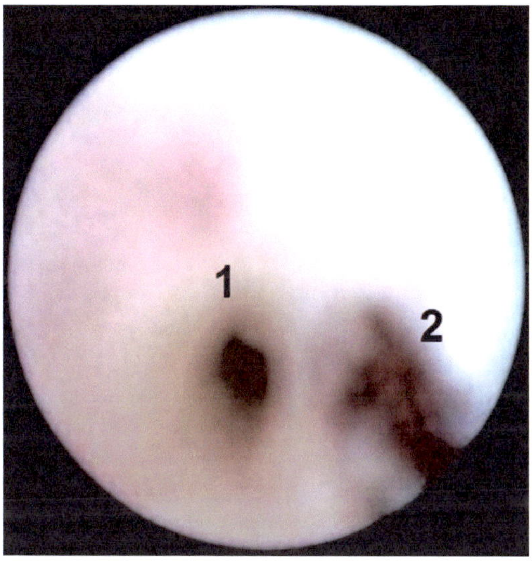

Fig. 8.23 The intraoperative view demonstrates perforation during sialoendoscopy of the parotid duct. *1*—the duct, *2*—the perforation

tified both in the parotid and the submandibular cases by continuous swelling of the gland following stone extraction without any evidence of remaining of additional stone or a stone particle in the duct, and the absence of saliva or reduced saliva secretion from the orifice of the affected gland. Most of the postoperative strictures are located near the orifice region and successful dilation is possible in the majority of cases [19, 36, 37, 39, 45].

The perforation (false rout) of the salivary duct occurs near the orifice of the duct because of separation of the ductal wall from the oral mucosa (Fig. 8.23). It can happen during sialoendoscopic mechanical intraductal procedures such as stone removal and stricture dilation [20, 22, 23]. The endoscopic identification of this pathology is possible, but the ductal structures of the lumen may be overlooked. Another sign is the excessive swelling in the region of the perforation due to the leakage of the irrigation solution to the surrounding tissue.

Postoperative *gland swelling* occurs when the main goal of the minimally invasive surgery was achieved, i.e., the gland was preserved. Excessive swelling following sialoendosopy usually occurs because of the obstruction of the main salivary duct, peroration of the duct, or excessive irrigation [19, 22, 45]. Such gland swelling usually resolves in approximately 24–48 h [20, 44, 46]. This usually minor complication may sometimes cause airway compromise after submandibular surgery [47]. To avoid such problem, in cases of bilateral submandibular interventions a surgeon should examine the gland and oral cavity after operating the first gland and assess whether it is safe for the patient to proceed with the second gland.

Ranula is a well-documented outcome of surgical procedures in the floor of the mouth (Fig. 8.24). Formation of such mucocele on the floor of the mouth can occur in patients following submandibular sialoendoscopy [39, 45, 48, 49]. In submandibular or sublingual endoscopic surgery, the risk is 1–2.45% [48–50]. The formation of ranula is proportional to the extensivity of the procedure and patients that underwent endoscopic assisted intervention like stretching procedure, have reasonable risk for this complication. Ranula is easily identified by swelling, mostly blue, in the floor of the oral cavity. Successful marsupialization occurs in majority of cases.

Lingual nerve paresthesia is a rare complication of sialoendoscopy of the submandibular gland (0.7–0.4%) [22, 24]. It can happen mainly in endoscopic assisted procedure—the stretching technique. During pure intraductal endoscopic procedure, it can happen only due to perforation of the salivary duct. Usually, the lesion is identified by the nerve assessment. Changing paresthesia into anesthesia is even rarer. If the nerve is damaged, steroid treatment should be administered immediately after the correct diagnosis. The currently analyzed cases show that the risk of this complication exists when the stones are located in the posterior third of the main duct [22, 36, 47].

The salivary fistulas, sialoceles, minor ductal tears, minor hemorrhage, and acute masseteric bend while having been reported should be considered as extremely rare complications [3, 36, 45, 47]. The large or recalcitrant parotid stones can leave a persistent stone fragment or produce obstructive symptoms due to a fibrous stricture that is also very rare.

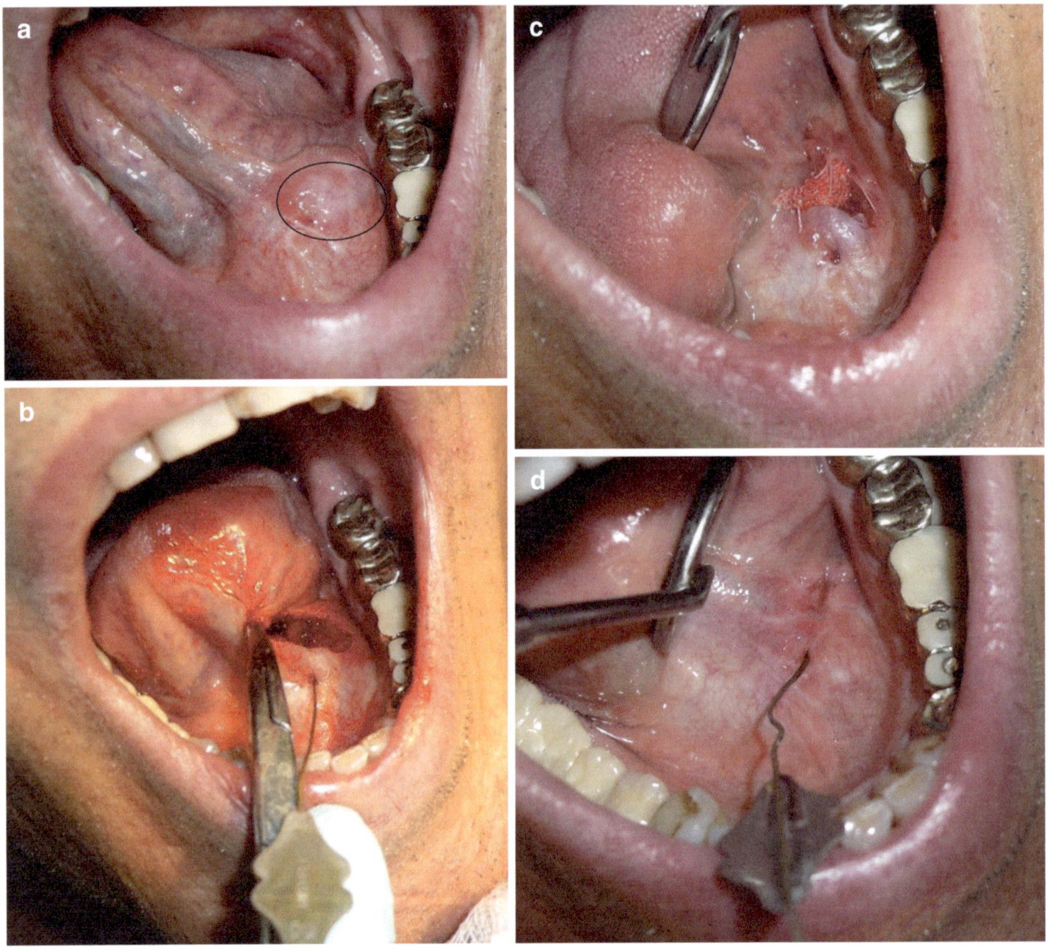

Fig. 8.24 (**a**) Ranula following sialoendoscopy of the left submandibular gland (in the oval); (**b**) the unroofing (marsupialization) procedure; a lachrymal probe is inserted into the Wharton's duct. (**c**) Iodoform gauze is packed into the cavity; (**d**) the postoperative view 2 weeks following the procedure

References

1. Buckenham T. Salivary duct intervention. Semin Intervent Radiol. 2004;21(3):143–8. https://doi.org/10.1055/s-2004-860872.
2. Zenk J, Zikarsky B, Hosemann WG, Iro H. The diameter of the Stenon and Wharton ducts. Significance for diagnosis and therapy. HNO. 1998;46(12):980–5.
3. Marchal F. Sialendoscopy. In: Myers E, editor. Salivary gland disorders. Berlin: Springer; 2007. p. 127–48.
4. Nahlieli O, Iro H, McGurk M, Caldart M. Minimally invasive methods and procedures for the treatment of salivary gland sialolithiasis. In: Nahlieli, et al., editors. Modern management preserving the salivary glands. Herzeliya: Isradon; 2006. p. 143–60.
5. Catalogue PolyDiagnost, version 2.6. Hallbergmoos: PolyDiagnost; 2015.
6. Drage NA, Brown JE, Escudier MP, Wilson RF, McGurk M. Balloon dilatation of salivary duct strictures: report on 36 treated glands. Cardiovasc Intervent Radiol. 2002;25:356–9.
7. Mandel L, Witek EL. Chronic parotitis diagnosis and treatment. J Am Dent Assoc. 2001;132:1707–11.
8. Rauch S, Gorlin RJ. Diseases of the salivary glands. In: Gorlin RJ, Goldman HM, editors. Oral pathology. St. Louis: Mosby; 1970. p. 962–1070.
9. Vitali C, Bombardieri S, Jonsson R, et al. Classification criteria for Sjögren's syndrome a revised version of the European criteria proposed by the American-European Consensus Group. Ann Rheum Dis. 2002;61:554–8.
10. Mok CC, Lau CS. Pathogenesis of systemic lupus erythematosus. J Clin Pathol. 2003;56:481–90.

11. Albilia JB, Lam DK, Clokie CM, Sándor GK. Systemic lupus erythematosus: a review for dentists. J Can Dent Assoc. 2007;73(9):823–8.
12. Karl Storz – Endoskope. Oral and Maxillofacial Surgery. Highlights 2016. Karl Storz; 2016.
13. PolyDiagnost. Operation manual: semi-rigid optics. PolyDiagnost; 2015.
14. Sialowave operating manual. Medispec, Germantown, MD, USA; 2014.
15. Kopeć T, Szyfter W, Wierzbicka M. Sialoendoscopy and combined approach for the management of salivary gland stones. Eur Arch Otorhinolaryngol. 2013;270(1):219–23. https://doi.org/10.1007/s00405-012-2145-x.
16. Boffano P, Gallesio C. Surgical treatment of a giant sialolith of the Wharton duct. J Craniofac Surg. 2010;21(1):134–5. https://doi.org/10.1097/SCS.0b013e3181c46bc4.
17. Capaccio P, Clemente IA, McGurk M, et al. Transoral removal of hiloparenchymal submandibular calculi: a long-term clinical experience. Eur Arch Otorhinolaryngol. 2011;268(7):1081–6. https://doi.org/10.1007/s00405-011-1508-z.
18. Zenk J, Gottwald F, Bozzato A, Iro H. Submandibular sialoliths. Stone removal with organ preservation. HNO. 2005;53(3):243–9.
19. Nahlieli O, Shacham R, Zagury A, Bar T, Yoffe B. The ductal stretching technique–endoscopic assisted technique for submandibular stones. Laryngoscope. 2007;117(6):1031–5.
20. Escudier MP. The development of salivary lithotripsy: it's role in the management of salivary calculi department of oral medicine. London: University of London; 2008.
21. Strychowsky JE, Sommer DD, Gupta MK, Cohen N, Nahlieli O. Sialendoscopy for the management of obstructive salivary gland disease: a systematic review and meta-analysis. Arch Otolaryngol Head Neck Surg. 2012;138(6):541–7. https://doi.org/10.1001/archoto.2012.856.
22. Witt RL, Iro H, Koch M, McGurk M, Nahlieli O, Zenk J. Minimally invasive options for salivary calculi. Laryngoscope. 2012;122(6):1306–11. https://doi.org/10.1002/lary.23272.
23. Parente Arias PL, Fernández Fernández MM, Varela Vázquez P, et al. Minimally invasive video-assisted submandibular sialadenectomy: surgical technique and results from two institutions. Surg Endosc. 2016;30(8):3314–20. https://doi.org/10.1007/s00464-015-4604-0.
24. Pitak-Arnnop P, Pausch NC, Dhanuthai K, Sappayatosok K, Ngamwannagul P, Bauer U, et al. Endoscope-assisted submandibular sialadenectomy: a review of outcomes, complications, and ethical concerns. Eplasty. 2010;10:e36.
25. Zenk J, Koch M, Iro H. Extracorporeal and intracorporeal lithotripsy of salivary gland stones: basic investigations. Otolaryngol Clin North Am. 2009;42(6):1115–37. https://doi.org/10.1016/j.otc.2009.08.005.
26. Zenk J, Koch M, Mantsopoulos K, Klintworth N, Schapher M, Iro H. The significance of extracorporeal shock wave lithotripsy in sialolithiasis therapy. HNO. 2013;61(4):306–11. https://doi.org/10.1007/s00106-013-2677-4.
27. Abdusalamov MR, Afanas'ev VV, Gamataev II. Shockwave lithotripsy in sialolithiasis patients. Stomatologiia (Mosk). 2014;93(2):31–2.
28. Desmots F, Chossegros C, Salles F, Gallucci A, Moulin G, Varoquaux A. Lithotripsy for salivary stones with prospective US assessment on our first 25 consecutive patients. J Craniomaxillofac Surg. 2014;42(5):577–82. https://doi.org/10.1016/j.jcms.2013.07.029.
29. Raif J, Vardi M, Nahlieli O, Gannot I. An Er:YAG laser endoscopic fiber delivery system for lithotripsy of salivary stones. Lasers Surg Med. 2006;38(6):580–7.
30. Schrötzlmair F, Müller M, Pongratz T, Eder M, Johnson T, Vogeser M, et al. Laser lithotripsy of salivary stones: correlation with physical and radiological parameters. Lasers Surg Med. 2015;47(4):342–9. https://doi.org/10.1002/lsm.22333.
31. Martellucci S, Pagliuca G, de Vincentiis M, Greco A, Fusconi M, De Virgilio A, et al. Ho:Yag laser for sialolithiasis of Wharton's duct. Otolaryngol Head Neck Surg. 2013;148(5):770–4. https://doi.org/10.1177/0194599813479914.
32. Koch M, Mantsopoulos K, Schapher M, von Scotti F, Iro H. Intraductal pneumatic lithotripsy for salivary stones with the StoneBreaker: preliminary experience. Laryngoscope. 2016;126(7):1545–50. https://doi.org/10.1002/lary.25849.
33. Nahlieli O, Shacham R, Zaguri A. Combined external lithotripsy and endoscopic techniques for advanced sialolithiasis cases. J Oral Maxillofac Surg. 2010;68(2):347–53. https://doi.org/10.1016/j.joms.2009.09.041.
34. Nahlieli O, London D, Zagury A, Eliav E. Combined approach to impacted parotid stones. J Oral Maxillofac Surg. 2002;60:1418–23.
35. Nahlieli O. Advanced sialoendoscopy techniques, rare findings, and complications. Otolaryngol Clin North Am. 2009;42(6):1053–72. https://doi.org/10.1016/j.otc.2009.08.007.
36. Iro H, Zenk J, Escudier MP, Nahlieli O, et al. Outcome of minimally invasive management of salivary calculi in 4,691 patients. Laryngoscope. 2009;119(2):263–8.
37. Bowen MA, Tauzin M, Kluka EA, Nuss DW, DiLeo M, McWhorter AJ, et al. Diagnostic and interventional sialendoscopy: a preliminary experience. Laryngoscope. 2010;121(2):299–303.
38. Lari N, Chossegros C, Thiery G, Guyot L, Blanc JL, Marchal F. Sialendoscopy of the salivary glands. Rev Stomatol Chir Maxillofac. 2008;109(3):167–71.
39. Walvekar RR, Razfar A, Carrau RL, Schaitkin B. Sialendosocopy and associated complications: a preliminary experience. Laryngoscope. 2008;118:776–9.
40. Marchal F, Chossegros C, Faure F, Delas B, Bizeau A, Mortensen B, et al. Salivary stones and stenosis. A comprehensive classification. Rev Stomatol Chir Maxillofac. 2008;109(4):233–6.

41. Nahlieli O, Bar T, Shacham R, Eliav E, Hecht-Nakar L. Management of chronic recurrent parotitis: current therapy. J Oral Maxillofac Surg. 2004;62(9):1150–5.
42. Nahlieli O, Nakar LH, Nazarian Y, Turner MD. Sialoendoscopy: a new approach to salivary gland obstructive pathology. J Am Dent Assoc. 2006;137(10):1394–400.
43. Atienza G, López-Cedrún JL. Management of obstructive salivary disorders by sialendoscopy: a systematic review. Br J Oral Maxillofac Surg. 2015;53(6):507–19. https://doi.org/10.1016/j.bjoms.2015.02.024.
44. Kroll T, Finkensieper M, Sharma SJ, Guntinas-Lichius O, Wittekindt C. Short-term outcome and patient satisfaction after sialendoscopy. Eur Arch Otorhinolaryngol. 2013;270(11):2939–45. https://doi.org/10.1007/s00405-013-2418-z.
45. Iwai T, Matsui Y, Yamagishi M, Hirota M, Mitsudo K, Maegawa J, et al. Simple technique for dilatation of the papilla in sialoendoscopy. J Oral Maxillofac Surg. 2009;67(3):681–2.
46. Nahlieli O, Droma EB, Eliav E, Zaguri A, Shacham R, Bar T. Salivary gland injury subsequent to implant surgery. Int J Oral Maxillofac Implants. 2008;23(3):556–60.
47. Mandel L. Plunging ranula following placement of mandibular implants: case report. J Oral Maxillofac Surg. 2008;66(8):1743–7.
48. Harrison JD, Kim A, Al-Ali S, Morton RP. Postmortem investigation of mylohyoid hiatus and hernia: aetiological factors of plunging ranula. Clin Anat. 2013;26(6):693–9. https://doi.org/10.1002/ca.22212.
49. Gary C, Kluka EA, Schaitkin B, Walvekar RR. Interventional sialendoscopy for treatment of juvenile recurrent parotitis. J Indian Assoc Pediatr Surg. 2011;16(4):132–6.
50. Al-Abri R, Marchal F. New era of endoscopic approach for sialolithiasis: sialendoscopy. Sultan Qaboos Univ Med J. 2010;10(3):382–7.

Extracapsular Dissection for Benign Parotid Tumours

9

Mark McGurk and Leandros-Vassilios Vassiliou

Abstract

Parotid tumours usually present in their majority as discrete lumps arising within the superficial portion of the gland. Histologically, the commonest type is the pleomorphic adenoma. Conventional teaching prescribes removal of these tumours by superficial parotidectomy (SP), which essentially requires facial nerve identification and excision of the superficial portion of the gland. Extracapsular dissection (ECD) comprises an alternative approach which is indicated for benign tumours. This chapter describes the origins of parotid surgery and its evolution to date. A step-by-step explanation of extracapsular dissection is illustrated. The outcomes of extracapsular dissection as demonstrated in all relevant studies and meta-analyses to date are presented. The tendency of pleomorphic adenomas to recur, as well as the possible underlying aetiology are discussed. Evidence support that extracapsular dissection comprises an oncologically valid procedure, with minimal complication rates.

9.1 History of Parotid Surgery

The standards of practice that prevailed 200 years ago have all but been forgotten. Surgery was not a dominant part of medicine for without anaesthesia, antibiotics, and blood transfusion the results were dire and only few patients submitted to surgery except in desperation.

M. McGurk, MD, BDS, FRCS, FDSRCS, DLO
L.-V. Vassiliou, DDS, MD, MSc, FRCS (✉)
Department of Oral and Maxillofacial Surgery, Guy's Hospital, London, UK
e-mail: leandros.vassiliou@nhs.net

The first reports of primitive parotidectomies appear in the eighteenth century [1, 2]. At that time, surgeons feared parotid surgery. This was because patients seldom presented with early disease but rather waited until the disease was advanced. Thus, tackling a large matted mass in the parotid inevitably meant having to secure the external carotid artery with the inevitable frightening bleeds. The facial nerve was not the worry but rather the uncontrollable bleeding.

In the nineteenth century, various surgeons attempted parotid surgery [3–5]. At the beginning of 1900s, the crude surgery of the pre-anaesthetic era gave way to more measured and refined

O. Nahlieli (ed.), *Minimally Invasive Oral and Maxillofacial Surgery*,
http://doi.org/10.1007/978-3-662-54592-8_9

procedures. Subsequently, consideration for the facial nerve started developing [5–8]. Parotidectomy improved along with the development of techniques to identify and preserve the facial nerve [9–13]. Even when the major problems such as control of haemorrhage and preservation of facial nerve were being overcome, a persistent issue arose—the high incidence of tumour recurrence.

Another factor complicating management was that the pathological nature of the salivary lesions was not understood. Confusion arose because approximately 40% of parotid cancers are indolent in nature and are easily mistaken for a benign lesion. Also the commonest lump displayed variable appearance and consistency, with cystic and cartilaginous components and consequently gained the name of pleomorphic adenoma. Initially, it was thought that these tumours represented hamartomas rather than neoplasms. It was not until 1953 that the first histological classification of parotid tumours was produced [14, 15].

The high rate of recurrence was masked by the time taken for a lump to reappear. Salivary tumours grow slowly and it took years for a recurrence to appear by which time the patient or the surgeon may have moved on. The association between parotid lumps and recurrence was first noticed by McFarland [16]. It was his practice to travel on horseback from hospital to hospital providing pathology reports. He compiled a register and noticed that the recurrence rates for parotid lumps were as high as 23%. In a different case series of the same time, the recurrence rate was reported to reach 43% [17]. Over time, this evidence made a profound impact on the surgical community and so the reputation of pleomorphic adenoma for recurrence was born.

At the turn of the 1900 until 1950, the approach to the parotid lump was by an incision directly over its surface. One approach was to enter the tumour and scoop its material out, leaving the capsule in situ—in essence an 'intracapsular enucleation'. Even if the surgeon's intention was to remove the tumour intact, the access provided by the incision was limited and rupture was common. Between the 1920s and 1950s salivary gland surgery became more topical and with it a drive for more careful surgery with preservation of the facial nerve developed.

Three surgeons started at this time—Janes [18] in Toronto, Bailey [9] in London, and Redon in Paris [19]. They wrote and lectured extensively on the topic of parotid surgery and between them advocated a new surgical approach which involved identifying the facial nerve as it entered the parotid gland and then tracing it through the parotid gland. As two-thirds of the parotid gland lies above the nerve, the majority of parotid tumours would lie in the superior lobe. Once the nerve was exposed and the dissection advanced in front of the lump, the gland bearing the lump could then be safely removed—so was born the superficial parotidectomy (which in reality is a nerve dissection). If the patient was unfortunate enough for the tumour to lie in the parotid tissue below the nerve (deep lobe), then the nerve had to be lifted off the underlying tissue and the remaining parotid gland bearing the lump was removed, hence the total parotidectomy. The nerve dissection technique was not accepted initially but stuttered through the 1940s and 1950s. A seminal piece of work undertaken by Professor Patey changed everything [20]. Patey and Thackray investigated the parotid specimens after superficial parotidectomy and demonstrated that the pleomorphic adenoma was surrounded by an incomplete connective tissue capsule [21, 22]. Little nodules of pleomorphic adenoma seemed to protrude outside the capsule. This seemed an obvious explanation for the high incidence of recurrence. Thackray gave the surgeons a biological explanation for tumour recurrence and this was grasped by the surgical community, and the superficial parotidectomy procedure was adopted universally. It now transpires that the real reason for the high recurrence rate was poor understanding of salivary tumour biology and poor surgical technique.

Paradoxically, the adoption of superficial parotidectomy inadvertently solved the issue of poor technique due to limited exposure as a large preauricular flap had to be raised to expose the gland. The incidence of recurrent disease dropped significantly and so seemed to confirm Patey and Thackray's supposition. The dogma that superficial and total parotidectomy were essential procedures for parotid lumps was now universally accepted.

However, Alan Nicholson, a surgeon practising at the Christie Hospital in Manchester, in the 1940–1960 was of the opinion that the high recurrence rate was due to poor exposure when an incision was made over the surface of the lump. He preferred to lift a preauricular skin flap and widely expose the gland. Rather than proceeding to nerve dissection, he made a cruciate incision over the lump and then proceeded to carefully dissect around the tumour a few millimetres from its surface (extracapsular dissection). By the time the debate was settled in 1957 as a result of Thackray's paper and Patey's authority, he had treated a large number of parotid tumours, quite successfully without recurrence. So rather than switching his practise, he persisted with his technique and taught it to a second surgeon (Neville Gleave) who continued with this approach through to the 1980s. By that time over 600 cases had been treated by extracapsular dissection and the analysis of the data showed that the recurrence rates were no more than those seen after superficial parotidectomy notably 1.5% at 10 years [23–25].

Coincidentally, it was about 1980s that Conley in the USA started to question the logic behind superficial parotidectomy. He noted 60% of parotid tumours lay on the facial nerve and in the process of a parotidectomy, the surgeon had to work directly on the capsule of the tumour [26]. These tumours did not recur and raised the question as to the relevance of the observations made by Thackray 30 years before.

Today, the majority of surgeons continue to use nerve dissection as their primary approach to parotid tumours. This is a very reliable and robust technique which was designed for the general surgeon whose surgical repertoire ranged from orthopaedic procedures, amputations, abdominal surgery, craniotomies, and where parotid gland surgery was relatively infrequently. Since this time, many of the robust and invasive surgical techniques have given away to minimally invasive approaches as surgeons have come to specialise in anatomical areas around the body. The march in surgery to embrace minimally invasive techniques is unfortunately conspicuous by its absence in parotid surgery. Modern extracapsular dissection is slow to be adopted apart from high volume surgical units that have the ability to choose suitable cases regularly and push their experience base forward. This is amply shown by experience in Erlangen (Fig. 9.1) where the number of extracapsular dissections performed rose from 2–3% to approximately 65% over a 10-year period [27]. Unfortunately, most surgeons undertaking parotid surgery only perform 10–15 operations a year which is insufficient for them to gain confidence in a technique that is based on completely different principles. Extracapsular dissection does not involve identifying the facial nerve—it is a non-nerve dissecting approach to parotid surgery.

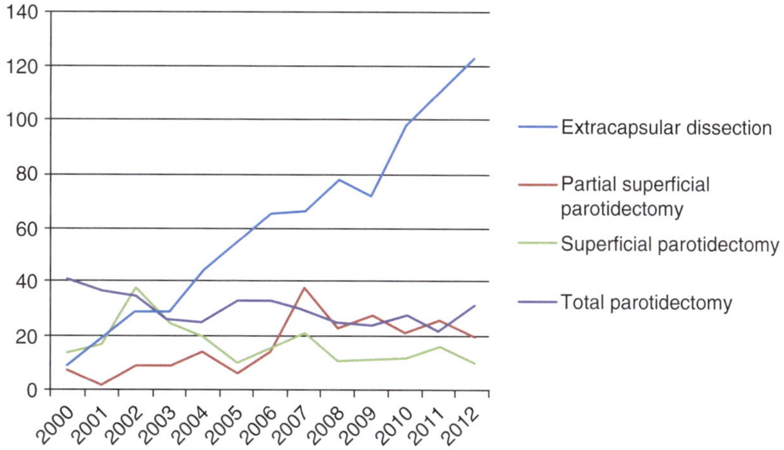

Fig. 9.1 Progression of parotid surgery modalities over the years. Courtesy of Mantsopoulos et al. [27]

9.2 Incidence of Parotid Tumours

Salivary gland neoplasms account for approximately 3–4% of all head and neck tumours [28, 29]. The incidence of all salivary gland tumours annually varies in different studies from 0.4 to 13.5 cases per 100,000 population [30]. It is estimated at 0.4 in Malawi [31], 0.7 in Uganda [32], 3.6 in Malaya [33], 4.2 in Scotland [34], and 13.5 in Canadian Eskimos [35].

The first salivary gland neoplasm classification was produced by Foote and Frazel [14, 15] in 1953 and later improved by Batsakis [36] and Seifert [37]. A World Health Organization (WHO) classification was reported in 1972 [38], revised in 1991 [30], and further updated in 2005 [39].

Traditionally, approximately 25% of parotid tumours were thought to be malignant, 50% in the submandibular, and 70% in the minor salivary glands [40]. A population-based study was undertaken by Professor Bradley of a discrete geographical area in England [41]. This region was served by only two hospitals in a single pathology department. Consequently, it was possible to identify all the salivary pathology specimens that had been processed in the population over a 20-year period. Armed with this information, Professor Bradley was able to work out the incidence of salivary neoplasms in the head and neck. He calculated that the annual incidence of combined benign and malignant salivary tumours ranged from 7.03 to 8.58 per 100,000 of population. The incidence of benign tumours alone ranged from 6.2 to 7.2, whereas for malignant neoplasms it ranged from 0.83 to 1.38 [41]. The risk of a malignant parotid tumour in this population was only 15%, 35% in the submandibular, and approximately 50% in the oral cavity with the risk increasing substantially as one moved from the soft palate through to the floor of mouth [41]. One hundred per cent of tumours in the sublingual gland prove to be malignant [40, 41].

Traditionally, the 100:10:10:1 ‘rule’ was used to explain the distribution of salivary tumours in that for every 100 parotid tumours there will be 10 tumours in the submandibular gland, 10 in minor salivary glands, and 1 in the sublingual gland [42]. This rule applied in the population studied by Bradley [41]. Almost four fifths (80%) of all salivary gland tumours arise in the parotid and amongst these more than 80% are benign [28, 43], with the pleomorphic adenoma being the most common type, followed by Warthin’s tumours [28, 41, 44, 45]. Pleomorphic adenomas comprise 45–60% of all neoplasms of salivary glands [40, 43–46]. Approximately 80% of all pleomorphic adenomas arise in the parotid gland [43]. These frequently occur in the inferior pole of the superficial lobe and less often in the deep lobe or in accessory parotid parenchyma [47, 48].

In the study of Bradley et al., approximately 90% of the parotid gland tumours were found benign, with pleomorphic adenomas in their majority (approximately 68%), followed by Warthin’s tumours (approximately 26%) [41]. The extracapsular dissection (ECD) is a conservative tumour extirpation technique that is intended for benign tumours and on the basis of the aforementioned statistics it may serve the majority of cases.

9.3 Surgical Technique Approaches and Traditional Nerve Dissection

Parotid surgery has two distinct aims: The first is tumour clearance and the second is to achieve this with the least possible morbidity. The latter includes facial nerve palsy (temporary or permanent), Frey’s syndrome, unsightly scar, paraesthesia, or anaesthesia of the ear lobe).

The current variants of parotidectomy are summarised in Table 9.1 and Fig. 9.1. There are two fundamentally different approaches; one is based on a nerve dissection and the second on a careful dissection of the tumour without focusing on the nerve. Snow proposed a simple classification that illustrates the numerous extensions of parotid surgery [49, 50].

The difference between two main approaches (superficial parotidectomy and its variations versus extracapsular dissection) is the dissection of the facial nerve. In superficial parotidectomy and its

Table 9.1 The current variants of parotidectomy

Nerve dissection (Identification of the main VII nerve trunk)	Superficial partial parotidectomy	Exposure of <2 branches running to tumour
	Superficial subtotal parotidectomy	Exposure of >2 branches running to tumour
	Superficial parotidectomy	Exposure of all 5 facial nerve branches
	Selective deep lobe parotidectomy	Exposure of all 5 facial nerve branches
	Total conservative parotidectomy	Skeletalisation of all 5 branches
No nerve dissection (no identification of the main VII nerve trunk)	Extracapsular dissection (ECD)	Dissection only of branches running around tumour
	Enucleation	Discredited procedure

variants, the identification and exposure of the main trunk and branches of the facial nerve is a prerequisite before commencing dissection of the parotid gland, irrespectively of the size or site of the tumour.

Traditionally, a superficial parotidectomy follows all the branches of the nerve and removes the portion of the parotid superficial to the nerve. Most surgeons today do not follow this approach slavishly, but, where appropriate, only remove a quadrant of the parotid gland in the vicinity of the tumour (partial superficial parotidectomy). This more conservative approach carries the benefit of less morbidity, but still the fundamental approach remains the identification and dissection of the facial nerve.

ECD focuses on careful blunt dissection around the periphery of the tumour. The nerve is close to the tumour then it is mobilised sufficiently to move it away from the surface of the tumour. No formal identification of the main trunk is required. This technique is oncologically sound (demonstrated by the low recurrence rates) and exhibits far lower morbidity comparing with the traditional approaches.

The incidence of facial nerve palsy, temporary or permanent, as well as Frey's syndrome is consistently lower when practising ECD in all studies. The explanation is that ECD does not expose a large portion of the nerve, only the branches in the vicinity of the tumour. Consequently, less nerve tissue is subjected to ischemia or injury as result of dissection and surgical manipulations.

Frey's syndrome can be avoided by sound closure of the parotid fascia [51]. In a partial or limited parotidectomy, a portion of the parotid gland with its overlapping fascia is removed, which makes it difficult to close the remaining surrounding parotid fascia primarily. ECD, on the contrary, incises through but does not remove any fascia. The cruciate incision facilitates access into the parenchyma, and it is only the tumour with a small cuff of surrounding normal parotid tissue which is excised. Subsequently, the fascia can be re-approximated and closed without tension, restoring the barrier between parotid parenchyma and skin, so all but eliminating the risk of Frey's.

Another common complication of parotid surgery is injury to the greater auricular nerve (GAN). This occurs so often that transection is considered to be 'acceptable' consequence of parotidectomy. In the majority of patients, the impact of the sensory deficit is acceptable but not in every case [52, 53]. The idea of preserving the GAN in parotid surgery was first proposed by Brown et al. and has been supported by other authors [53–59]. The GAN usually has an anterior and a posterior branch, the latter supplying the earlobe via the lobular branch and in 23% of the cases the nerve trifurcates in posterior, lobular, and anterior branch, of which the lobular branch is of primary sensory importance [55]. Extracapsular dissection favours preservation of the GAN in 60–99% of the cases, as the superficial parotid pole is not being mobilised in its entirety [60, 61]. But preservation of the nerve is guaranteed by this technique for it depends to a large extent on the position of the tumour. If the lesion lies in the superficial lobe, for example, in the tail or in the region of the accessory parotid gland, then the GAN can be avoided in its entirety. But if the tumour lies close to the tragus or posterior boarder of the mandible, then to facilitate an optimum approach to the ECD the parotid gland had to be freed from its attachment to the sternocleidomastoid muscle and tragus. This means the posterior branch and in many cases most of the GAN has to be cut. So ECD offers greater opportunity to preserve the GAN but is not a solution to GAN injury.

The final sequela of surgery that concerns the patient is the cosmetic impact of treatment with regard to the scar and contour of the cheek. Historically, access for parotidectomy has evolved from initially transverse incisions directly over the lump to vertical incisions over the mastoid process [18]. A lazy 'S' incision was proposed by Blair [62], which was further modified by Bailey [10] into a J-shaped incision beginning at the level of the zygomatic arch and proceeding downwards as close as possible to the pinna and tragus, then gently curving round the root of the lobule to end over the tip of the mastoid process. The modified Blair incision remains the standard parotid access incision to date. ECD, by definition, does not require the full exposure of the parotid gland as is required by superficial parotidectomy but just an area 1–2 cm peripheral to the tumour in question. So with experience the incision and skin flap can be reduced significant compared to the traditional parotidectomy approach. But a word of caution in that a wide exposure should be practised with ECD until the surgeon becomes experienced with the technique. Otherwise, limited exposure can lead to risk of rupture and tumour spillage. The fact that the parotid gland is not removed but rather parted with the ECD technique means that there is no contour change or hollowing of the retromandibular space as commonly occurs post superficial and very obviously after total parotidectomy.

Currently in the West, there is a shift in emphasis to more aesthetically sensitive surgical approaches to the parotid in the adoption of the rhytidectomy (facelift) incisions [63–74], but this dictates a very wide exposure and elevation of skin flaps with its attendant risks. In contrast, Chinese surgeons have pioneered the introduction of endoscopic ECD [75] and robot-assisted parotid surgery is in evolution [76].

9.4 Extracapsular Dissection

9.4.1 Indications: Case Selection

The intention of the extracapsular dissection technique is for the surgeon to be working within 2–3 mm of tumour. It is therefore important to avoid encountering low grade malignant tumour masquerading as a benign lump.

There is a natural inclination when adopting a new technique to select what appears to be a simple case on which to gain experience. Intuitively small parotid lumps seem to be the optimum choice. However, approximately 40% of the malignant salivary gland tumours are low grade and indolent in nature and particularly when small they are difficult to distinguish from simple benign parotid lump. They have not had time to express their underlying malignant nature in the form of clinical signs. Once they have grown to 2–3 cm, it becomes quite clear that they have an infiltrative nature due to lack of mobility or pain. These features are not evident in small lesions that masquerade as benign lumps. The message to the surgeon commencing ECD is to be wary of small lumps and to favour large freely mobile tumours in the first instance. With experience mall parotid lumps should be excised with a minimum of 5 mm of normal tissue.

Clinical examination of the parotid lumps is quite effective in distinguishing benign from malignant lumps (almost 90%) and fine needle aspiration cytology (FNAC) improves the diagnostic yield even further but never to 100% [77, 78]. In the context of small lumps, FNAC is less reliable as the needle may miss the target and sample apparently benign tissue. FNAC results can be uninformative or misleading in up to 20% of cases [79–82]. If there is any discordance between the clinical picture and the FNAC result, then back clinical judgement and re-investigate where appropriate. All benign parotid neoplasms can be addressed by extracapsular dissection. The 2 cm well-defined mobile lump is the ideal choice when starting this technique.

Similarly, Warthin's tumours are another obvious pathological entity that can be addressed by extracapsular dissection. Warthin's tumour is not a neoplasm but rather an inflammatory cyst. If it is spilt, it has no implication on the health of the patient or risk of recurrence. They can be multifocal (multicentric occurrence) in up to 50% of the cases and may occur bilaterally (4–10%) [83, 84]. In the senior author's experience, this does not preclude extracapsular dissection, because if a new lump develops, it can be dealt with quite simply by a further extracapsular dissection as the facial nerve has not been exposed or disturbed in the original surgery. The presence of a Warthin's tumour is not a valid excuse to proceed to total parotidectomy!

9.4.2 ECD Technique

There are a number of steps which should be followed when undertaking ECD. Use of magnification and facial nerve monitoring are useful adjuncts. Meticulous attention should be paid to haemostasis; otherwise, it may be difficult to identify the shiny white facial nerve when it enters the surgical field. Before preparing the patient in the operating theatre, the tumour is marked on the skin surface and the area infiltrated with 1:200,000 adrenaline. This gives time for the adrenaline to take effect. Hypotensive anaesthesia is not required, haemostasis being the responsibility of the surgeon, not the anaesthetist.

A preauricular incision is made, the length and position of which is adapted to the size and site of the tumour (Fig. 9.2a). When first practising extracapsular dissection, the preauricular skin incision should be approximately the same size (large) as that employed for superficial parotidectomy. With experience the incision can then be reduced. The dissection proceeds in the plane immediately above the white parotid fascia (SMAS) layer which lies in continuity with the platysma muscle. The skin flap should extend past the lump for at least 1 cm and ideally 2 cm. Now that the skin flap is raised and before commencing surgery the lump should be palpated again one last time. If there is any doubt as to its nature, then an ECD can be abandoned in favour of a superficial parotidectomy.

The circumference of the tumour is marked with ink and a cruciate incision marked over the surface (Fig. 9.2b). The legs of the cruciate incision should extend 1 cm past the edge of the tumour. This is an essential part of the technique. Four small artery clips are then placed where the two lines bisect. The artery clips are used to tent up the parotid fascia which is then divided along the cruciate lines (Fig. 9.2c). Small rounded end scissors are then used to commence a blunt dissection through the parotid gland. This careful dissection is identical to that undertaken when parting the parotid tissue to identify the trunk of the facial nerve (Fig. 9.3).

The rule is that no tissue can be cut unless once can see through the fascia. The dissection advances in a blunt fashion and only when the scissors blades are visible through the fascia may the tissue bridge be divided. This can seem a tedious exercise, however after a short period the flaps of the cruciate incision are freed exposing the tumour below. The advantage extended by applying traction to the sounding facial through the attached artery clips cannot be over emphasised. The parotid tissue is frequently pulled away from the vicinity of the lump revealing valuable planes for dissection outside the tumour capsule.

As the blunt dissection proceeds around the periphery of the tumour, if a branch of the facial nerve is in the vicinity it is easy to discern both clinically and by way of the continual nerve monitor (Fig. 9.4). It is prudent to use continuous facial monitoring as an additional layer of security for the surgeon. But it is emphasised that it is not difficult to recognise a branch of the nerve as long as the basic principle is adhered to: this is that no parotid parenchyma is diathermised or cut, unless one can see through the tissues.

In circumnavigating the lump, if the dissection becomes difficult at any one point then the rule is to move to another site, in so doing tissues are freed and invariably the original problem is

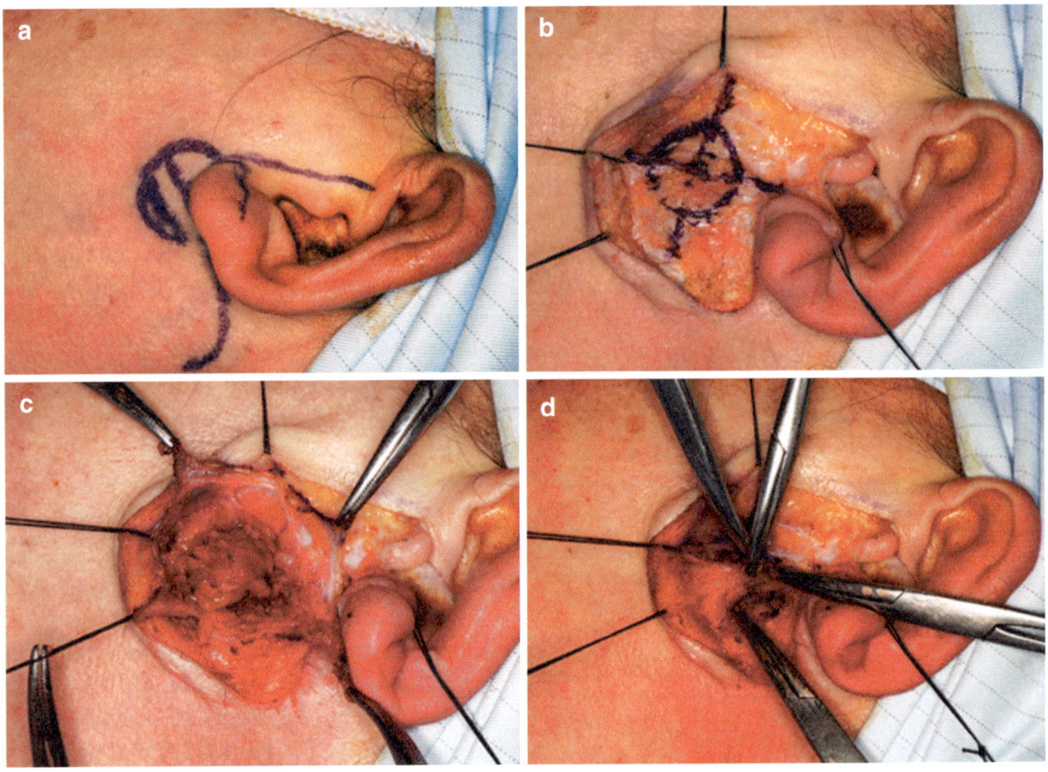

Fig. 9.2 Steps of extracapsular Extracapsular dissection (ECD)dissection: (**a**) Surface markings; preauricular incision and tumour location. (**b**) Markings of cruciate incision on parotid fascia. (**c**) Parotid fascia is lifted and lateral pole of tumour is mobilised. (**d**) Repair of fascia after tumour extirpation

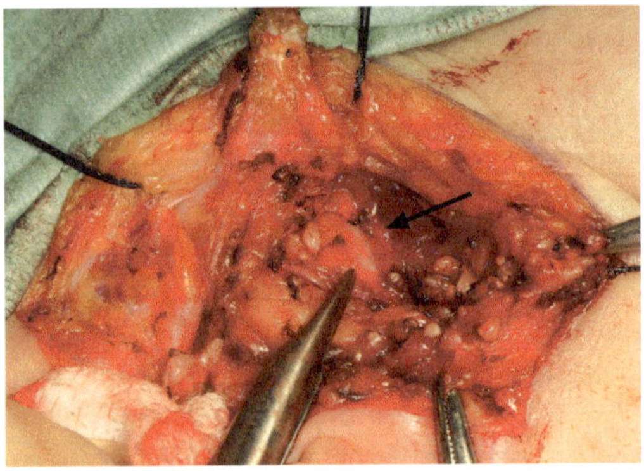

Fig. 9.3 Trunk of facial nerve (*arrow*) identified overlapping the inferior aspect of a pleomorphic adenoma

easily overcome when approached from a different angle. The key to the extracapsular dissection technique is to place traction on the artery clips which pulls the parotid tissue away from the lump and normally reveals a plane through which the surgeon can work 2–3 mm away from the tumour. When a branch of the facial nerve is observed, it is not necessarily dissected unless in close vicinity to the tumour capsule. Retractors can be used on the normal parotid gland to improve exposure of the tumour but never on the lump. The latter should only be handled by finger traction.

As the tissues around the parotid tumour are slowly released, the cruciate incision opens up much like the petals of a flower to reveal the tumour at its centre. The tumour is removed, leaving a parted but essentially intact parotid gland. Depending on the depth of the tumour, a suction drain can be used at the surgeon's discretion. The cruciate incision is re-approximated and the skin incision closed. It is advised that a mastoid-type pressure dressing is always applied at the end of the procedure otherwise sialoceles can occur. The pressure dressing is kept for about 48 h.

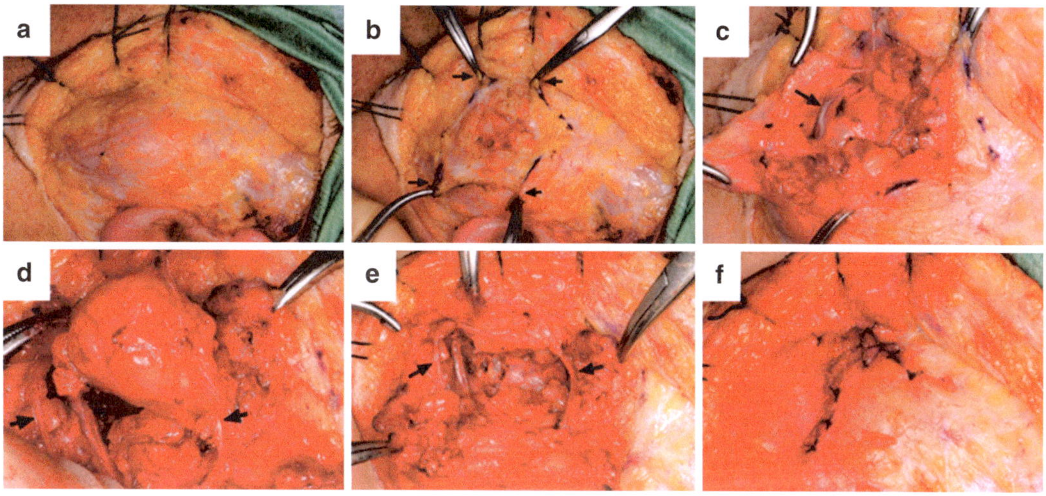

Fig. 9.4 Extracapsular dissection for a large parotid gland pleomorphic adenoma: (**a**) Development of skin flap and exposure of parotid fascia—note the tumour bulge. (**b**) Dissection of parotid fascia. Note the clips lifting the corners of the cruciate incision (*arrows*). (**c**) Lateral pole of tumour identified. A branch of the facial nerve (*arrow*) is crossing over the tumour. (**d**) Mobilisation of the tumour with a small margin of parotid parenchyma. Note the two branches of the facial nerve (*arrows*) that have been identified and dissected off the tumour. (**e**) Cavity after tumour extirpation. *Arrows* show the facial nerve branches. The masseter fascia is seen at the deep aspect of the wound. (**f**) Closure of the parotid fascia

An important adaption to the extracapsular technique which is particularly relevant to tumours wedged between the mandible and the mastoid is to free the parotid gland from local structures prior to undertaking an extracapsular dissection. Once the skin is lifted the parotid is freed from the pretragal pointer, mastoid process, and then along the sternocleidomastoid muscle to the depth of the accessory nerve. Once freed, the gland is surprisingly mobile and it can be rotated forward such that tumours that would normally be wedged between the mandible and the mastoid are now superficial and easy to access. Also tumours lying on the deep surface of the gland can be accessed extremely easily by ECD without having to pass through the full depth of the parotid gland (Fig. 9.5). Rather a thin film of parotid tissue lying under the lump can be incised giving quick access to the lesion.

9.4.3 Results and Meta-Analysis

Extracapsular dissection is now an alternative to superficial parotidectomy that is applicable to solitary benign parotid tumours. It is a less invasive procedure that achieves sound oncological results with reduced morbidity, as long as it is utilised is appropriate cases.

A series of studies and meta-analyses have been undertaken to date to compare the recurrence rates of pleomorphic adenomas after extracapsular dissection and partial or superficial parotidectomy. The overall results show no statistical significance and even favour ECD. The recurrence rates as demonstrated in different series are summarised in Table 9.2.

In a meta-analysis done by Albergotti et al. in 2012, pooled data from nine studies included 1882 patients and the recurrence rates following ECD and SP were 1.5% and 2.4%, respectively, in a median follow-up time of 12 years (range 2–32 years) [82]. The results were similar in another meta-analysis by Foresta et al., who included 19 studies and assessed the recurrence incidence in a total of 1907 patients with parotid pleomorphic adenoma [108]. The pooled recurrence rate was 1.3 per 1000 person-years for extracapsular dissection and 2.0 per 1000 person-years for superficial parotidectomy [108]. In the most recent meta-analysis from

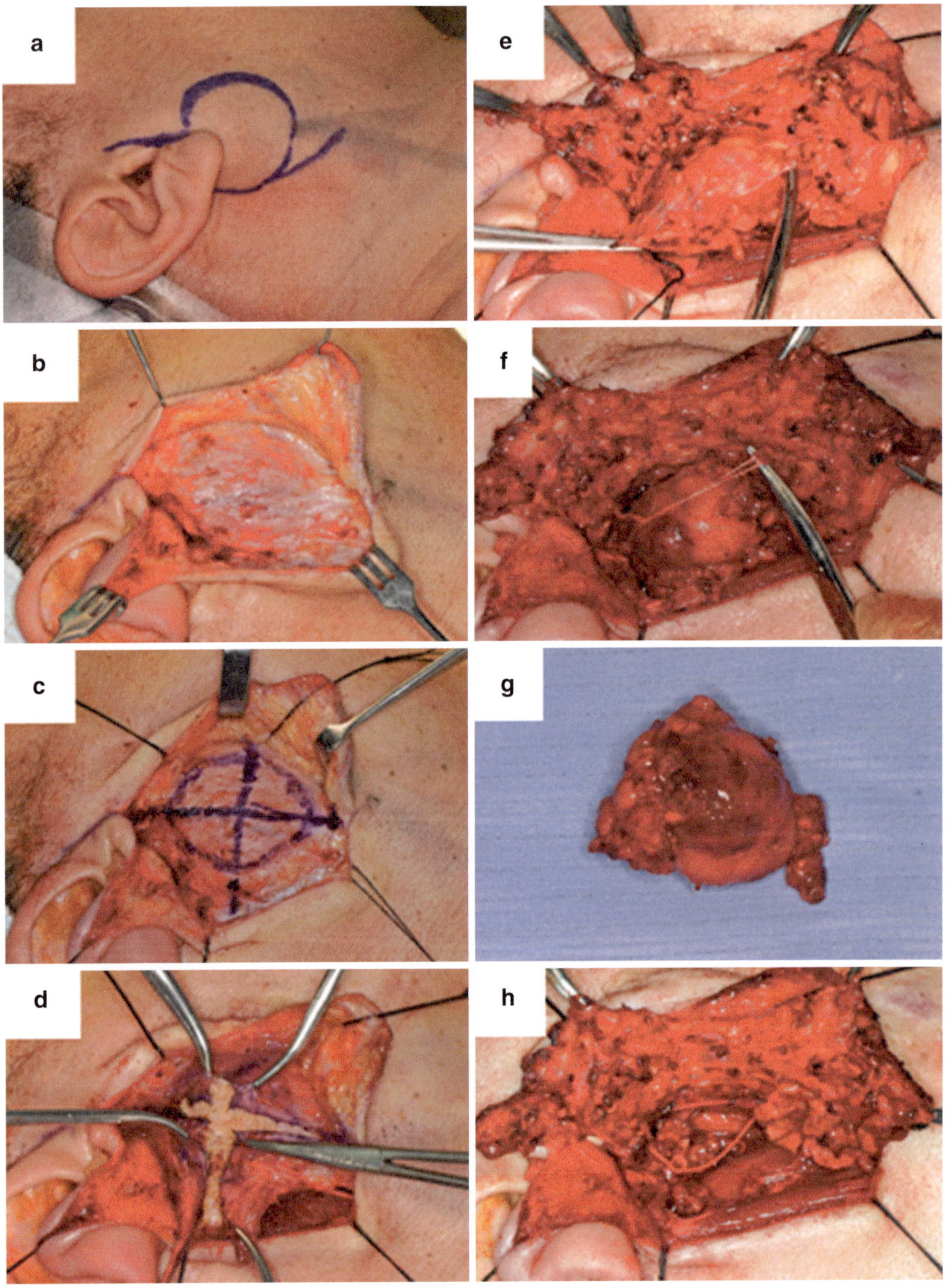

Fig. 9.5 Extracapsular dissection for a parotid gland deep lobe pleomorphic adenoma: (**a**) Surface markings. (**b**) Development of skin flap and exposure of parotid fascia. (**c**) Markings of the cruciate incision over the tumour. The lines are long enough to allow adequate exposure. (**d**) Incision through the parotid fascia. Note the clips lifting the corners of the cruciate incision. (**e**) Lateral pole of tumour identified. A branch of the facial nerve (clip) is crossing over the tumour. (**f**) Mobilisation of the tumour. Note the branch of the facial nerve (clip) that has been dissected off the tumour. (**g**) Tumour extirpated with a small cuff of parotid parenchyma. (**h**) Cavity after tumour extirpation with the facial nerve in the middle

Table 9.2 Incidence of parotid gland pleomorphic adenoma recurrence in relation to surgical procedure (F/U: follow-up time in years)

Study		Extracapsular dissection			Partial parotidectomy			Superficial parotidectomy		
Year	First author	*N*	F/U	Recurrence (%)	*N*	F/U	Recurrence (%)	*N*	F/U	Recurrence (%)
1979	Gleave [23]							188	n.s.	12 (6.4%)
1992	Prichard [85]							15	3–13	1 (6.7%)
1994	Natvig [86]	5	18	0 (0%)				268	18	5 (2.6%)
1994	Federspil [87]							130	3–26	6 (4.6%)
1996	Laskawi [88]							139	5	1 (0.7%)
1996	McGurk [89]	380	12.5	7 (1.8%)				95	12.5	2 (2.1%)
1997	Leverstein [25]	131	8	0 (0%)				61	8	0 (0%)
1998	Henriksson [90]							181	10.5	8 (4.4%)
1998	Rehberg [91]							26	1–24	0 (0%)
1999	Hancock [92]	28	10.3	0 (0%)				73	8.3	0 (0%)
2003	Ghosh [93]	30	12.5	1 (3.3%)				49	12.5	3 (6.1%)
2003	O'Brien [94]				254	6	0 (0%)			
2004	Piekarski [95]	98	2.9	8 (8.2%)						
2004	Guntinas [96]							171	6	0 (0%)
2005	Ferreira [97]							69	3–15	4 (5.5%)
2005	Witt [98]				30	10	0 (0%)			
2007	Roh [99]				52	2–5	0 (0%)	45	2–5	0 (0%)
2007	Smith [100]	27	0.5–6	0 (0%)						
2007	Zernial [101]							28	2–20	0 (0%)
2010	Chan [102]	104	10.6	0 (0%)				2	10.6	0 (0%)
2011	Riad [103]							164	4.7	5 (3.0%)
2012	Barzan [104]	332	7	7 (2.3%)				52	7	5 (12%)
2012	Riffat [105]	46	4.6	0%						
2013	Orabona [106]	176	3.8	8 (4.5%)				56	4.4	2 (3.6%)
2014	Christofaro [107]	153	5	5 (3.3%)				45	5.5	1 (2.2%)

2015, Collela et al. have included 16 studies, pooling together the outcomes of 580 patients who underwent extracapsular dissection and 1049 patients who had superficial parotidectomy and the recurrence rates were found to be 0.01 and 0.02, respectively [109]. The preponderance of pleomorphic adenoma to recur is discussed in detail in Sect. 9.5.

With regard to the morbidity of parotid surgery, a number of reports have demonstrated that the incidence of temporal and permanent facial nerve palsy is decreased in extracapsular dissection (Table 9.3).

The numbers compare favourably for extracapsular dissection as shown in large meta-analyses with a temporary facial nerve palsy rate almost three times less, comparing to superficial parotidectomy (8% for ECD versus 20.4% for SP) [82]. The rate of permanent facial nerve palsy was not statistically significant in (1.4% for ECD versus 1.1% for SP). Foresta et al. pooled together the data of 19 studies in a more recent meta-analysis and calculated the rate of permanent facial nerve paralysis to 1.1% after ECD and 2.2% after superficial parotidectomy [108].

Perhaps amongst all the strengths of extracapsular dissection in comparison to superficial or partial parotidectomy, the most striking is its significantly low rates of Frey's syndrome (Table 9.4). Again the relevant meta-analyses have shown the superiority of ECD, with Albergotti et al. reporting rates as low as 4.5% after ECD in comparison to 26.1% after superficial

Table 9.3 Incidence of temporary facial nerve palsy (tFNP) and permanent facial nerve palsy (pFNP) in relation to surgical approach

Study		Extracapsular dissection			Partial parotidectomy			Superficial parotidectomy		
Year	First author	*N*	tFNP	pFNP	*N*	tFNP	pFNP	*N*	tFNP	pFNP
1989	Owen [110]							96	43 (44.8%)	10 (10.4%)
1992	Prichard [85]	31	1 (3.2%)	0 (0%)				15	2 (13.3%)	1 (6.7%)
1996	McGurk [89]	380	41 (10.8%)	7 (1.8%)				95	30 (31.6%)	1 (1.1%)
1998	Rehberg [91]				270	5 (1.9%)	2 (0.7%)	50	11 (22.0%)	1 (2.0%)
1999	Witt [111]							53	9 (17.0%)	0 (0%)
1999	Hancock [92]	28	2 (7%)	0 (0%)						
2004	Papadogeorgakis [112]	3	0 (0%)	0 (0%)	42	3 (7.1%)	0 (0%)			
2005	Iwai [113]				49	7 (14.3%)	0 (0%)			
2005	Witt [98]				30	5 (16.7%)	0 (0%)			
2006	Guntinas-Lichius [96]							587	129 (22.0%)	35 (6.0%)
2007	Roh [99]				52	6 (11.5%)	0 (0%)			
2007	Zernial [101]							28	5 (17.9%)	0 (0%)
2010	Klintworth [61]	377	23 (6.1%)	8 (2.1%)						
2010	Koch [114]							134	34 (25.6%)	1 (0.7%)
2011	George [60]	156	5 (3%)	2 (1%)						
2012	Barzan [104]	299	n.s.	4 (1.3%)				50	n.s.	3 (6%)
2012	Riffat [105]	46	0 (0%)	0 (0%)						
2013	Orabona [106]	176	7 (3.9%)	0 (0%)				56	15 (26.8%)	5 (8.9%)
2014	Christofaro [107]	153	7 (4.5%)	0 (0%)				45	9 (20%)	1 (2.2%)

Table 9.4 Incidence of Frey's syndrome in relation to surgical approach

	Study	Extracapsular dissection		Partial parotidectomy		Superficial parotidectomy	
Year	First author	*N*	Frey's syndrome	*N*	Frey's syndrome	*N*	Frey's syndrome
1992	Prichard [85]	31	0 (0%)			15	6 (40.0%)
1996	Laskawi [88]					139	20 (14.4%)
1996	McGurk [89]	380	18 (4.7%)			95	36 (37.9%)
1997	Helmus [115]			146	2 (1.4%)		
1997	Leverstein [25]			131	9 (6.9%)		
1998	Rehberg [91]					59	5 (9.1%)
1999	Witt [111]					53	9 (17.0%)
1999	Hancock [92]	28	0 (0%)			73	18 (25.0%)
2001	Kuttner [51]					69	43 (62.0%)
2005	Witt [98]			30	2 (6.7%)		
2006	Guntinas-Lichius [96]					376	13 (3.5%)
2007	Smith [100]	27	0 (0%)				
2007	Roh [99]			52	3 (5.8%)		
2008	Giannone [116]			34	0 (0%)		
2010	Koch [114]					134	73 (54.5%)
2011	George [60]	156	1 (0.6%)				
2012	Barzan [104]	299	4 (1.3%)			50	22 (44%)
2012	Riffat [105]	46	0 (0%)				
2013	Orabona [106]	176	0 (0%)			56	3 (5.3%)
2014	Christofaro [107]	153	0 (0%)			45	0 (%)

parotidectomy in a total of 889 patients [82]. Similarly, Foresta et al. reported Frey's syndrome rates almost six times less in cases of extracapsular dissection (5% after ECD versus 28% after SP) [108]. It is clear that traditional parotid surgery by way of superficial, partial superficial, and total parotidectomy is plagued by Frey's syndrome. This is an inherent weakness of this approach from its basic principle; the downfall is that following the facial nerve, one develops the medial (deep) plane of resection that inevitably mobilises and detaches the superficial lobe with the parotid facia included. The remaining fascia cannot be closed, leaving behind inevitably a defect where the residual parotid parenchyma closes in direct contact with the skin, thus predisposing to Frey's.

In summary, extracapsular dissection is a less invasive parotid surgery approach intended to treat benign parotid gland tumours. In the hands of a trained surgeon, it represents an effective technique from oncological standpoint with far less associated complications [117–119].

9.5 Recurrence in Pleomorphic Adenoma

The recurrence rate of pleomorphic adenomas ranged from 23 to 43% in the period of enucleation [16, 17]. It was considered that inadequate removal and possible implantation from ruptured adenoma accounted for the recurrences.

The seminal work of Patey and Thackray on the capsular characteristics of pleomorphic adenomas built on this concept and demonstrated capsular incompleteness and also focal infiltration of tumour cells through the capsule. Intuitively factors could be explained why marginal excision of pleomorphic adenomas may leave tumour cells behind [22]. The capsule thickness varies from 0.015 to 1.75 mm thickness [119–122]. In reality, these biological features were not the explanation for the high recurrence rate but rather inappropriate surgical technique and on occasion intentional tumour rupture. The results of ECD demonstrate quite clearly that a careful dissection can be undertaken in close apposition to the tumour capsule with little consequence. The recurrence rate is similar to that expected by traditional superficial parotidectomy; ~1.5% at 10 years [82, 108, 109, 117, 119, 123, 124]. If a tumour is ruptured during a dissection, the evidence suggests that this raises the prospect of recurrence from 1 to 8% at 20 years [86].

The recurrent PA is almost always multifocal. Originally proposed hypotheses included tumour capsule rupture and subsequent seeding in the operative bed and multicentricity of the primary tumour [20, 28]. The latter hypothesis has been disregarded [14, 22].

What was interpreted in Patey's initial studies as satellite tumour nodules in the vicinity of the main tumour was later proven to represent finger-like projections (pseudopodia) in continuity with the main tumour. Unless serial sections are performed to exhibit the connection of these pedunculated outgrowths with the main tumour, they may misleadingly appear as separate islands [22]. One third of pleomorphic adenomas demonstrate capsular incompleteness and more than half have pseudopodia [120, 123].

Slowly over time, the concept of compulsory 'lateral lobectomy' or superficial parotidectomy that prevailed through to the 1980s was reduced to 2 cm margin of normal parotid parenchyma around the tumour and subsequently to 1 cm by Witt [124–126]. In reality, most surgeons nowadays are practising partial parotidectomies for pleomorphic adenomas. Even so in over 60% of cases, the facial nerve lies on the tumour capsule (bare area [119]) and in the most extreme cases the nerve can be tented so tightly over the surface of a tumour as to be hardly visible. These nerves are released with no tissue safety margin what so ever. Yet tumour recurrence is not the norm [25, 86]. In reality, the surgeon practising traditional parotidectomy is undertaking an ECD at some point in the procedure in >60% of patients treated. This is irrespective of the technique adopted (SP, PP) and how the nerve has been approached right from its exit point and followed on the pes anserinus or firstly encountered on the deep aspect of the lump, both will end in a bare area [124].

The question is why there is a stubborn recurrence rate of about 1.5% at 10 years. That does not seem remedial to modern surgical techniques. Also in the author's experience, the appearance of recurrent lesions is fickle and recurrence occurs in an arbitrary manner. They occur when totally unexpected in cases where the surgery was totally uneventful even considered exemplary and yet in another case with the nerve pealed from the tumour capsule no recurrence is forthcoming. In various studies, capsular exposure in the nerve interface area did not correlate with recurrence [26, 119, 122, 124]. Ghosh et al. showed that in 91% of pleomorphic adenomas the tumour was abutting the facial nerve; however, no positive excision margins were found and no recurrences in a mean follow-up period of 12.5 years [93].

A harrowing event is to have a patient return with miliary spread of tumour throughout the surgical wound. In one such case which occurred inexplicably the original pathological specimen was retrieved and serially sectioned in our pathology laboratory. The subsequent analysis revealed a small tear in the capsule which may have allowed an imperceptive leak of fluid from within the tumour into the wound bed during surgery. Natvig and Soberg extensively analysed the pathological specimens of 6 PA and in only two managed to identify the potential cause, namely ruptured and incomplete capsule with positive margins, respectively [86].

The evidence suggests that recurrent disease is more common in younger patients. Based on the proportions between stroma (myxoid component) and parenchyma (tumour cells), pleomorphic adenomas have been divided into three variants [37, 127]:

- Stroma-rich or myxoid with a stroma content of 80% and above
- Classic with a stroma content of 30–50%
- Parenchyma-rich (cellular) type with a stroma content of 30% or less

The structural composition of the tumours has been associated with the thickness of the capsule, with the stroma-rich adenomas demonstrating thinner and in areas widely incomplete capsules (69–71%), whereas the cellular types tend to have more complete and thick capsules (focal absence of capsule in 11%) [120, 121].

It could be speculated that these three subtypes represent different stages of the tumour's natural history, with the tumour starting as hypocellular with stromal abundance (myxoid type) and gradually evolving into the classic and more solid (cellular) variant with concomitant gradual capsular maturation. This could be the explanation of why recurrences are more often in younger patients—when the tumour capsule is immature and incomplete. The senior author has experience of three patients who developed recurrence after ECD. They were all young adults but the advantage of the ECD technique was that the recurrent nodules were contained in the small surgical compartment used for ECD and were not spread throughout the tissue planes. In one case presenting to a surgical colleague, a superficial parotidectomy was performed without mishap as the nerve and surrounding tissue was unblemished. In the two remaining cases, the recurrent nodule was removed by further ECD, but giving the nodules a wider margin.

References

1. Allen E, Turk JL, Murley R. The case books of John Hunter FRS. London: Royal Society of Medicine; 1993.
2. Heister L. Commercium Litterarium Norimbergae. Nuremberg; 1788.
3. Carmichael C. Extirpation of a tumour of the neck. Trans Assoc Kings Queens College Physicians Ireland. 1818;ii:101.
4. Kirby JT. The history of a case in which an enlarged parotid gland was successfully removed. Dublin: Hodges and McArthur; 1825.
5. Velpeau A. New elements of operative surgery with an atlas of nearly three hundred engravings. Washington, DC: Duff Green; 1835.
6. Nahlieli O, Iro H, McGurk M, Zenk J, editors. Modern management preserving the salivary glands. Tel Aviv: Publishing House Isradon; 2007.
7. Brunetti F, Fiori-Ratti L, Rossi G, De Campora E. La Ghiandole Salivari; 1969.
8. Erichsen GE. La scienza e l'arte della chirurgia. Milan: Vallardi; 1869.
9. Bailey H. The treatment of tumours of the parotid gland with special reference to total parotidectomy. Br J Surg. 1941;28:337–46.
10. Bailey H. Parotidectomy: indications and results. Br Med J. 1947;1(4499):404–7.
11. Bailey H. The technique of parotidectomy. J Int Coll Surg. 1949;12(2):103–10.
12. Kidd HA. Complete excision of the parotid gland with preservation of the facial nerve. Br Med J. 1950;1:898–991.
13. Martin H. The operative removal tumors of the parotid salivary gland. Surgery. 1952;31(5):670–82.
14. Foote FW Jr, Frazell EL. Tumors of the major salivary glands. Cancer. 1953;6(6):1065–133.
15. Foote FW Jr, Frazell EL. Tumors of the major salivary glands. Atlas of tumor pathology. Washington, DC: The Armed Forces Institute of Pathology; 1954.
16. McFarland J. Three hundred mixed tumours of the salivary gland of which 69 recurred. Surg Gynecol Obstet. 1936;63:457–68.
17. Benedict EB, Meigs JV. Tumours of the parotid gland—a study of 225 cases with complete end-results in 80 cases. Surg Gynecol Obstet. 1930;51:626–47.
18. Janes RM. The treatment of tumours of the salivary glands by radical excision. Can Med Assoc J. 1940;43(6):554–9.
19. Redon H. Discussion on the surgical treatment of parotid tumours. Proc R Soc Med. 1953;46:1013–20.
20. Patey DH. The mixed tumours of the salivary glands. Br J Surg. 1930;18:241–58.
21. Patey DH, Thackray AC. British Empire Cancer Campaign. Annu Rep. 1953;31:74.
22. Patey DH, Thackray AC. The treatment of parotid tumours in the light of a pathological study of parotidectomy material. Br J Surg. 1958;45(193):477–87.
23. Gleave EN, Whittaker JS, Nicholson A. Salivary tumours—experience over thirty years. Clin Otolaryngol Allied Sci. 1979;4(4):247–57.
24. Gleave EN. Tumours of the parotid gland. In: Rob C, Smith R, editors. Operative surgery. Fundamental international techniques. Head and neck part II. 3rd ed. London: Butterworths; 1981. p. 848–61.
25. Leverstein H, van der Wal JE, Tiwari RM, van der Waal I, Snow GB. Surgical management of 246 previously untreated pleomorphic adenomas of the parotid gland. Br J Surg. 1997;84(3):399–403.
26. Donovan DT, Conley JJ. Capsular significance in parotid tumor surgery: reality and myths of lateral lobectomy. Laryngoscope. 1984;94(3):324–9.
27. Mantsopoulos K, Koch M, Klintworth N, Zenk J, Iro H. Evolution and changing trends in surgery for benign parotid tumors. Laryngoscope. 2015;125(1):122–7.
28. Eneroth CM. Histological and clinical aspects of parotid tumors. Acta Otolaryngol Suppl. 1964;188:Suppl-99.
29. Leegaard T, Lindeman H. Salivary-gland tumours. Clinical picture and treatment. Acta Otolaryngol Suppl. 1969;263:155–9.
30. Ellis GL, Auclair PL, Gnepp DR. Surgical pathology of the salivary glands. Philadelphia, PA: W.B. Saunders; 1991.

31. Thomas KM, Hutt MS, Borgstein J. Salivary gland tumors in Malawi. Cancer. 1980;46(10):2328–34.
32. Davies JN, Burkitt DP, Dodge OG. Salivary-gland tumors in Uganda. Cancer. 1964;17:1310–22.
33. Loke YW. Salivary gland tumours in Malaya. Br J Cancer. 1967;21(4):665–74.
34. Gunn A, Parrott NR. Parotid tumours: a review of parotid tumour surgery in the Northern Regional Health Authority of the United Kingdom 1978-1982. Br J Surg. 1988;75(11):1144–6.
35. Wallace AC, MacDougall JT, Hildes JA, Lederman JM. Salivary gland tumors in Canadian Eskimos. Cancer. 1963;16:1338–53.
36. Batsakis JG. Tumours of the head and neck; clinical and pathological considerations. 2nd ed. Baltimore, MD: Williams & Wilkins; 1979.
37. Seifert SG, Sobin LH. World Health Organization international histological classification of tumours: histological classification of salivary gland tumours. 2nd ed. Berlin: Springer; 1991.
38. Thackray A, Sobin L. Histological typing of salivary gland tumours. WHO international classification of tumours, no 4. Geneva: World Health Organization; 1972.
39. Barnes L, Eveson JW, Reichart L, Sidransky D. World Health Organization classification of tumours: pathology and genetics of head and neck tumours. Lyon: IARC Press; 2005.
40. Spiro RH. Salivary neoplasms: overview of a 35-year experience with 2,807 patients. Head Neck Surg. 1986;8(3):177–84.
41. Bradley PJ, McGurk M. Incidence of salivary gland neoplasms in a defined UK population. Br J Oral Maxillofac Surg. 2013;51(5):399–403.
42. Thackray AC. Salivary gland tumours [abridged]. Proc R Soc Med. 1968;61(11 Pt 1):1089–90.
43. Eveson JW, Cawson RA. Salivary gland tumours. A review of 2410 cases with particular reference to histological types, site, age and sex distribution. J Pathol. 1985;146(1):51–8.
44. Jones AV, Craig GT, Speight PM, Franklin CD. The range and demographics of salivary gland tumours diagnosed in a UK population. Oral Oncol. 2008;44(4):407–17.
45. Tian Z, Li L, Wang L, Hu Y, Li J. Salivary gland neoplasms in oral and maxillofacial regions: a 23-year retrospective study of 6982 cases in an eastern Chinese population. Int J Oral Maxillofac Surg. 2010;39(3):235–42.
46. Woods JE, Chong GC, Beahrs OH. Experience with 1,360 primary parotid tumors. Am J Surg. 1975;130(4):460–2.
47. Batsakis JG. Deep-lobe parotid gland tumors. Ann Otol Rhinol Laryngol. 1984;93(4):415–6.
48. Lin DT, Coppit GL, Burkey BB, Netterville JL. Tumors of the accessory lobe of the parotid gland: a 10-year experience. Laryngoscope. 2004;114(9):1652–5.
49. Snow G. The surgical approaches to the treatment of parotid pleomorphic adenomas. In: McGurk M, Renehan A, editors. Controversies in the management of salivary gland disease. Oxford: Oxford University Press; 2001. p. 57–66.
50. Tweedie DJ, Jacob A. Surgery of the parotid gland: evolution of techniques, nomenclature and a revised classification system. Clin Otolaryngol. 2009;34(4):303–8.
51. Kuttner C, Berens A, Troger M, Keil C, Eckardt A. [Frey syndrome after lateral parotidectomy. Follow-up and therapeutic outlook]. Mund Kiefer Gesichtschir. 2001;5(2):144–9.
52. Patel N, Har-El G, Rosenfeld R. Quality of life after great auricular nerve sacrifice during parotidectomy. Arch Otolaryngol Head Neck Surg. 2001;127(7):884–8.
53. Yokoshima K, Nakamizo M, Ozu C, Fukumoto A, Inai S, Baba S, et al. Significance of preserving the posterior branch of the great auricular nerve in parotidectomy. J Nippon Med Sch. 2004;71(5):323–7.
54. Brown JS, Ord RA. Preserving the great auricular nerve in parotid surgery. Br J Oral Maxillofac Surg. 1989;27(6):459–66.
55. Hu J, Ye W, Zheng J, Zhu H, Zhang Z. The feasibility and significance of preservation of the lobular branch of the great auricular nerve in parotidectomy. Int J Oral Maxillofac Surg. 2010;39(7):684–9.
56. Min HJ, Lee HS, Lee YS, Jeong JH, Cho SH, Lee SH, et al. Is it necessary to preserve the posterior branch of the great auricular nerve in parotidectomy? Otolaryngol Head Neck Surg. 2007;137(4): 636–41.
57. Becelli R, Morello R, Renzi G, Matarazzo G. Great auricular nerve preservation during parotidectomy for benign tumors. J Craniofac Surg. 2014;25(2):422–4.
58. Vieira MB, Maia AF, Ribeiro JC. Randomized prospective study of the validity of the great auricular nerve preservation in parotidectomy. Arch Otolaryngol Head Neck Surg. 2002;128(10): 1191–5.
59. Christensen NR, Jacobsen SD. Parotidectomy. Preserving the posterior branch of the great auricular nerve. J Laryngol Otol. 1997;111(6):556–9.
60. George KS, McGurk M. Extracapsular dissection—minimal resection for benign parotid tumours. Br J Oral Maxillofac Surg. 2011;49(6):451–4.
61. Klintworth N, Zenk J, Koch M, Iro H. Postoperative complications after extracapsular dissection of benign parotid lesions with particular reference to facial nerve function. Laryngoscope. 2010;120(3):484–90.
62. Blair VP. Surgery and diseases of the mouth and jaws. 3rd ed. St. Louis: C. V. Mosby; 1918.
63. Hagan WE, Anderson JR. Rhytidectomy techniques utilized for benign parotid surgery. Laryngoscope. 1980;90(4):711–5.
64. Amin A, Mostafa A, Rifaat M, Nabawi A, Shallan M, Rabie A, et al. Parotidectomy for benign parotid tumors: an aesthetic approach. J Egypt Natl Canc Inst. 2011;23(2):67–72.

65. Grover N, D'Souza A. Facelift approach for parotidectomy: an evolving aesthetic technique. Otolaryngol Head Neck Surg. 2013;148(4):548–56.
66. de Vicente JC, González-Garcia M, de Villalein L, Fernández-Valle A. Modified facelift approach combined with a superficial musculoaponeurotic system flap in the treatment of benign parotid tumors. J Craniomaxillofac Surg. 2015;43(8):1655–61. https://doi.org/10.1016/j.jcms.2015.06.049.
67. Kyrgidis A, Triaridis S. Facelift approach in benign parotid surgery, Frey syndrome, and total superficial parotidectomy. J Oral Maxillofac Surg. 2011;69(10):2486–7.
68. Bianchi B, Ferri A, Ferrari S, Copelli C, Sesenna E. Improving esthetic results in benign parotid surgery: statistical evaluation of facelift approach, sternocleidomastoid flap, and superficial musculoaponeurotic system flap application. J Oral Maxillofac Surg. 2011;69(4):1235–41.
69. Dabrowska-Bien J, Pietniczka-Zaleska M, Rowicki T. [Facelift incision parotidectomy: preliminary report]. Otolaryngol Pol. 2009;63(6):485–9.
70. Lohuis PJ, Tan ML, Bonte K, van den Brekel MW, Balm AJ, Vermeersch HB. Superficial parotidectomy via facelift incision. Ann Otol Rhinol Laryngol. 2009;118(4):276–80.
71. To EW, Pang PC, Chu GM. The use of modified rhytidectomy for parotidectomy. Br J Plast Surg. 2000;53(1):80.
72. Charakorn C. The scarless rhytidectomy incision in superficial parotidectomy. J Med Assoc Thail. 1998;81(9):705–7.
73. Murthy P, Hussain A, McLay KA. Parotidectomy through a rhytidectomy incision. Clin Otolaryngol Allied Sci. 1997;22(3):206–8.
74. Terris DJ, Tuffo KM, Fee WE Jr. Modified facelift incision for parotidectomy. J Laryngol Otol. 1994;108(7):574–8.
75. Woo SH, Kim JP, Baek CH. Endoscope-assisted extracapsular dissection of benign parotid tumors using hairline incision. Head Neck. 2016;38(3):375–9. https://doi.org/10.1002/hed.23901.
76. Shin YS, Choi EC, Kim CH, Koh YW. Robot-assisted selective neck dissection combined with facelift parotidectomy in parotid cancer. Head Neck. 2014;36(4):592–5.
77. McGurk M, Hussain K. Role of fine needle aspiration cytology in the management of the discrete parotid lump. Ann R Coll Surg Engl. 1997;79(3):198–202.
78. Shaha AR, Webber C, DiMaio T, Jaffe BM. Needle aspiration biopsy in salivary gland lesions. Am J Surg. 1990;160(4):373–6.
79. Geisinger KR, Weidner N. Aspiration cytology of salivary glands. Semin Diagn Pathol. 1986;3(3):219–26.
80. Palombini L. Challenges in the interpretation of FNAs from the salivary glands. Diagn Cytopathol. 1997;17(6):417–21.
81. Schindler S, Nayar R, Dutra J, Bedrossian CW. Diagnostic challenges in aspiration cytology of the salivary glands. Semin Diagn Pathol. 2001;18(2):124–46.
82. Albergotti WG, Nguyen SA, Zenk J, Gillespie MB. Extracapsular dissection for benign parotid tumors: a meta-analysis. Laryngoscope. 2012;122(9):1954–60.
83. Chung YF, Khoo ML, Heng MK, Hong GS, Soo KC. Epidemiology of Warthin's tumour of the parotid gland in an Asian population. Br J Surg. 1999;86(5):661–4.
84. Seifert G, Bull HG, Donath K. Histologic subclassification of the cystadenolymphoma of the parotid gland. Analysis of 275 cases. Virchows Arch A Pathol Anat Histol. 1980;388(1):13–38.
85. Prichard AJ, Barton RP, Narula AA. Complications of superficial parotidectomy versus extracapsular lumpectomy in the treatment of benign parotid lesions. J R Coll Surg Edinb. 1992;37(3):155–8.
86. Natvig K, Soberg R. Relationship of intraoperative rupture of pleomorphic adenomas to recurrence: an 11-25 year follow-up study. Head Neck. 1994;16(3):213–7.
87. Federspil PA, Federspil P, Schatzle W. [Pleomorphic parotid adenomas and their recurrence]. HNO. 1994;42(1):28–35.
88. Laskawi R, Schott T, Mirzaie-Petri M, Schroeder M. Surgical management of pleomorphic adenomas of the parotid gland: a follow-up study of three methods. J Oral Maxillofac Surg. 1996;54(10):1176–9.
89. McGurk M, Renehan A, Gleave EN, Hancock BD. Clinical significance of the tumour capsule in the treatment of parotid pleomorphic adenomas. Br J Surg. 1996;83(12):1747–9.
90. Henriksson G, Westrin KM, Carlsoo B, Silfversward C. Recurrent primary pleomorphic adenomas of salivary gland origin: intrasurgical rupture, histopathologic features, and pseudopodia. Cancer. 1998;82(4):617–20.
91. Rehberg E, Schroeder HG, Kleinsasser O. [Surgery in benign parotid tumors: individually adapted or standardized radical interventions?]. Laryngorhinootologie. 1998;77(5):283–8.
92. Hancock BD. Clinically benign parotid tumours: local dissection as an alternative to superficial parotidectomy in selected cases. Ann R Coll Surg Engl. 1999;81(5):299–301.
93. Ghosh S, Panarese A, Bull PD, Lee JA. Marginally excised parotid pleomorphic salivary adenomas: risk factors for recurrence and management. A 12.5-year mean follow-up study of histologically marginal excisions. Clin Otolaryngol Allied Sci. 2003;28(3):262–6.
94. O'Brien CJ. Current management of benign parotid tumors—the role of limited superficial parotidectomy. Head Neck. 2003;25(11):946–52.
95. Piekarski J, Nejc D, Szymczak W, Wronski K, Jeziorski A. Results of extracapsular dissection of pleomorphic adenoma of parotid gland. J Oral Maxillofac Surg. 2004;62(10):1198–202.

96. Guntinas-Lichius O, Klussmann JP, Wittekindt C, Stennert E. Parotidectomy for benign parotid disease at a university teaching hospital: outcome of 963 operations. Laryngoscope. 2006;116(4):534–40.
97. Ferreira PC, Amarante JM, Rodrigues JM, Pinho CJ, Cardoso MA, Reis JC. Parotid surgery: review of 107 tumors (1990-2002). Int Surg. 2005;90(3):160–6.
98. Witt RL. Minimally invasive surgery for parotid pleomorphic adenoma. Ear Nose Throat J. 2005;84(5):308, 310, 310-08, 311.
99. Roh JL, Kim HS, Park CI. Randomized clinical trial comparing partial parotidectomy versus superficial or total parotidectomy. Br J Surg. 2007;94(9):1081–7.
100. Smith SL, Komisar A. Limited parotidectomy: the role of extracapsular dissection in parotid gland neoplasms. Laryngoscope. 2007;117(7):1163–7.
101. Zernial O, Springer IN, Warnke P, Harle F, Risick C, Wiltfang J. Long-term recurrence rate of pleomorphic adenoma and postoperative facial nerve paresis (in parotid surgery). J Craniomaxillofac Surg. 2007;35(3):189–92.
102. Chan WH, Lee KW, Chiang FY, Ho KY, Chai CY, Kuo WR. Features of parotid gland diseases and surgical results in southern Taiwan. Kaohsiung J Med Sci. 2010;26(9):483–92.
103. Riad MA, Abdel-Rahman H, Ezzat WF, Adly A, Dessouky O, Shehata M. Variables related to recurrence of pleomorphic adenomas: outcome of parotid surgery in 182 cases. Laryngoscope. 2011;121(7):1467–72.
104. Barzan L, Pin M. Extra-capsular dissection in benign parotid tumors. Oral Oncol. 2012;48(10):977–9.
105. Riffat F, Mahrous AK, Buchanan MA, Fish BM, Jani P. Safety of extracapsular dissection in benign superficial parotid lesions. J Maxillofac Oral Surg. 2012;11(4):407–10.
106. Dell'Aversana OG, Bonavolonta P, Iaconetta G, Forte R, Califano L. Surgical management of benign tumors of the parotid gland: extracapsular dissection versus superficial parotidectomy—our experience in 232 cases. J Oral Maxillofac Surg. 2013;71(2):410–3.
107. Cristofaro MG, Allegra E, Giudice A, Colangeli W, Caruso D, Barca I, et al. Pleomorphic adenoma of the parotid: extracapsular dissection compared with superficial parotidectomy—a 10-year retrospective cohort study. Scientific World J. 2014;2014:564053.
108. Foresta E, Torroni A, Di NF, de WC, Poscia A, Gasparini G, et al. Pleomorphic adenoma and benign parotid tumors: extracapsular dissection vs superficial parotidectomy—review of literature and meta-analysis. Oral Surg Oral Med Oral Pathol Oral Radiol. 2014;117(6):663–76.
109. Colella G, Cannavale R, Chiodini P. Meta-analysis of surgical approaches to the treatment of parotid pleomorphic adenomas and recurrence rates. J Craniomaxillofac Surg. 2015;43(6):738–45.
110. Owen ER, Banerjee AK, Kissin M, Kark AE. Complications of parotid surgery: the need for selectivity. Br J Surg. 1989;76(10):1034–5.
111. Witt RL. Facial nerve function after partial superficial parotidectomy: an 11-year review (1987-1997). Otolaryngol Head Neck Surg. 1999;121(3):210–3.
112. Papadogeorgakis N, Skouteris CA, Mylonas AI, Angelopoulos AP. Superficial parotidectomy: technical modifications based on tumour characteristics. J Craniomaxillofac Surg. 2004;32(6):350–3.
113. Iwai H, Yamashita T. Local excision procedure for Warthin's tumor of the parotid gland. Otolaryngol Head Neck Surg. 2005;132(4):577–80.
114. Koch M, Zenk J, Iro H. Long-term results of morbidity after parotid gland surgery in benign disease. Laryngoscope. 2010;120(4):724–30.
115. Helmus C. Subtotal parotidectomy: a 10-year review (1985 to 1994). Laryngoscope. 1997;107(8):1024–7.
116. Giannone N, Lo ML, Politi M. Extracapsular lumpectomy and SMAS flap for benign parotid tumours: an early outcome in a small number of cases on Frey's syndrome and facial nerve dysfunction. J Craniomaxillofac Surg. 2008;36(4):239–43.
117. Iro H, Zenk J. Role of extracapsular dissection in surgical management of benign parotid tumors. JAMA Otolaryngol Head Neck Surg. 2014;140(8):768–9.
118. Mehta V, Nathan CA. Extracapsular dissection versus superficial parotidectomy for benign parotid tumors. Laryngoscope. 2015;125(5):1039–40.
119. Zbaren P, Vander PV, Witt RL, Woolgar JA, Shaha AR, Triantafyllou A, et al. Pleomorphic adenoma of the parotid: formal parotidectomy or limited surgery? Am J Surg. 2013;205(1):109–18.
120. Stennert E, Guntinas-Lichius O, Klussmann JP, Arnold G. Histopathology of pleomorphic adenoma in the parotid gland: a prospective unselected series of 100 cases. Laryngoscope. 2001;111(12):2195–200.
121. Webb AJ, Eveson JW. Pleomorphic adenomas of the major salivary glands: a study of the capsular form in relation to surgical management. Clin Otolaryngol Allied Sci. 2001;26(2):134–42.
122. Naeim F, Forsberg MI, Waisman J, Coulson WF. Mixed tumors of the salivary glands. Growth pattern and recurrence. Arch Pathol Lab Med. 1976;100(5):271–5.
123. Lam KH, Wei WI, Ho HC, Ho CM. Whole organ sectioning of mixed parotid tumors. Am J Surg. 1990;160(4):377–81.
124. Witt RL, Iacocca M. Comparing capsule exposure using extracapsular dissection with partial superficial parotidectomy for pleomorphic adenoma. Am J Otolaryngol. 2012;33(5):581–4.
125. Iizuka K, Ishikawa K. Surgical techniques for benign parotid tumors: segmental resection vs extracapsular lumpectomy. Acta Otolaryngol Suppl. 1998;537:75–81.
126. Witt RL. The significance of the margin in parotid surgery for pleomorphic adenoma. Laryngoscope. 2002;112(12):2141–54.
127. Zbaren P, Stauffer E. Pleomorphic adenoma of the parotid gland: histopathologic analysis of the capsular characteristics of 218 tumors. Head Neck. 2007;29(8):751–7.

10 Minimally Invasive Implant Surgery with and Without Sinus Floor Elevation

Oded Nahlieli and Awfa Abu-Nimer

Abstract

The minimally invasive (MI) implant surgery is based on two innovations: the endoscopic approach to the implantation procedure and the endoscopy-friendly smart implant. The proper changes in the construction of the dental implant may solve three problems, i.e., (1) to reduce risk of complications; (2) to improve the maxillary sinus lifting procedure; and (3) to secure proper management of inflammatory diseases, bone loss, and low-density bone. Having these three problems in mind, we developed the dynamic implant valve approach (DIVA) for the dental implant procedures that uses an implant with an inner sealing screw (Upheal Dental Ltd. Netanya, Israel). This innovation was combined to the previously used endoscopic assistance during the dental implant placements and revolutionized the maxillary sinus lifting procedure itself. The innovation was put to test more than 7 years ago, and this chapter describes the results that we obtained and provides general instructions to use DIVA in the dental implantology.

O. Nahlieli, DMD (✉)
Department of Oral and Maxillofacial Surgery, The Barzilai Medical Center, Ashkelon, Israel

The Faculty of Medicine, Ben Gurion University of the Negev, Beer Sheva, Israel

Department of Oral and Maxillofacial Surgery, Eastman Institute for Oral Health University of Rochester, Rochester, NY, USA

Department of Oral and Maxillofacial Surgery, University of Michigan Health System, Ann Arbor, Michigan, USA
e-mail: nahlieli@yahoo.com

A. Abu-Nimer, DMD
Department of Oral and Maxillofacial Surgery, Barzilai Medical Center, Ashkelon, Israel

10.1 Introduction

Implantation techniques in dentistry have gradually developed from blind drilling and insertion procedures to the computerized guided surgery (stereolithographic stents). Later on, navigation equipment was introduced to assist in accurate and precise implant placement, so overcoming the shortcomings of the blind technique. An intraoperative examination of implant sites was presented in the 2000s. Initially, the examination of implant cavities was performed with immersion endoscopy. In 2006, a micro-endoscope (Visio Scope) was intro-

O. Nahlieli (ed.), *Minimally Invasive Oral and Maxillofacial Surgery*,
http://doi.org/10.1007/978-3-662-54592-8_10

duced for multidisciplinary use in dentistry, including dental implantology. It was just a next logical step after introduction of the root canal endoscopy. The second logical step was to design an endoscopy-friendly implant that also was introduced. The main goal of the endoscopic assisted dental implantation is to increase the longevity of oral implants by securing proper implant placement into bone of sufficient density. For the planning of surgery, bone conditions can be accurately evaluated endoscopically without causing any pressure necrosis of the bone. In complementary procedures, the endoscope can assist in sinus lifting intervention, and during the operation, endoscopic observation can further assess bone density and implant stability. In this chapter, we will describe

- General endoscopy-assisted implant surgery
- Endoscopy-assisted implantation procedure with the maxillary sinus lift surgery
- The use of the smart implant for the minimally invasive sinus lift procedure

10.2 The Tools: The Dental Endoscope and the DIVA Smart Implant

10.2.1 The Dental Endoscope

The Modular Dental Endoscope (POLYDIAGNOST GmbH, Hallbergmoos, Germany) is a medical device intended to allow visualization of the root canal or the implantation site and provide access for accessories used in dental implantology [1–3]. The device is a semi-rigid endoscope with a diameter smaller than 1 mm. It has high resolution optics with a 0.55 or 0.9 mm diameter, allowing easy introduction into the endoscopic cannula without being damaged. The optic element is covered with a Nitinol tube protecting it from the instruments which run through the same endoscopic cannula besides the optic element. For easy use, the optic element has an optic shifter adjustable to the cannulas of different length and keeping the optic element at the distal end of the endoscopic cannula all the time (Fig. 10.1).

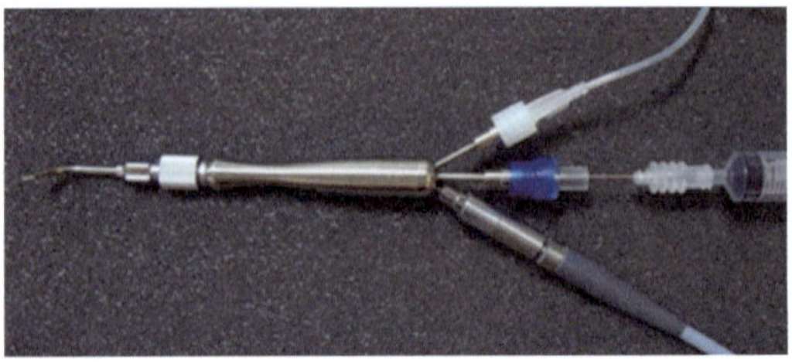

Fig. 10.1 The irrigation and injection cannula enables direct injection of saline and low viscosity material via the instrument channel under direct vision. The cannula can be advanced

Diagnostic and treatment procedures can be performed with the same endoscope by changing the disposable cannula only. Such endoscopes are usually available with an optic system of 6000 pixel or 10,000 pixel and wide field lens (120°). The dental endoscope is used with a Xenon light source, camera, and monitor. The additional instruments for such endoscopes include an irrigation device, injection cannula, mini forceps, microdrills, needles, and brushes.

The semi-rigid endoscope combines the advantages of flexible and rigid mini endoscopes: it has a clear view, a small diameter, stiffness, and good "pushability"; hence, it may be the best instrument available. Miniature endoscope for implantation procedures basically consists of three segments:

- A semi-flexible examination probe, to be inserted into the implantation site or the inner hole of the implant (see below), including an ergonomic handle
- Flexible optical fiber connections for light transmission (toward distal) and image transmission (toward proximal)
- Rigid eyepiece with a cold light source connection and coupler for a high-quality CCD camera.

The flexible optical fiber connection enables the decoupling of the examination probe from the rigid eyepiece, which gains in weight due to the CCD camera and the connected cold light cable. The work can be carried out using minimal effort while maintaining excellent precision, just as with a purely hand-held instrument. For dental clinics and medical centers, the integrated all-in-one laptop-like system, having a light source, camera, and monitor (Model SIA-COM-01, PolyDiagnost or similar) is recommended.

10.2.2 The DIVA Smart Implant (Upheal Dental Ltd., Netanya, Israel)

The Titanium-Aluminum-Vanadium implant (Ti-6Al-4V ELI) was designed with an internal central port with and dedicated sealing screw [4–7] (Fig. 10.2). This internal channel is essential for endoscopic observation during the implantation procedure and visual assessment of the bone quality, the sinus floor elevation (SFE) during the procedure, and might serve for endoscopic direct observation after the placement of an implant in cases complicated with infection, as well as for grafting material delivery or delivery of medications above the implant (Fig. 10.3). It means that the construction of the implant solves at least three problems, i.e., (1) reduces the risk of complications; (2) improves the maxillary sinus lifting procedure; and (3) secures proper management of inflammatory diseases, bone loss, and low-density bone. Naturally, there is no need to use endoscopy in each and every case and many implantations could be performed routinely. Yet, in complicated cases the DIVA implant provides additional means for observation and/or medical intervention above the implant.

The implants have external standard platform diameters of 3.75 mm and 4.2 mm and were tested in the ISRAC—Israel Laboratory Accreditation Authority for dynamic fatigue test as requested for endosseous dental implants (ISO 14801:2007). They were successfully tested on the animal model [5]. The additional fatigue test (EndoLab Mechanical Engineering) revealed that the run-out bending moment for the newly proposed implant was above the range reached by dental implants of the predicate devices (metal dental implants with a diameter of 3.75 mm were chosen for comparison). The implants were successfully tested for a possible inner screw leakage during screw-unscrew procedures (leakage sealing test, ISO 11737-2:2009; ISO 11737-1:2006; Milouda SOPs – 200.04.0116). In this test, no bacteria growth was detected and the test group and control group met the test's acceptance criteria [4, 5]. The implant was designed that way to make it possible to serve as an implant and at the same time as a drug delivery system. This newly designed implant is actually a two-component system (implant body + inner screw). The inner sealing screw was designed to serve in augmentation procedures, periapical lesion treatment, and for intra-osseous feedback via implant.

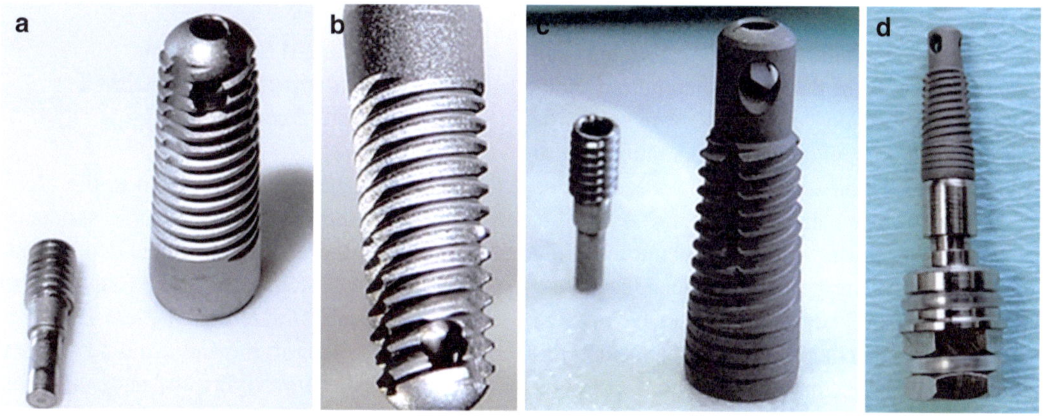

Fig. 10.2 The DIVA implants with the internal sealing screw

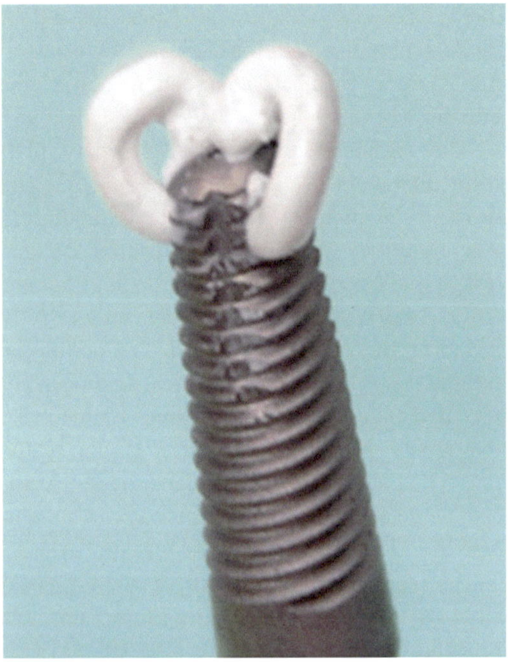

Fig. 10.3 An injection of a bony substitute via the inner channel of the implant

10.3 Endoscopy in the Implant Surgery Without Sinus Floor Elevation

Even if no intervention to the maxillary sinus is planned, the dental endoscopy assists implantation to increase the longevity of oral implants by securing proper implant placement into bone of sufficient density. To meet this objective, the dental implant endoscope can perform various tasks. For the planning of surgery, bone conditions can be accurately evaluated without causing any pressure necrosis of the bone. In complementary procedures, the endoscope can assist in sinus lifting intervention, and during the operation, endoscopic observation can further assess bone density and implant stability.

Endoscopy during routine implantology and during implant site preparation depends on the timing of the procedure. In immediate implant placement, endoscopic evaluation of socket condition can be performed in real time. The irrigation procedure allows observing the cavity walls of the immersed bleeding alveolar socket under variable magnification. Irrigation is crucial in every endoscopic procedure since the implant's locus must be filled with fluid to allow free and full visualization of the 120°-wide field. To maintain good visibility, the area must be lavaged, preferably with isotonic saline. Thus, intravenous tubing containing isotonic saline is connected to the irrigation port, and the endoscope's move forward is accompanied by a gentle flow of saline. Cortical and cancellous bone structures can be differentiated in situ, and pathologies are detectable even with capillary bleeding.

In late implantations, a pilot hole is drilled into the recipient site and expanded by using progressively wider drills. Before each drill is used, endoscopic observation assures that anatomical structures, like the inferior alveolar nerve, maxillary sinus are avoided [4–7].

Irrigation and suction are possible through small diameter cannula that irrigate and connect the suction to the side port of the endoscope. After assuming the form of the implant site, the tip of the irrigation cannula should be fixed one or two millimeters in front of the tip of the suction cannula, using the endoscope's control module, to prevent premature removal of the rinsing saline.

During surgery itself, endoscopic inspection of perforations and of other drilling and implant preparation errors can be performed, and endoscopic assistance in flapless implant procedures is possible.

10.3.1 Combined Endoscopic and Computerized Guided Implant Surgery

On our experience and in addition to the aforementioned benefits, when endoscopic assistance was added to the computerized guided implant surgery (surgical stent usage), we found further advantages, such as safe and flapless implantation surgery by identifying and avoiding anatomical structures and verifying the surgical stents position, preoperative planning of implant and prosthetic location, predictable procedure with possible immediate loading, shorter surgical and prosthetic procedure and improved postoperative morbidity.

10.3.2 Future Perspective

We hypothesize that future studies will find that endoscopic implant techniques can also significantly reduce the associated complication rate. Nevertheless, the need for intensive training might be considered a disadvantage. We envision that additional applications of modular dental implant endoscope will be developed in the future. These include assistance in implant planning and design, development of a membrane suitable for endoscopic application for the closure of perforations, and endoscopic nerve repositioning.

10.4 When and Why the Maxillary Sinus Floor Elevation/Augmentation Is Needed?

Endoscopically guided implant placements of the implants with internal port can be performed at any dental location both in the maxillae bones and the mandible. Yet, certain locations in the maxilla might require additional procedure known in various publications as maxillary sinus lift surgery, subantral augmentation, maxillary sinus floor elevation, maxillary sinus augmentation, or maxillary ridge augmentation. Regardless of dental implants installation, Philip Boyne was the first to report the elevation of the maxillary sinus floor for preprosthetic reasons in 1960. The maxillary sinus was augmented prior to a tuberosity reduction to increase the interarch distance and create a more symmetric maxillary arch for denture prosthesis [8]. Before we go further, let us recall general anatomy of the area.

10.4.1 Anatomy and Physiology of the Maxillary Sinuses

Humans have four-paired air-filled spaces that surround the nasal cavity called paranasal sinuses, these include: frontal and ethmoid sinuses between the eyes, sphenoid sinuses behind the ethmoid bone, and maxillary sinuses surrounding the nasal cavity. The maxillary sinuses are the largest of the paranasal sinuses. According to the existing theory, the biological roles of sinuses include decreasing the relative weight of skull, increasing voice resonance, providing a buffer against blows to face, insulating structures, and humidifying/heating inhaled air [9].

The maxillary sinus is a pyramid-shaped cavity, with an anterio-lateral wall corresponding to the facial surface of the maxilla (Fig. 10.4). Its size remains minimal until the eruption of permanent teeth. The average dimensions of the adult maxillary sinus are a width of 25–35 mm, a height of 36–45 mm, and a length of 38–45 mm. Its convex floor is approximately 1 cm below the nasal floor, with its deepest point usually being in the first molar region. Roots of the maxillary teeth frequently cause convolutions in the floor of the sinus [10]. Anteriorly, the sinus extends to the canine or premolar region. The maxillary sinus will maintain its overall size while the posterior teeth remain in function, but tends to expand with

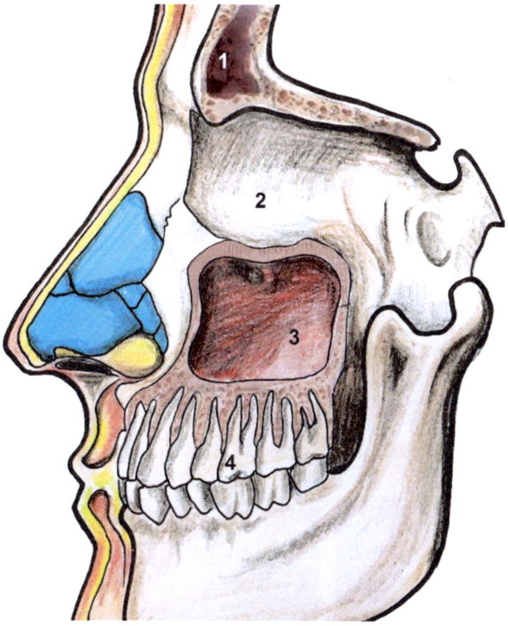

Fig. 10.4 The maxillary sinus and the teeth. *1*—the frontal sinus, *2*—the medial wall of the orbit, *3*—the maxillary sinus, *4*—the maxillary teeth

age and especially when posterior teeth are lost. The extent of this pneumatization varies from person to person and from side to side, with direction being both inferiorly and laterally. At the edentate stage, expansion often continues until only a paper-thin bony wall on the lateral and occlusal sides are left. One theory for this expansion is that the alveolar bone exhibits atrophy as the strain from occlusal function is reduced [9].

The inner walls of the maxillary sinus are lined with the sinus membrane, also known as the *Schneiderian membrane*. This membrane consists of ciliated epithelium cells resting of the basement membrane. It is continuous with, and connects to, the nasal epithelium through the ostium in the middle meatus. The blood circulation to the maxillary sinus is primarily obtained from the posterior superior alveolar artery and the infraorbital artery, both being branches of the maxillary artery. Many anastomoses are occurred between these two arteries in the lateral antral wall. The nerve supply to the sinus is derived from the superior alveolar branch of the maxillary division of the trigeminal nerve (CN-V).

10.4.2 The Bone Quantity/Bone Quality Issues

Compared with laboratory animals, the lowest bone density and fracture stress values were found in the human samples. The fundamental cause for differences in the survival of dental implants is bone quality. Currently, the assessment of bone quality is based on radiographic evaluation and on the subjective sensation of resistance experienced by the surgeon when preparing the implant site. The bone quality of the patients should be initially assessed by the cone-beam CT (CBCT) and CT images. The bone density can be measured at the CT images. At the same time, additional qualitative objective methods for evaluating bone quality are needed, and indeed, endoscopic observation of the site can determine the quality of bone density. Both anterior and posterior parts of the maxilla initially have poor bone quality, but the poorer one can be found in the posterior maxilla.

As for bone quantity, in 1981 Kayser attracted attention to the *atrophic posterior maxilla* by reporting that with maxillary premolar occlusion (shortened upper dental arch) 50–80% of chewing capacity is maintained [11]. Implant placement to reconstruct missing dentition in the posterior maxillary alveolar ridges is well accepted in the modern prosthetic dentistry, but it is often challengeable because of anatomical limitations and peculiarities as well as technical ones, of these:

- The absence of adequate *bone quantity* especially when inadequate vertical height of the residual/native alveolar bone is observed in the presurgical imaging. This bone loss is due to one or more of the following factors:
  - Rapid sinus pneumatization: caused by an increase in osteoclastic activity of the periosteum [12] results in loss of vertical bone height.
  - Ridge resorption (post extraction)
  - Periodontal disease
  - Trauma
  - Pathology and resection/surgery
- Poor *bone quality*, usually a Class III (porous cortical and fine trabecular "balsa wood" type) or Class IV (fine trabecular "Styrofoam" type) according to Lekholm and Zarb [13–16] (Fig. 10.5).
- Difficult hygiene accessibility
- Difficult surgical accessibility
- Higher occlusal loading in the molar regions in comparison with other areas, resulting in a lower success rate than elsewhere in the maxillary or the mandible [17]

To overcome these limitations, a variety of procedures have been reported in the literature: ridge bone grafts; sinus lifts (also designated as sinus floor elevation—SFE); and tilted, short, zygomatic, and pterygoid implants. Each method has its advantages and disadvantages, when the former two ones—separately or in combined—enables placing implants of adequate height as well as axial orientation. SFE is discussed in detail below. It can be performed with or without sequential subantral augmentation, while ridge

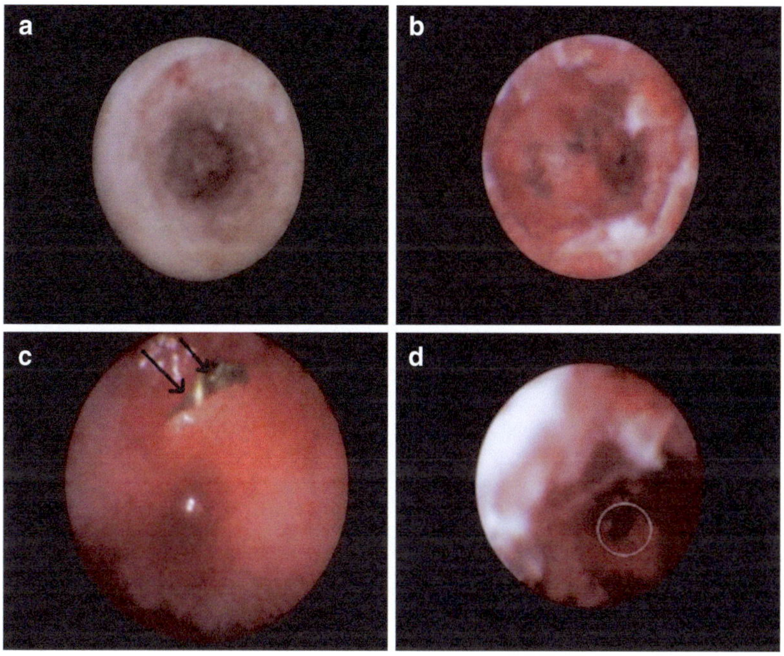

Fig. 10.5 Endoscopic observation of the drilling site can determine the quality of bone density. (**a**) Endoscopic demonstration of high-density bone quality. (**b**) Endo. scopic demonstration of low-density bone quality. (**c**) Endoscopic view of socket immediately after extraction. Note (*arrows*) fenestration in the cortical wall. (**d**) Intraoperative view during drilling for implant in the location of the first lower molar. Due to the poor bone quality, the inferior alveolar nerve can be observed (*yellow circle*) (Nahlieli et al. 2011)

bone grafting in this area can be done in either one of these fashions:

- Onlay grafting [18, 19], depends on the interarch distance in the area of lost teeth
- Guided bone regeneration [20, 21]
- Appositional bone graft or saddle-graft [22]
- A combination of two or more of the abovementioned procedures [23]

10.5 Indications and Contraindications for the Sinus Floor Elevation

As with any therapeutic procedure, treatment success depends on appropriate patient selection, careful evaluation of the anatomy, surgery planning, identification and management of any pathology, sound surgical procedures, and appropriate postsurgical management both by the healthcare team and patient himself.

Since the main goal of the sinus floor elevation (SFE) is to restore the posterior maxillary dentition by placement of endosseous dental implants, deficient of alveolar bone height in this area is the primary indication for the procedure, especially when less than 7 mm of vertical bone height exists. Other factors that must be considered include: the patient health, the dental and periodontal statuses, and the likelihood of a beneficial outcome. A thorough evaluation of the patient and the judgment of the clinician ultimately determine whether the procedure is indicated for any particular individual.

Contraindications to maxillary sinus floor elevation surgery are similar to that of other surgical procedures in the maxillofacial field in terms of the systemic health status, with the addition of some local consideration of the maxillary sinus itself, so that patients must be in good general health and free of diseases that affect the maxilla or maxillary sinus.

In short summary, the contraindications are:

Local factors	Systemic contraindications
Presence of tumors	Radiation therapy
Maxillary sinus infection	Uncontrolled metabolic disease (e.g., diabetes)
Severe chronic sinusitis	Excessive tobacco use
Scar or deformity of the sinus cavity (usually from previous surgery)	Drug or alcohol abuse
Dental infection	Psychologic or mental impairment
Severe allergic rhinitis	CF (yet questionable)
Chronic use of topical steroids	History of fungal infection (yet questionable)

10.6 Endoscopy and the DIVA Implant in the Implant Surgery with the Maxillary Sinus Floor Elevation

With a well-established long-term success [24–26], SFE is a currently well-accepted procedure to treat bone atrophy in posterior maxilla in purpose to compensate the bone loss by creating increased bone volume and thus permitting the installation of implants with adequate length as well as ideal axial orientation. Yet, high incidence of intraoperative complications also has been reported [27]. Thus, attempts were continually made to find a less-invasive approach, and SFE continues to be an important part of the implant surgeon's repertoire.

For the purpose of dental implantation, the procedure was first introduced orally by Hilt Tatum at the Alabama Implant Congress in 1976 [28, 29], but first published in the literature by Boyne and James in 1980 in a report on maxillary sinus floor augmentation [30], where they described a two-stage implant surgery of a lateral window osteotomy with sinus floor preservation and elevation superiorly, and simultaneous subantral bone augmentation (particulate autogenous bone graft harvested from the iliac crest was used); 3 months later, *blade implants* were placed to support removable or fixed reconstructions. In 1986, Tatum suggested and reported a less-invasive one-stage sinus floor elevation with subsequent augmentation and implant placement, a method that involved raising the membrane using an inferior crestal approach through the implant preparation site [31]. A "socket former" was used to prepare the implant site and create green-stick fracture of the sinus floor. A *root-formed implant* was placed and allowed to heal in a submerged way.

The crestal approach was refined later by Robert Summers, the change/transition which can be attributed to the so-called minimal invasive sinus lift surgery [32]. Summers actually described another crestal approach designated *the osteotome sinus floor elevation* (OSFE) using tapered osteotomes with increasing diameters, each with concave tip (Fig. 10.6) in attempt to gain vertical bone height by retaining and relocating all the existing bone. Thus, when the osteotome is pushed toward the sinus floor, bone shavings from the lateral walls of the osteotomy are collected in its concave part before being pushed upward into the subantral plane elevating the sinus floor and membrane with minimal risk. Using this approach, Summers reported a 96% success rate at 18 months after loading 143 press-fit submerged implants in type IV bone [33]. Advantages of this approach are well reported in the literature, citing reduced morbidity and postoperative discomfort as well as shortened surgical time [34–36]. Our opinion is that the minimal drilling for osteotomy preparation may be required before introducing the osteotome in some cases (such as in type III bone quality). Summers further modified the OSFE technique by adding bone graft into the osteotomy prior to sinus elevation [36]. This was referred to as the *bone-added osteotome sinus floor elevation* (BAOSFE) technique. Autogenous, allogenic, and/or xenogenic bone grafts were added to increase the volume below the elevated sinus membrane. Using the BAOSFE technique, consistent sinus membrane elevation of 4–5 mm was described by Summers. Other reports have demonstrated a wide variation in the amount of sinus elevation that could be predictably achieved [37–39].

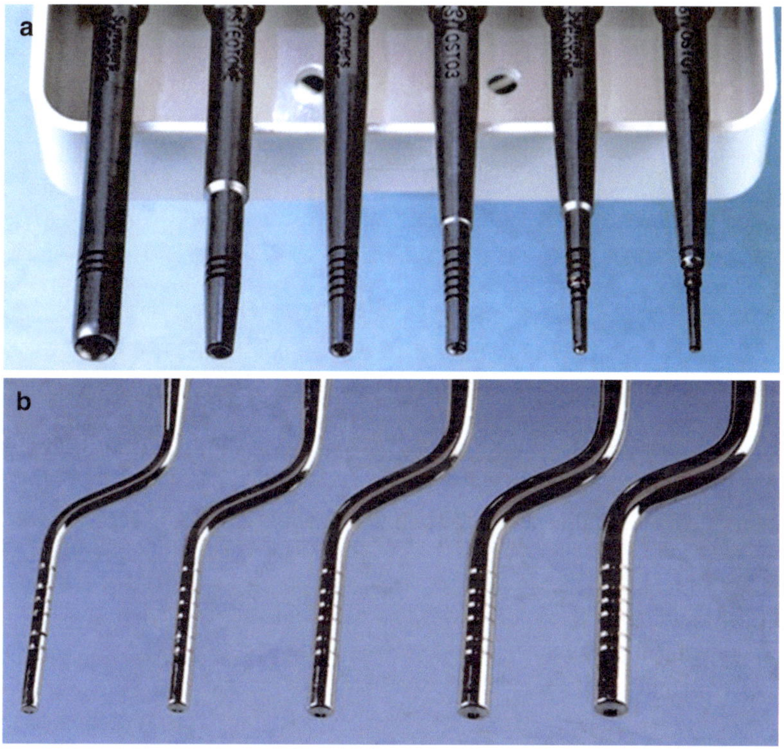

Fig. 10.6 The osteotome instruments used for the implantation procedures. (**a**) Straight osteotomes, (**b**) offset osteotomes

While the osteotome sinus floor elevation or the OSFE technique is considered to be a "conservative" approach to sinus lifting, it is, unfortunately, a "blind" technique because it does not allow a surgeon to visualize the Schneiderian membrane during the osteotomy. Limitation of the augmentation amount as well as the difficulty to control the osteotome tapping force—to avoid perforation—were reported [40, 41]. In addition, verification of success according to this technique can only be observed with postoperative radiographs. For these reasons, it considered a technique-sensitive procedure. Using an endoscope during the BAOSFE procedure has been recommended to overcome these limitations will be discussed later.

10.6.1 Techniques and Modifications of Sinus Lift Surgery

The concept of sinus lift surgery was established and confirmed in many retrospective and prospective controlled studies in the literature [42]. In general, there are two major well-accepted approaches to elevate the sinus floor: lateral window approach and transalveolar (transcrestal) approach, each with lots of modifications being evolved around. The lateral window approach can be one- or two-stage techniques for the implant placement; while the latter is a one-stage technique, mainly based on available residual bone and the possibility of achieving the primary stability of the implant.

As would be expected for such a popular procedure, various technical modifications reported to the both original "lateral window" and "transcrestal" sinus floor elevation approaches, such as:

- Membrane elevation by inflation of a balloon catheter such as MIAMBE technique [43, 44]
- The use of hydraulic pressure [45]
- The use of negative pressure [46]
- Gel-pressure technique [47]
- Reamer-mediated transalveolar SFE [48]
- Implants with internal port (iRaise [49, 50], DIVA [5–7])

Although the effect of these alterations on the outcome is still questionable, some of these surgical techniques can ease and fasten the surgical procedure as well as minimize the postsurgical morbidity.

10.7 Endoscopic-Assisted SFE

Baumann and Ewers in their cadaver study reported an impressive bone gain of 13 mm when osteotome sinus floor elevation was performed under endoscopic control [51]. Intraoperative visualization of membrane integrity using an endoscope during the BAOSFE procedure has been recommended especially when anticipated sinus elevation is greater than 3 mm [52]. The SFE can be controlled by the use of endoscope, whether by direct subantral endoscopy or indirectly using intra-antral endoscopy (sinuscopy) [2–7, 53].

10.7.1 The Dynamic Implant Valve Approach

High demand for minimally invasive procedures led us to invent the implant for a one-stage transcrestal-approached surgery, so that the implant placement is enabled along with sinus floor elevation with or without subantral augmentation as preferred, all these benefits at the same minimal invasive procedure. We have developed the "DIVA—dynamic implant valve approach," an upheal dental system based on the idea of an implant with internal central port and inner sealing screw. This innovation facilitates and expedites the minimally invasive time-saving sinus lift procedure, increases success rates, and reduces complications (particularly the risk for inadvertently tearing the Schneiderian membrane and a nerve damage).

This system was tested in vitro, and later its feasibility was tested in a large animal model (swine), and the first successive results were published in 2014 [4–6]. The testing revealed that the DIVA can be successfully used for augmentation procedures, especially of the maxillary sinus, in a standard fashion, as well as for intra- or postoperative delivery of therapeutic agents, and in combination with a dental endoscope for direct vision during the procedure. To date, more than 250 patients were treated with DIVA so that each patient underwent SFE with subsequent implant insertion, and more than 600 implants were inserted. The implants were inserted in the maxilla both with bone level < 5 mm and with bone level > 5 mm (in lesser number of cases). The number of implants per patients varied from one to eight. The failure happened in 4% without further complications. No correlation was found between failure cases and the bone density or quality. Follow-up (4–24 months) showed that in majority of cases (96%), the implantation was totally successful from objective clinical view, radiographic findings, and subjective patients' viewpoints [6].

The DIVA implants were successful in patients with atrophic posterior maxilla and native vertical bone range 3–9 mm. All patients were augmented subantrally using jelly alloplastic material injected via the implant port. There was no significant difference ($p = 0.32$) in the complication rate between implants inserted in bone level < 5 mm and those in bone level > 5 mm [7]. It was concluded that DIVA is a predictable one-stage implant surgery technique for implantation in posterior atrophic maxilla. By which, SFE becomes less invasive and with lower morbidity, the surgical field view is optimized during the procedure, adequate bone height can be achieved with long-term stability, and high acceptance by patients.

Depending on the preference of the surgeon, this approach can be used with gingival flap elevation or flapless, and endoscopically controlled if warranted. In our opinion, it is highly recommended to expose the alveolar ridge bone by performing a mid-crestal gingival incision with buccopalatal gentle elevation of the gingiva, even with the use of release incisions if needed as well, in order to assess both adequate mesiodistal location and axial orientation of the implants, and for direct visualization of bony bounders of the implantation site to avoid and manage cortical perforation or cracks while inserting the implant, the thing that cannot be done without exposure and direct visualization of the surgical field. The following describes our modification for SFE and outlines the basic surgical technique using the DIVA system, which is a minimally invasive approach procedure that requires one surgeon.

10.8 Preoperative Planning

Presurgical evaluation of the maxillary sinus should be primarily accomplished using radiographic examination. Cone-beam CT (CBCT) scan is the authors' modality of choice for this purpose although several observations about the anatomy can be made with a periapical or panoramic projection. The maxillary sinus should be evaluated for any pathology, masses, or the presence of septa (Figs. 10.7 and 10.8). Immediately prior to surgery, a practitioner should ask a patient to rinse the oral cavity with a chlorhexidine digluconate solution 0.2% for 1 min.

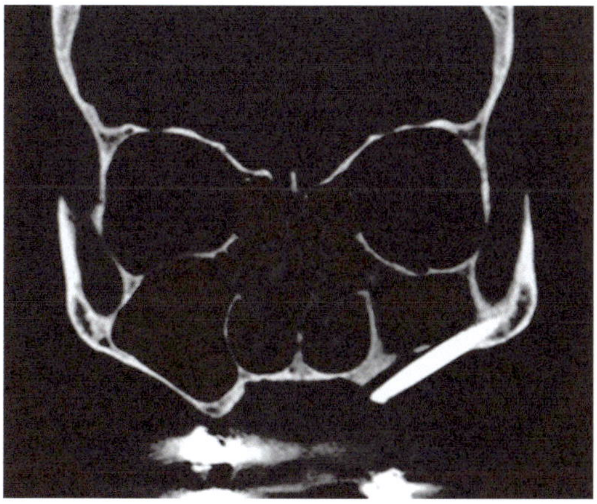

Fig. 10.7 Cone beam CT (CBCT) scan is the modality of choice for observations about the anatomy of the sinuses, a periapical or panoramic projection also can be of help. Note the difference between the left and the right maxillary sinuses

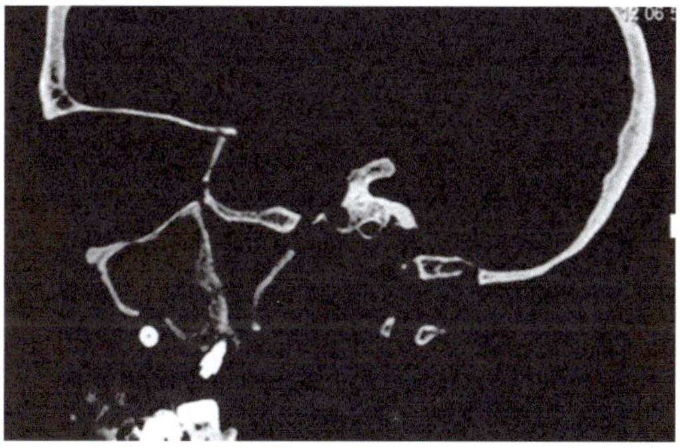

Fig. 10.8 The maxillary sinus should be evaluated for any pathology, masses, or the presence of septa

10.9 The Crestal Incision

As the first step, make an antero-posterior crestal incision placed slightly toward the palatal aspect of the edentulous area and supplemented by buccal releasing incisions at the anterior and posterior ends of the horizontal incisions when necessary. Elevate a full-thickness flap to expose and access the alveolar crest in the planned implant sites.

10.10 Osteotome Technique (OSFE)/Transalveolar Approach/Crestal

The crestal approach for the osteotomy is initiated by marking the site with a small round bur, followed by a 2-mm twist drill for the osteotomy preparation ending within 1 mm short of the sinus floor as suggested by Reiser et al. for predictable SFE [39].

Following the drilling, we apply the osteotome technique (OSFE technique) differently from that described originally by Summers [36], using a 2.7 mm curved osteotome into the drilling site to reach the left subantral 1 mm cortical bone, and to rupture it along with its adherent sinus membrane, so that the cortical bone is still connected to the sinus membrane above (Fig. 10.9a–c). This technique compresses the crestal bone and creates a bone disk that further

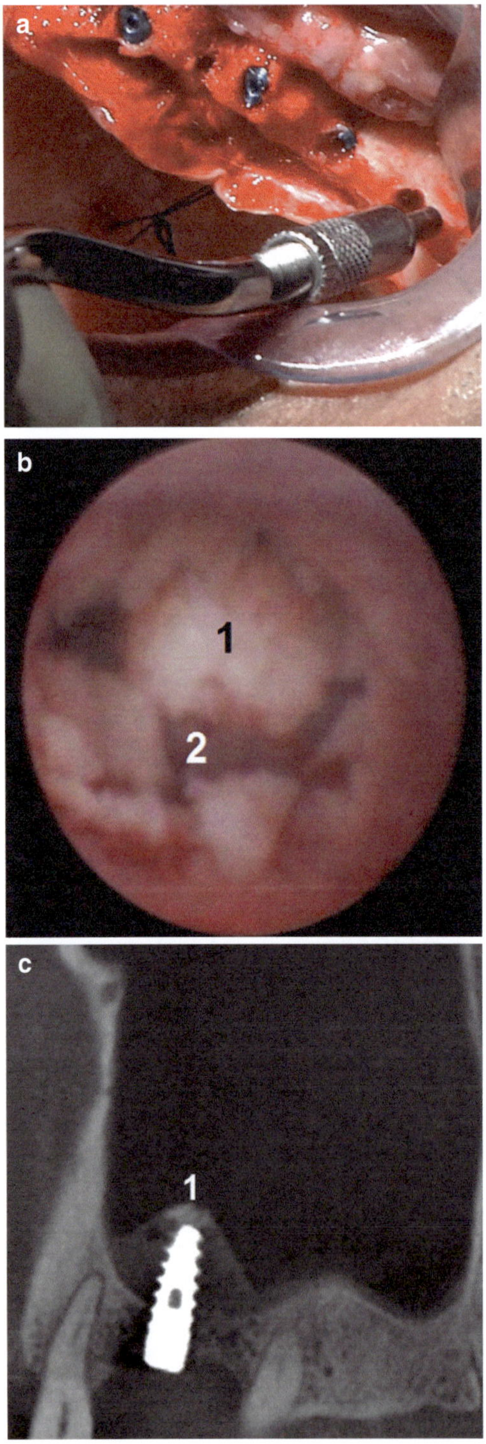

Fig. 10.9 (**a**) The osteotome technique—preparation of the implant site with 2.7 mm curved osteotome; (**b**) the endoscopic view following the osteotome procedure indicates the bony disk (*1*) and the Schneiderian membrane (*2*); (**c**) CBCT image demonstrates the creation of the stable tent with the bony disk (*1*) supported by the implant

being transferred subantrally to the sinus by the implant slow ratcheting will be performed later. The patient should be instructed to perform the Valsalva maneuver multiple times during the procedure to ensure membrane integrity.

In cases of the bone level being smaller than 5 mm, the osteotome technique enables primary stability for the implant, stable subantral tent and bone connected to the sinus membrane (bone disk).

10.11 Direct Endoscopic Evaluation (Optional)

In complicated cases, after the bone plate is split (transalveolar osteotomy) and before primary stability insertion of the dental DIVA implant, the surgeon can insert the tip of the endoscope beyond the existing sinus floor to verify the bony disk separation/fracture and its cephalic connection the sinus membrane (Fig. 10.10a, b).

10.12 Implant Insertion and Sinus Membrane Elevation

After the bone plate is split, the implant (diameter: 3.75 mm; length: 13 mm) can be inserted till, primary stability is reached (Fig. 10.11a). Then, the internal screw should be removed (Fig. 10.11b), bleeding from the caudal implant opening is usually seen in this stage due to the bone fracture and membrane separation around its apex (Fig. 10.11c). Now, begin saline irrigation via the internal port, introduce 1 cm^3 of saline followed by 1 mm of slow ratcheting (Fig. 10.11d), and keep on performed this until reaching the implant length level needed. We prefer performing this irrigation by using a non-hermetically sealed flexible plastic tube connected to syringe. The integrity of the Schneiderian membrane can be evaluated by the respiratory movement of the saline level via the implant caudal opening (Fig. 10.11e).

Thus, the authors suggest that membrane elevation by water injection as discussed above as hydraulic/diffuse pressure is preferable over using the blunt elevator in the margins to dissect the sinus membrane and to elevate it. The

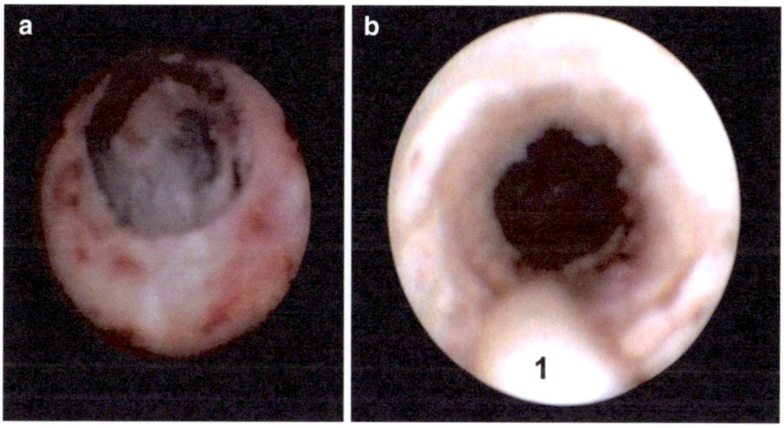

Fig. 10.10 (**a**) Endoscopic closed sinus elevation: intraoperative endoscopic view, note the intact sinus membrane after the endoscopic procedure. (**b**) Intraoperative endoscopic view during closed sinus elevation, note the jet cannula (*1*) during the membrane elevation

latter is more likely to jeopardize the sinus membrane integrity. The results of the procedure should be evaluated after the implantation (Fig. 10.11f).

10.13 Injection of Grafting Material as Needed

After completion of the sinus floor elevation, either liquid or jelly bony substitute can be optionally injected via the inner channel of the implant in order to stabilize the tent formation. Remember that the vital periosteum alone initiates bone regeneration and production in the absence of any calcified structure or augmentation material, as Srouji et al. [54] were able to prove; only a stable subantral blood coagulum is needed. We use 0.5–1 mL of βTCP with Hylanoronic acid (Cerasorb Paste Curasan AG Kleinostheim, Germany) for tent stabilization for each implant. Another good options is to inject the collagen paste (OsteoBiol, Tecnoss, Giaveno, Italy) around the implant or PRF/PRP. The DIVA injection adaptor can also be used. Then, and regardless of your choice, insert the internal sealing screw which comes as additional part within the DIVA kit and tighten it.

The authors suggest that liquid or jelly materials are preferable to the sharp-edged autogenous bone mass or bone substitute chips, which are more likely to jeopardize sinus membrane integrity when directly placed in contact with the sinus membrane (Fig. 10.12).

Following graft placement and final ratcheting of the implants, the mucoperiosteal flaps can be repositioned and sutured with 4-0 monofilament sutures without tension.

10.14 Postoperative Care and Follow-Up

Patients should be instructed not to wear their dentures for 2 weeks postoperatively until the prosthesis is relined with a soft liner as accepted. Antibiotics should be prescribed for 7–10 days and analgesics as required. Sutures should be removed 2 weeks following surgery and postsurgical visits can be scheduled at monthly intervals to check the course of healing (Fig. 10.13).

10.15 Second-Stage Surgery and Prosthetic Loading

After a healing period of 4–6 months, second-stage surgery can be carried out, stability of the fixtures should be verified, and healing abutments can be connected to the implants on the way for definitive prosthetic rehabilitation by fixed bridges.

10.15.1 Complications

The complications encountered in all minimally invasive sinus lift procedures and their modifications are dramatically less than those encountered in the lateral window approach and its

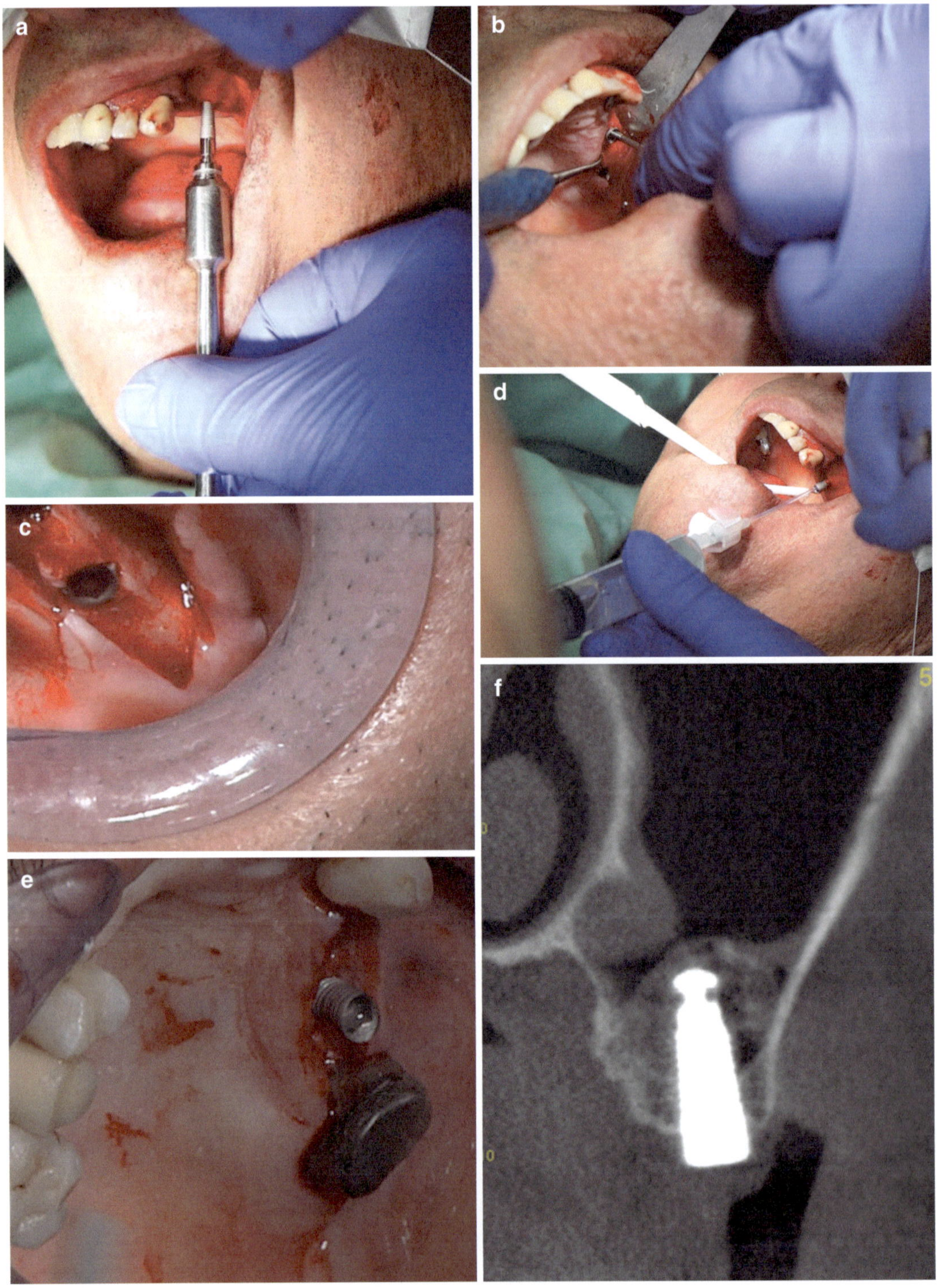

Fig. 10.11 Implant insertion and sinus membrane elevation: (**a**) the implant is inserted till primary the stability is reached; (**b**) the internal screw should be removed; (**c**) bleeding from the caudal implant opening is to be assessed; (**d**) saline irrigation via the internal port includes 1 cm^3 of saline followed by 1 mm of slow ratcheting; (**e**) the integrity of the Schneiderian membrane is evaluated by the respiratory movement of the saline level via the implant caudal opening; (**f**) the results of the procedure should be evaluated after the implantation. CBCT demonstrates a selective sinus floor elevation

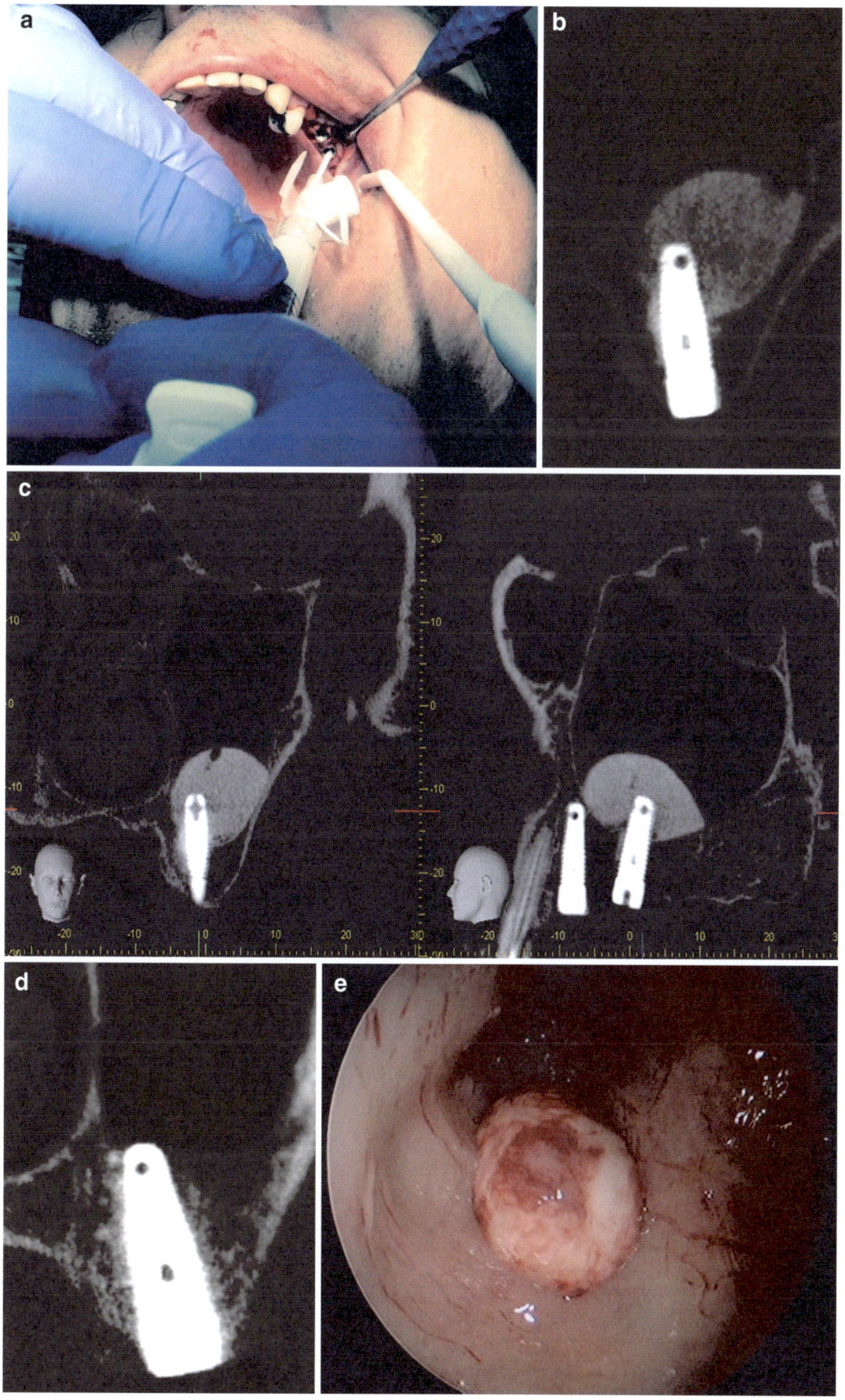

Fig. 10.12 (**a**) βTCP Paste (Cerasorb Curasan AG Kleinostheim Germany) injection via the DIVA channel; (**b**, **c**) immediate CBCT imaging; (**d**) 16 weeks postoperative CBCT demonstrating bone regeneration around the DIVA implant; (**e**) endoscopic view of the sinus site of the selective sinus elevation with the DIVA implant, note the 360° coverage of the implant with the βTCP paste (*white*). The bone disk is in the center of the picture

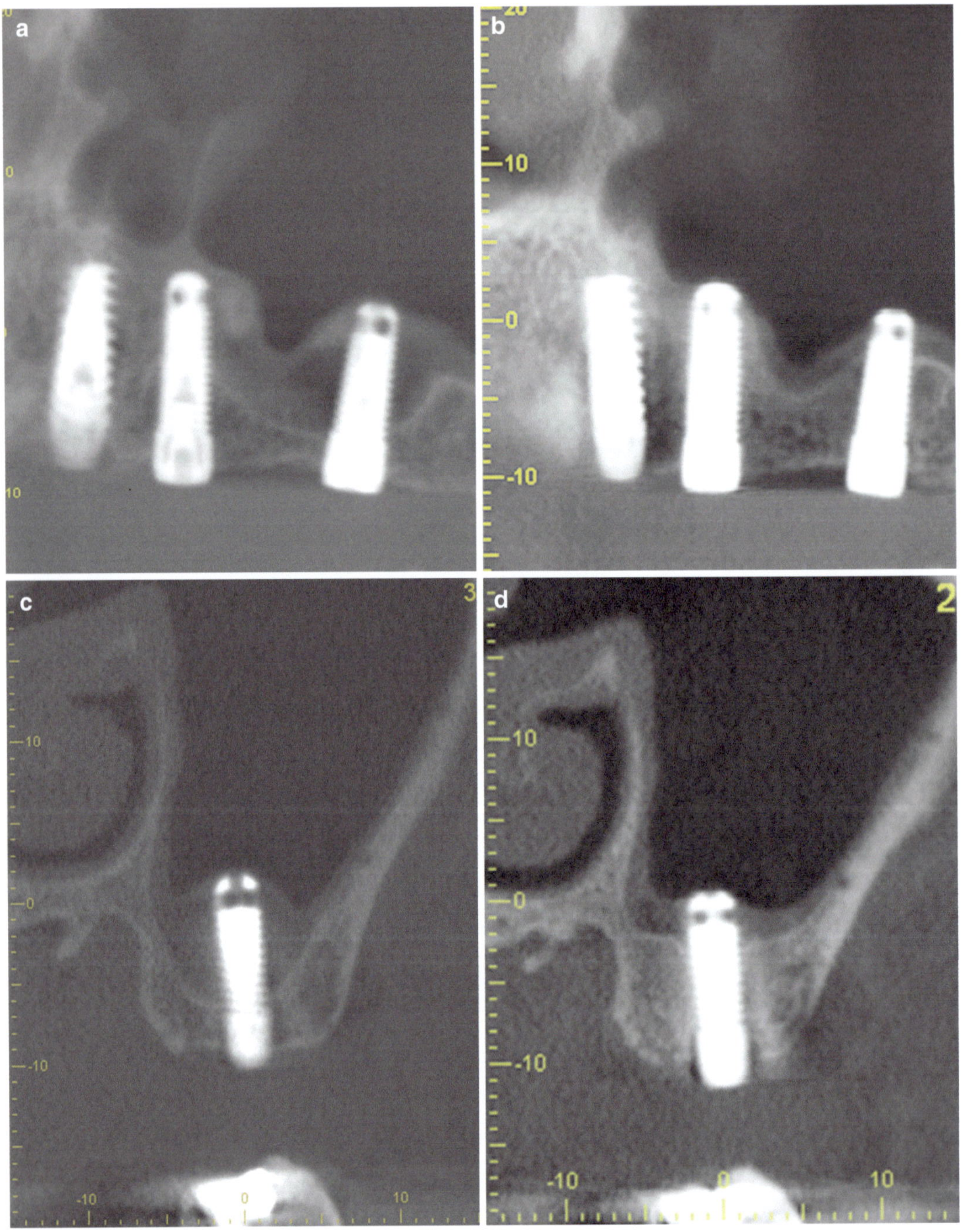

Fig. 10.13 Follow-up assessment. (**a**) CBCT image (sagittal section view) of 56-year-old female taken immediately after the selective sinus elevation, insertion of two DIVA implants, and creation of the stable tent; (**b**) the same patient 16-week follow-up demonstrates the formation of the bone in the tent; (**c**) the immediate coronal section view image of the same patient; (**d**) the 16-week follow-up coronal section view of the same patient; (**e**) CBCT image (coronal section view) of 60-year-old female taken immediately after the similar procedure; (**f**) the same patient 16-week follow-up demonstrates the formation of the bone in the tent

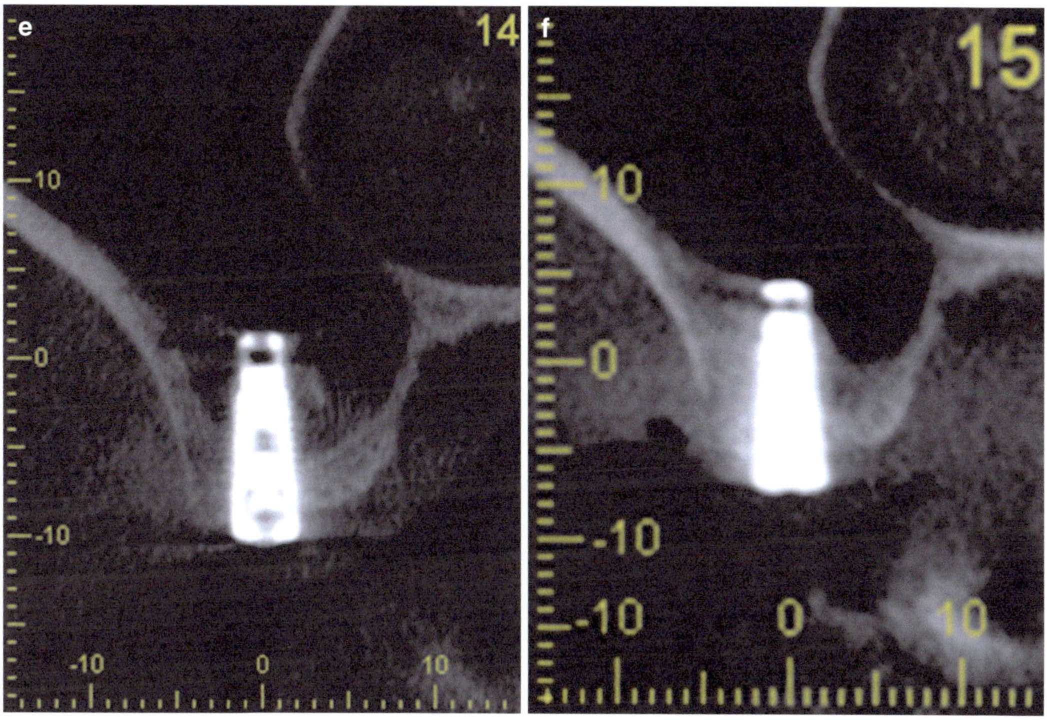

Fig. 10.13 (continued)

modifications. Owing to techniques, similarities in MI-SFE, the complication encountered are almost the same, and include membrane perforation, bleeding, sinusitis, sinus cavity obliteration, implant dislodgement, and sequestration and infection of one graft material [55]. Specifically in OSFE, and because of osteotome tapping, a benign paroxysmal positional vertigo (the so-called OSFE-BPPV) can occur in incidence less than 3% as was reported [56, 57]. Paraesthesia is also a rare complication reported in MI-SFE.

Membrane perforation during the MI-SFE techniques can be minimized using sound clinical planning and accurate determination of available preoperative bone height. Research has found that implants can heal uneventfully if a small perforation without graft dispersion occurs [58]. The incidence and management of these complications is well discussed in the above-mentioned literature.

10.16 Alternatives to Performing a Sinus Lift

When SFE is contraindicated, and for achieving the prosthetic/prosthodontic goal mentioned, there are several alternative techniques available by which the surgeon can avoid manipulation of the sinus floor.

10.16.1 Short Implants

The simplest solution is placing short implants which greatly reduce the chances of entering the sinus cavity upon insertion. Short implants, ≤8 mm in length, when placed without grafting offer the opportunity of a less complex, cheaper, and faster treatment. Reports of the successful use of shorter implants to avoid encroachment of pneumatized sinuses are available [59, 60].

However, an analysis of longitudinal studies, which included 16,344 implants, demonstrated that along with other risk factors, poor bone quality in connection with short implants seemed to be associated with failure [61].

In general, and regardless the implantation site, reports also have shown implants shorter than 10 mm are less successful than longer implants [13, 62–65].

Although there is a paucity of data comparing short implants in the posterior maxilla with long implants in grafted sinuses, it is possible that in the future the improved implant surface topography may further raise the survival rates for these shorter implants.

10.16.2 Tilted Implants

Another option without a compromise in the optimal implant length is placement of the implants in a tilted fashion either mesially or distally in a way that they do not penetrate the maxillary sinus. By this alternative treatment option, longer implants, with lengths of up to 15 mm, can be placed and anchored with larger cortical bone contact [66]. Nevertheless, long-term data regarding tilted implants success are still limited [66–68].

10.16.3 Zygomatic and Pterygoid Implants

Either passes through the sinus cavity or laterally, zygomatic implants can be used. Although these implants yield high survival rates, when infection occurs their removal is difficult [69–71]. As it is with tilted implants, non-axial implants prone to significant crestal bone loss after remodeling are complete, leading to increased probing depths and peri-implant pathologies.

The pterygoid implant passes through the maxillary tuberosity, pyramidal process of palatine bone, and then engages the pterygoid process of the sphenoid bone. However, in some studies they are placed in a more anterior position, in the pterigomaxillary area and parallel to the posterior wall of the sinus [72–75]. Such implants avoid the need for bone grafting in the atrophied or resorbed maxilla, eliminate prosthetic cantilevering, improve axial loading, and achieve stability and high rates of long-term success.

10.16.4 Onlay Bone Graft

Onlay bone grafts may be used for a horizontal or vertical augmentation of the residual ridge; however, vertical ridge augmentation using block grafting does not achieve a predictable bone height gain [75]. Although horizontal ridge augmentation by way of guided bone regeneration is predictable, augmentation in a vertical direction is not.

Conclusion

We see the DIVA contribution to MI-SFE surgery as follows:

- More quantity of elevation and the implant's height
- Less perforations
- Less discomfort and PBBV during the surgical procedure
- Reduced operative time
- Intraoperative option for control and intervention by an endoscope

References

1. Moshonov J, Michaeli E, Nahlieli O. Endoscopic root canal treatment. Quintessence Int. 2009;40(9):739–44.
2. Nahlieli O, Moshonov J, Zagury A, Michaeli E, Casap N. Endoscopic approach to dental implantology. J Oral Maxillofac Surg. 2011;69(1):186–91. https://doi.org/10.1016/j.joms.2010.07.071.
3. Moshonov J, Nahlieli O. Endoscopy in endodontics. Alpha Omegan. 2011;104(1–2):26–34.
4. Nahlieli O. Dynamic implant valve approach for dental implant procedures. Chin J Dent Res. 2014;17(1):15–21.
5. Nahlieli O, Casap N, Moshonov J, Zagury A, Michali E, Samuni Y. A novel dental implant system with an internal port for endoscopic closed sinus augmentation: a feasibility study in pigs. Int J Oral Maxillofac Implants. 2013;28(6):e556–61. 10.11607/jomi.te36.

6. Nahlieli O, Zagury A, Michaeli E, Bruck N, Nahlieli DD, Casap N. Four-years' experience with dynamic implants with internal port for minimally invasive sinus elevation. Quintessence Int. 2016;47(8):669–75. https://doi.org/10.3290/j.qi.a36328.
7. Bruck N, Zagury A, Nahlieli O. Minimal invasive implantology. Refuat Hapeh Vehashinayim (1993). 2015;32(3):44–51, 70.
8. Boyne PJ. Restoration of osseous defects maxillofacial causalities. J Am Dent Assoc. 1969;78:767–76.
9. Pjetursson BE, Lang NP. Elevation of the maxillary sinus floor. In: Lang NP, Lindhe J, editors. Clinical periodontology and implant dentistry. 6th ed. Oxford: Wiley-Blackwell; 2015. p. 1120–9.
10. van den Bergh J, Bruggenkate ten CM, Disch F, Tuinzing DB. Anatomical aspects of sinus floor elevations. Clin Oral Implants Res. 2000;11:256–65.
11. Kayser AF. Shortened dental arches and oral function. J Oral Rehabil. 1981;8(5):457–62.
12. Misch C. Contemporary implant dentistry. 2nd ed. St. Louis, MO: Mosby; 1999. p. 469–95.
13. Sennerby L, Roos J. Surgical determinants of clinical success of osseointegrated oral implants: a review of the literature. Int J Prosthodont. 1998;11(5):408–20.
14. Esposito M, Hirsh JM, Lekholm U, et al. Biological factors contributing to failures of osseointegrated oral implants. (II). Etiopathogenesis. Eur J Oral Sci. 1998;106(3):721–64.
15. Bryant SR. The effects of age, jaw site, and bone condition on oral implant outcomes. Int J Prosthodont. 1998;11(5):470–90.
16. Lekholm U, Zarb GA. Patient selection and preparation. In: Branemark PI, Zarb GA, Albrektsson T, editors. Tissue integrated prostheses: osseointegration in clinical dentistry. Chicago: Quintessence Publishing Company; 1985. p. 199–209.
17. Ridell A, Gröndahl K, Sennerby L. Placement of Brånemark implants in the maxillary tuber region: anatomical considerations, surgical technique and long-term results. Clin Oral Implants Res. 2009;20:94–8.
18. Smiler DG. Surgical solutions to prosthetic problems. J Dent Symp. 1993;1:44–9.
19. Jensen J, Sindet-Pedersen S. Autogenous mandibular bone grafts and osseointegrated implants for reconstruction of the severely atrophied maxilla: a preliminary report. J Oral Maxillofac Surg. 1991;49(12):1277–87.
20. Buser D, Dula K, Belser U, et al. Localized ridge augmentation using guided bone regeneration. 1. Surgical procedure in the maxilla. Int J Periodontics Restorative Dent. 1993;13(1):29–45.
21. Artzi Z. Coronal ridge augmentation in the absence of bilateral bony plates around a pathologically denuded implant surface. Int J Periodontics Restorative Dent. 2000;20(2):191–7.
22. Bahat O, Fontanessi RV. Efficacy of implant placement after bone grafting for three-dimensional reconstruction of the posterior jaw. Int J Periodontics Restorative Dent. 2001;21(3):220–31.
23. McFadden DD. Pre-prosthetic surgery options for fixed dental implant reconstruction of the atrophic maxilla. Ann R Australas Coll Dent Surg. 2000;15:61–4.
24. Tong DC, Rioux K, Dragsholt M, et al. A review of survival rates for implants placed in grafted maxillary sinuses using meta-analysis. Int J Oral Maxillofac Implants. 1998;13(2):175–82.
25. Jensen OT, Shulman LB, Block MS, et al. Report of the Sinus Consensus Conference of 1996. Int J Oral Maxillofac Implants. 1998;13(Suppl):11–45.
26. Wallace SS, Froum SJ. Effect of maxillary sinus augmentation on the survival or endosseous dental implants. A systematic review. Ann Periodontol. 2003;8(1):328–43.
27. Schwartz-Arad D, Herzberg R, Dolev E. The prevalence of surgical complications of the sinus graft procedure and their impact on implant survival. J Periodontol. 2004;75(4):511–6.
28. Tatum OH. Lecture presented to the Alabama Implant Congress. Birmingham; 1976.
29. Smiler DG, Johnson PW, Lozada JL, et al. Sinus lift grafts and endosseous implants. Treatment of the atrophic posterior maxilla. Dent Clin N Am. 1992;36(1):151–86.
30. Boyne PJ, James RA. Grafting of the maxillary sinus floor with autogenous marrow and bone. J Oral Surg. 1980;38(8):613–6.
31. Tatum H Jr. Maxillary and sinus implant reconstructions. Dent Clin N Am. 1986;30(2):207–29.
32. Summers RB. A new concept in maxillary implant surgery: the osteotome technique. Compend Contin Educ Dent. 1994;15(2):152–62.
33. Davarpanah M, Martinez H, Tecucianu JF, et al. The modified osteotome technique. Int J Periodontics Restorative Dent. 2001;21(6):599–607.
34. Zitzmann NU, Schärer P. Sinus elevation procedures in the resorbed posterior maxilla. Comparison of the crestal and lateral approaches. Oral Surg Oral Med Oral Pathol Oral Radiol Endod. 1998;85(1):8–17.
35. Coatoam GW, Krieger JT. A four-year study examining the results of indirect sinus augmentation procedures. J Oral Implantol. 1997;23(3):117–27.
36. Summers RB. The osteotome technique: part 3: less invasive methods of elevating the sinus floor. Compend Contin Educ Dent. 1994;15(6):698–704.
37. Fugazzotto PA. Augmentation of the posterior maxilla: a proposed hierarchy of treatment selection. J Periodontol. 2003;74(11):1682–91.
38. Komarnyckyj OG, London RM. Osteotome single-stage dental implant placement with and without sinus elevation: a clinical report. Int J Oral Maxillofac Implants. 1998;13(6):799–804.
39. Reiser GM, Rabinovitz Z, Bruno J, et al. Evaluation of maxillary sinus membrane response following elevation with the crestal osteotome technique in human cadavers. Int J Oral Maxillofac Implants. 2001;16(6):833–40.
40. Ahn SH, Park EJ, Kim ES. Reamer mediated sinus floor elevation without osteotome and simultaneous

implant placement in the maxillary molar area: clinical outcomes of 391 implants in 380 patients. Clin Oral Implants Res. 2012;23(7):866–72.
41. Yamada JM, Park HJ. Internal sinus manipulation (ISM) procedure a technical report. Clin Implant Dentistry Related Res. 2007;9(3):128–35.
42. Pjetursson BE, Tan WC, Zwahlen M, Lang NP. A systematic review of the success of sinus floor elevation and survival of implants inserted in combination with sinus floor elevation. J Clin Periodontol. 2008;35(8 Suppl):216–40.
43. Soltan M, Smiler DG. Antral membrane balloon elevation. J Oral Implantol. 2005;31:85–90.
44. Kfir E, Kfir V, Mijiritsky E, Rafaeloff R, Kaluski E. Minimally invasive antral membrane balloon elevation followed by maxillary bone augmentation and implant fixation. J Oral Implantol. 2006;32:26–33.
45. Chen L, Cha J. An 8-year retrospective study: 1,100 patients receiving 1,557 implants using the minimally invasive hydraulic sinus condensing technique. J Periodontol. 2005;76:482–91.
46. Suguimoto RM, Trindade IK, Carvalho RM. The use of negative pressure for the sinus lift procedure: a technical note. Int J Oral Maxillofac Implants. 2006;21:455–8.
47. Pommer B, Watzek G. Gel-pressure technique for flapless transcrestal maxillary sinus floor elevation: a preliminary cadaveric study of a new surgical technique. Int J Oral Maxillofac Implants. 2009;24:817–22.
48. Better H, Slavescu D, Barbu H, Cochran DL, Chaushu G. Minimally invasive sinus lift implant device: a multicenter safety and efficacy trial preliminary results. Clin Implant Dent Relat Res. 2014;16:520–6. https://doi.org/10.1111/cid.12021.
49. Tallarico M, Better H, De Riu G, Meloni SM. A novel implant system dedicate to hydraulic Schneiderian membrane elevation and simultaneously bone graft augmentation: an up-to 45 months retrospective clinical study. J Craniomaxillofac Surg. 2016;44(8):1089–94. https://doi.org/10.1016/j.jcms.2016.05.016.
50. Tallarico M, Meloni SM, Xhanari E, Pisano M, Cochran DL. Minimally invasive sinus augmentation procedure using a dedicated hydraulic sinus lift implant device: a prospective case series study on clinical, radiologic, and patient-centered outcomes. Int J Periodontics Restorative Dent. 2017;37(1):125–35. 10.11607/prd.2914.
51. Baumann A, Ewers R. Minimally invasive sinus lift. Limits and possibilities in the atrophic maxilla. Mund Kiefer Gesichtschir. 1999;3(Suppl 1):S70–3.
52. Nkenke E, Schlegel A, Schultze-Mosgau S, et al. The endoscopically controlled osteotome sinus floor elevation: a preliminary prospective study. Int J Oral Maxillofac Implants. 2002;17(4):557–66.
53. Engelke W, Deckwer I. Endoscopically controlled sinus floor augmentation. A preliminary report. Clin Oral Implants Res. 1997;8:527–31.
54. Srouji S, Ben-David D, Lotan R, Riminucci M, Livne E, Bianco P. The innate osteogenic potential of the maxillary sinus (Schneiderian) membrane: an ectopic tissue transplant model simulating sinus lifting. Int J Oral Maxillofac Surg. 2010;39(8):793–801.
55. Katranji A, Fotek P, Wang HL. Sinus augmentation complications: etiology and treatment. Implant Dent. 2008;17:339–49.
56. Penarrocha-Diago M, Rambla-Ferrer J, Perez V, Perez-Garrigues H. Benign paroxysmal vertigo secondary to placement of maxillary implants using the alveolar expansion technique with osteotomes: a study of 4 cases. Int J Oral Maxillofac Implants. 2008;23:129–32.
57. Di Girolamo M, Napolitano B, Arullani CA, Bruno E, Di Girolamo S. Paroxysmal positional vertigo as a complication of osteotome sinus floor elevation. Eur Arch Otorhinolaryngol. 2005;262:631–3.
58. Berengo M, Sivolella S, Majzoub Z, et al. Endoscopic evaluation of the bone-added osteotome sinus floor elevation procedure. Int J Oral Maxillofac Surg. 2004;33(2):189–94.
59. Renouard F, Nisand D. Short implants in the severely resorbed maxilla: a 2-year retrospective clinical study. Clin Implant Dent Relat Res. 2005;7(Suppl 1):s104–10.
60. Fugazzotto PA. Shorter implants in clinical practice: rationale and treatment results. Int J Oral Maxillofac Implants. 2008;23(3):487–96.
61. das Neves FD, Fones D, Bernardes SR, et al. Short implants—an analysis of longitudinal studies. Int J Oral Maxillofac Implants. 2006;21(1):86–93.
62. Beschnidt SM, Muche R, Krausse A, et al. Implant survival and success rates in partially edentulous patients—part I. Schweiz Monatsschr Zahnmed. 2003;113(4):396–403.
63. Buser D, Mericske-Stern R, Bernard JP, et al. Long-term evaluation of non-submerged ITI implants. Part 1: 8-year life table analysis of a prospective multi-center study with 2359 implants. Clin Oral Implants Res. 1997;8(3):161–72.
64. Guttenberg SA. Longitudinal report on hydroxyapatite-coated implants and advanced surgical techniques in a private practice. Compend Suppl. 1993;15:S549–53.
65. Jemt T, Lekholm U. Implant treatment in edentulous maxillae: a 5-year follow-up report on patients with different degrees of jaw resorption. Int J Oral Maxillofac Implants. 1995;10(3):303–11.
66. Aparicio C, Perales P, Rangert B. Tilted implants as an alternative to maxillary sinus grafting: a clinical, radiologic, and periotest study. Clin Implant Dent Relat Res. 2001;3(1):39–49.
67. Krekmanov L, Kahn M, Rangert B, et al. Tilting of posterior mandibular and maxillary implants for improved prosthesis support. Int J Oral Maxillofac Implants. 2000;15(3):405–14.
68. Testori T, Del Fabbro M, Capelli M, et al. Immediate occlusal loading and tilted implants for the rehabilitation of the atrophic edentulous maxilla: 1-year interim results of a multicenter prospective study. Clin Oral Implants Res. 2008;19(3):227–32.

69. Atalay B, Doğanay Ö, Saraçoğlu BK, Bultan Ö, Hafiz G. Clinical evaluation of zygomatic implant-supported fixed and removable prosthesis. J Craniofac Surg. 2016 Nov 23. [Epub ahead of print].
70. Faot F, Thomé G, Bielemann AM, Hermann C, Melo AC, Padovan LE, de Mattias Sartori IA. Simplifying the treatment of bone atrophy in the posterior regions: combination of zygomatic and wide-short implants-a case report with 2 years of follow-up. Case Rep Dent. 2016;2016:5328598.
71. Araújo RT, Sverzut AT, Trivellato AE, Sverzut CE. Retrospective analysis of 129 consecutive zygomatic implants used to rehabilitate severely resorbed maxillae in a two-stage protocol. Int J Oral Maxillofac Implants. 2017;32(2):377–84. 10.11607/jomi.5136.
72. Curi MM, Cardoso CL, Ribeiro Kde C. Retrospective study of pterygoid implants in the atrophic posterior maxilla: implant and prosthesis survival rates up to 3 years. Int J Oral Maxillofac Implants. 2015;30(2):378–83. 10.11607/jomi.3665.
73. Jokstad A, Sanz M, Ogawa T, Bassi F, Levin L, Wennerberg A, Romanos GE. A systematic review of the role of implant design in the rehabilitation of the edentulous maxilla. Int J Oral Maxillofac Implants. 2016;31(Suppl):s43–99. 10.11607/jomi.16suppl.g2.
74. Rodríguez X, Lucas-Taulé E, Elnayef B, et al. Anatomical and radiological approach to pterygoid implants: a cross-sectional study of 202 cone beam computed tomography examinations. Int J Oral Maxillofac Surg. 2016;45(5):636–40. https://doi.org/10.1016/j.ijom.2015.12.009.
75. Penarrocha M, Carrillo C, Boronat A, Peñarrocha M. Retrospective study of 68 implants placed in the pterygomaxillary region using drills and osteotomes. Int J Oral Maxillofac Implants. 2009;24:720–6.

11 Tissue Engineering as a Minimally Invasive Method

Sara A. Hinds and Stephen E. Feinberg

Abstract

As the field of tissue engineering enters a phase of clinical translation, there is a need to consider the surgical principles for transplantation of engineered biologic organs and tissues, which have traditionally been constructed with harvested cells seed on scaffolds and cultured in laboratory bioreactors. The methods of minimally invasive surgery should be an important component of clinical translation of tissue engineering techniques, which have been verified in vitro. This chapter will serve to illustrate how in situ tissue engineering can be used to harness the body's ability to regenerate through the process of cell homing, an innate self-healing mechanism to recruit stem cells to injured or diseased tissues. By employing the body as a bioreactor, this technique of tissue engineering can be considered a minimally invasive method.

11.1 Introduction

Tissue engineering evolved from the field of biomaterials and refers to the practice of combining scaffolds, cells, and biologically active molecules to create tissue equivalents. The goal of tissue engineering (TE) is to assemble biologic constructs that restore function and dimension to damaged native tissues. Regenerative medicine (RM) is a broader field that encompasses tissue engineering but also incorporates research on self-healing, which describes the body's ability to use intrinsic cellular processes, sometimes with help from foreign biological material, to rebuild tissues and organs. The aim of minimally invasive (MI) surgery is to reduce iatrogenic trauma to the body. Traditionally preformed with small surgical incisions, MI surgery employs thin needles and an endoscope to visually guide the surgery. The advantages of minimally invasive surgery are reduced perioperative blood loss and postoperative pain, decreased recovery time and minimal scarring.

S.A. Hinds, MS, DDS • S.E. Feinberg, DDS, MS, PhD (✉)
Department of Oral and Maxillofacial Surgery, University of Michigan, Ann Arbor, MI, USA
e-mail: hindss@med.umich.edu ; sefein@umich.edu

O. Nahlieli (ed.), *Minimally Invasive Oral and Maxillofacial Surgery*,
http://doi.org/10.1007/978-3-662-54592-8_11

The authors propose that there is significant potential for tissue engineering and regenerative medicine (TE/RM) to augment the armamentarium of minimally invasive therapy. TE/RM has the potential to reduce the significant morbidity associated with tissue harvesting in surgeries that require a tissue donor (i.e., organ transplantation) or donor site (i.e., autologous grafting or microvascular free flaps). Advances in the field of TE/RM will usher in a new era of less invasive microtransplantation. The classical techniques and instruments of MI surgery will require modification and adaptation to the microsurgical scale. New methods and technologies will have to be developed requiring collaboration between scientists and clinicians from the disciplines of both TE/RM and MI [1].

In this chapter, we will briefly review the state of the art for TE/RM as it applies to minimally invasive surgery. It is important to note that these techniques are rapidly evolving with frequent modifications and improvements.

11.2 The Concept of Cell Homing and Endogenous Tissue Engineering

Homing is the process by which cells migrate to and engraft in a tissue matrix, where they can exert local, functional, and reparative effects. Cell homing is an innate self-healing mechanism that can be employed by tissue engineering techniques to recruit stem cells to injured or diseased tissues and direct their migration to specific target niches following mobilization [2]. The classical tissue engineering strategy involves cell isolation from tissue biopsy followed by the seeding of culture-expanded cells on scaffolds that mature and differentiate in bioreactors (Fig. 11.1a). The end product of this technique, a functional bioengineered tissue construct, would then be transplanted in vivo. Although this approach has been validated, it involves extensive cell expansion and tissue culture steps, requiring a large amount of time and laborious effort before implantation. To bypass this ex vivo process, a new approach has been introduced [3]. In situ tissue regeneration utilizes cell homing and the body's own regenerating capacity by mobilizing host endogenous stem cells or tissue-specific progenitor cells to the site of injury (Fig. 11.1b). This approach relies on development of a target-specific biomaterial scaffolding system that can effectively control the host microenvironment and mobilize the appropriate cells [2, 3].

Prospective progenitor cells can be targeted from either a hematologic or interstitial cell population. Cells homed from a distant or disseminated hematologic source must first be mobilized intravascular and arrive at the desired location where they interact with the endothelial cells at the target site. A coordinated multistep extravasation occurs involving cell rolling, adhesion, transepithelial migration, invasion, and chemotaxis (Fig. 11.2a). Similarly, interstitial stem cells can migrate to the target site via extravascular guidance cues. This process is distinct in that it requires amoeboid movements and is seen independent of blood flow (Fig. 11.2b). Regulation of cell homing is complex and involves chemokines, cytokines, adhesion molecules, and proteases expressed in spatial and temporal gradients. Importantly, once the cells have arrived at the target location the cells must proliferate to amplify the population prior to differentiation. This is especially true for elderly or diseased patients with depleted or inactive stem cell populations.

The delivery of biological cues has been the subject of extensive research that demonstrates the ability for molecular factors to be encapsulated in biocompatible microparticles such as injectables or loaded into preformed matrices with tissue-specific architecture depending on the regenerative requirements of various tissues [4]. These products can be prepackaged and made available in a medical or dental office at the time of clinical need. The use of these products may eliminate the need for autologous tissue grafting, which is concordant with the goal of cell homing as a minimally invasive TE therapy by reducing surgical trauma while yielding long lasting esthetic and functional outcomes.

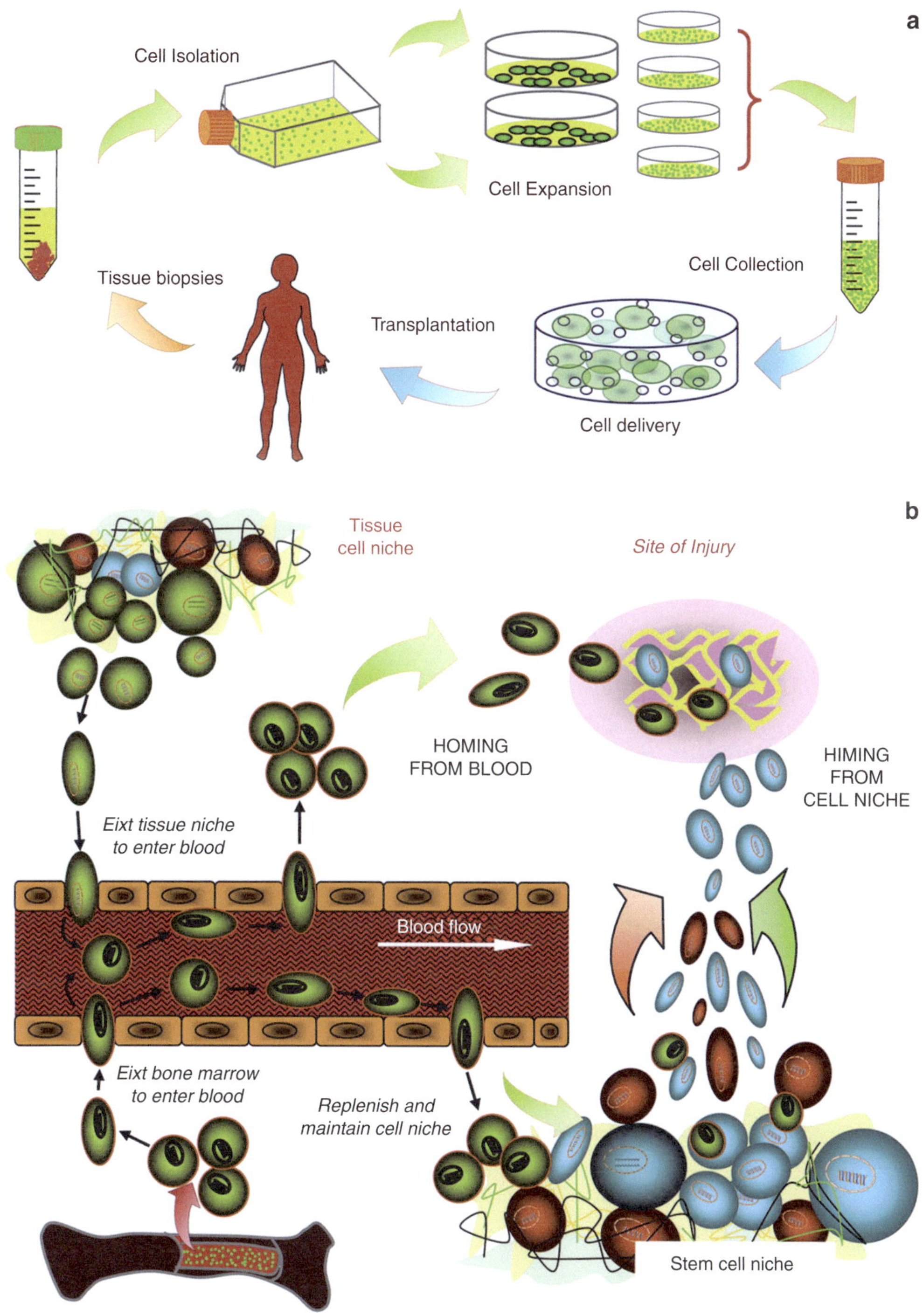

Fig. 11.1 Tissue engineering strategy schematic demonstrating the difference between the classic approach (**a**) involving tissue biopsy, ex vivo cell isolation and expansion followed by cell collection, and transplantation compared with the self-healing/cell homing approach (**b**) whereby host stem cells are recruited from the blood or tissue cell niches and then migrate to and engraft in a tissue matrix at the sight of injury. Cost and complexity are lower for the cell homing method, which holds great promise for minimally invasive techniques in tissue engineering. (Reproduced with permission from Chen et al. [2])

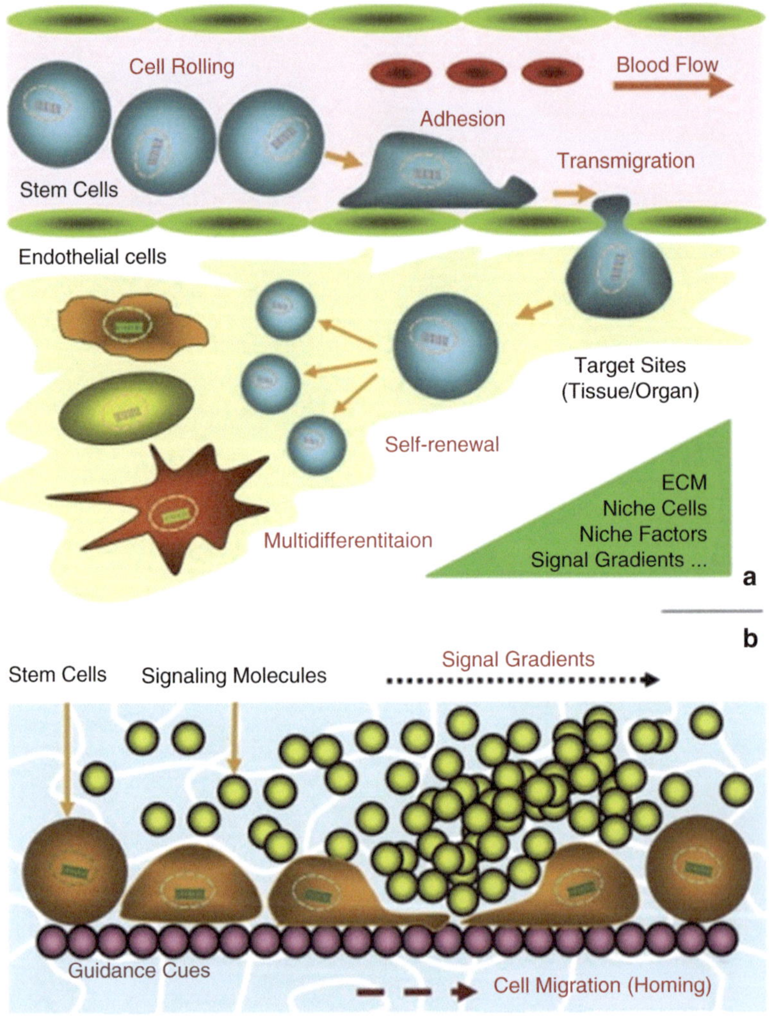

Fig. 11.2 Cell homing techniques for tissue engineering can target either hematologic or interstitial stem cell populations. (**a**) Hematologic stem cells disseminated throughout the body are recruited to the site of tissue injury by interactions with the endothelial cells and a coordinated process of cell rolling, adhesion, and transmigration. The stem cells then undergo self-renewal and differentiation depending upon interactions with ECM and growth factors. (**b**) Cell homing of interstitial cells involves guidance cues expressed in a signal gradient. (Reproduced with permission from Chen et al. [2])

11.3 Current Applications of Therapeutic Tissue Regeneration by Endogenous Stem Cell Homing

11.3.1 Periodontal Regeneration

Periodontitis is a highly prevalent chronic inflammatory condition that causes the progressive destruction of periodontal tissues often resulting in tooth loss. The significant burden of this disease has inspired research efforts to regenerate lost periodontium, namely the periodontal ligament, alveolar bone, and root cementum. These techniques have had varying results owing to the complexity of rebuilding three distinct tissue layers in the setting of localized infection and inflammation. Clinically, the standard of care for periodontal disease includes open flap debridement, after which epithelial cells migrate to and "repair" the periodontal defect by creating a fibro-epithelial attachment. Due to the rapid migration of epithelial cells, other tissue-specific progenitor cells are not able to reach the defect in time, thereby precluding orderly regeneration of the hybrid periodontium. Membranes have been utilized with some success to serve as a physical barrier to the swift ingrowth of epithelial cells and theoretically afford time for nearby undifferentiated progenitor cells to migrate to the defect. Termed guided tissue regeneration, this technique is often used in combination with particulate bone grafting and localized large bolus delivery of tissue growth factors such as bone morphogenetic protein (BMP).

Current research efforts, which go a step farther than traditional guided tissue regeneration of utilizing a physical barrier or membrane to exclude non-osteoprogenitor cells, are aimed to harness the self-healing potential of the hosts periodontal ligament (PDL) with tools such as patient-derived growth factors and biopolymer scaffolds in combination with commercially available products including Emdogain® and Bio-Oss®. TE/RM of the periodontal tissue must successfully recruit progenitor stem cells to a biomimetic material niche with appropriate levels and sequencing of regulatory signals (Fig. 11.3). This is in contrast to the single large bolus delivery of a growth factor such as BMP.

Candidates for biomaterials, which have been reviewed extensively elsewhere, include platelet-rich plasma (PRP) suspended in a fibrin matrix both derived from autologous blood [5]–[7]. PRP is centrifuged blood plasma that contains a high concentration of platelets and growth factors released from alpha granules. PRP in combination with bone grafts has demonstrated significant clinical success in bone reconstruction of mandibular defects with a radiographic maturation rate 1.62–2.16 times the control bone grafts [6]. Homologous fibrin sealants have been used in surgery for hemostasis and wound sealing for many years and recently autologous fibrin sealants have become commercially available with devices such as CryoSeals® and Vivostats® systems. It is important to note that autologous biologic products often have high batch variability and as such clinical studies may have variable and sometimes with inconclusive results. Future

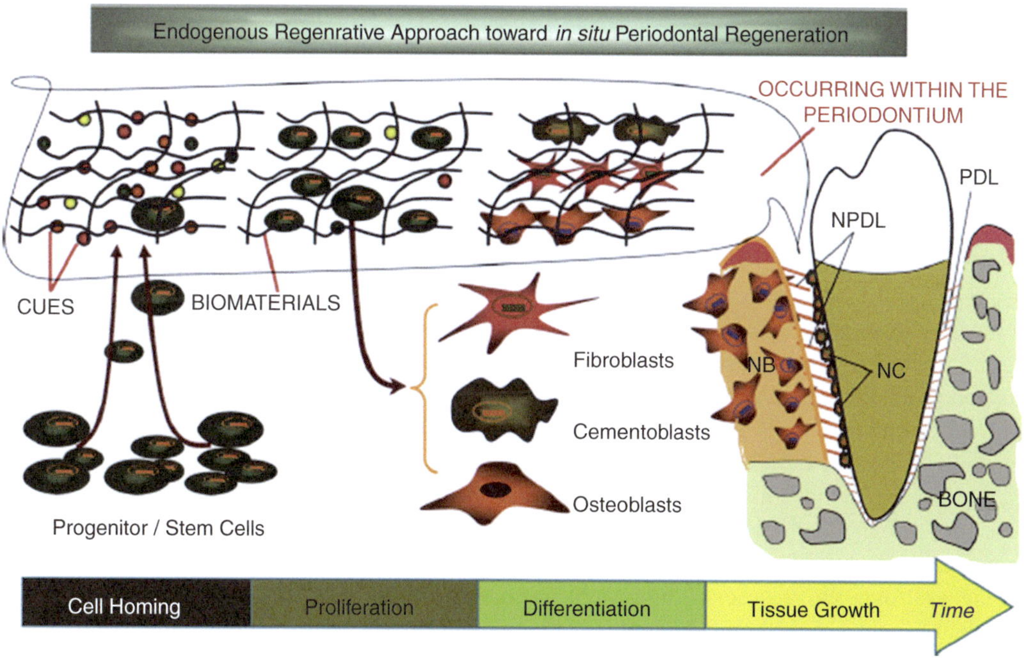

Fig. 11.3 Schematic representation of the application of cell homing for in situ periodontal regeneration. Bioactive cues can be incorporated into biomaterial tissue matrix implanted in the periodontal matrix. Stem cells are recruited to this matrix where they proliferate and differentiate into fibroblasts cementoblasts and osteoblasts. The hybrid periodontium including alveolar bone, periodontal ligament, and cementum is regenerated. (*NB* new bone, *NPDL* new periodontal ligament, *PDL* periodontal ligament, NC new cementum). (Reproduced with permission from Chen et al. [5])

studies should aim to standardize harvesting, concentration, and delivery techniques.

In addition to PRP and fibrin, Emdogain® can be incorporated into the tissue niche to promote formation of root cementum, a critical component of functional periodontal tissue. Emdogain® is an enamel matrix derivative that contains enamel matrix proteins that play a key role in the development of tooth supporting tissues during embryogenesis. Overall, endogenous regenerative therapy is a promising clinical tool that utilizes commercially available products and minimally invasive surgically intervention to regenerate periodontal tissue resulting in clinically significant reduction in pocket probing depths and restoration of tooth stability [5].

11.3.2 Musculoskeletal Tissue Regeneration

Musculoskeletal (MSK) defects can occur as a consequence of trauma, surgical ablation, congenital syndromes, or degenerative disease. There is an innate ability for muscle and bone to regenerate, these cellular processes cannot be utilized in critical-size defects, and tissue engineering is required for functional and structural restoration of MSK systems. Bone marrow hematopoietic cells, vascular pericytes, and muscle-specific stem cells (i.e., satellite cells) are a ready source of stem cells that can be used for muscle, bone, and cartilage regeneration. By homing these cells to biomimetic matrices, endogenous tissue engineering of MSK tissue can take advantage of the bodies replenishing stem cell population and uses the body as an in situ bioreactor creating a microenvironment and utilizing the existing blood supply for tissue regeneration. Because the MSK system is load-bearing scaffolds are a crucial component to regeneration and should serve as both a biochemical and biophysical signaling construct. Angiogenesis is an important component for MSK regeneration particularly for highly metabolic tissues like muscle. Furthermore, muscle requires that motor unit innervation for functionality and tissue maintenance. Therefore, ERT for MSK tissue requires physical, biochemical, and electrical integration into the host system [8].

11.3.3 Treatment of Cardiovascular Diseases

Valvular heart disease, characterized by damage to one of the four heart valves, can have significant morbidity when severe and associated with congestive heart disease. Valve replacement surgery is often performed with minimally invasive transvascular, catheter-based implantation of biosynthetic valves. These biosynthetic valves are often plagued with calcification and progressive dysfunction. Schmidt and others demonstrated the feasibility of combining the novel heart valve replacement technologies of: (1) tissue engineering and (2) minimally invasive implantation based on autologous cells and composite self-expandable biodegradable biomaterials [9]. Trileaflet heart valves were fabricated from biodegradable synthetic scaffolds, integrated in self-expanding stents, and seeded with autologous vascular or stem cells (bone marrow and peripheral blood) that were generated in vitro using dynamic bioreactors (Fig. 11.4a). The tissue-engineered heart valves (TEHV) were minimally invasively implanted as pulmonary valve replacements in sheep (Fig. 11.4b). They assessed in vivo functionality using echocardiography and angiography up to 8 weeks. The transapical implantations were successful in all animals. The TEHV demonstrated in vivo functionality with mobile but thickened leaflets. Histology revealed layered neotissues with endothelialized surfaces. Quantitative extracellular matrix analysis at 8 weeks showed higher values for deoxyribonucleic acid, collagen, and glycosaminoglycans compared to native valves. Mechanical profiles demonstrated sufficient tissue strength, but less pliability independent of the cell source. The study demonstrated the principal feasibility of merging tissue engineering and minimally invasive valve replacement technologies and may enable a valid alternative to current bioprosthetic devices [9].

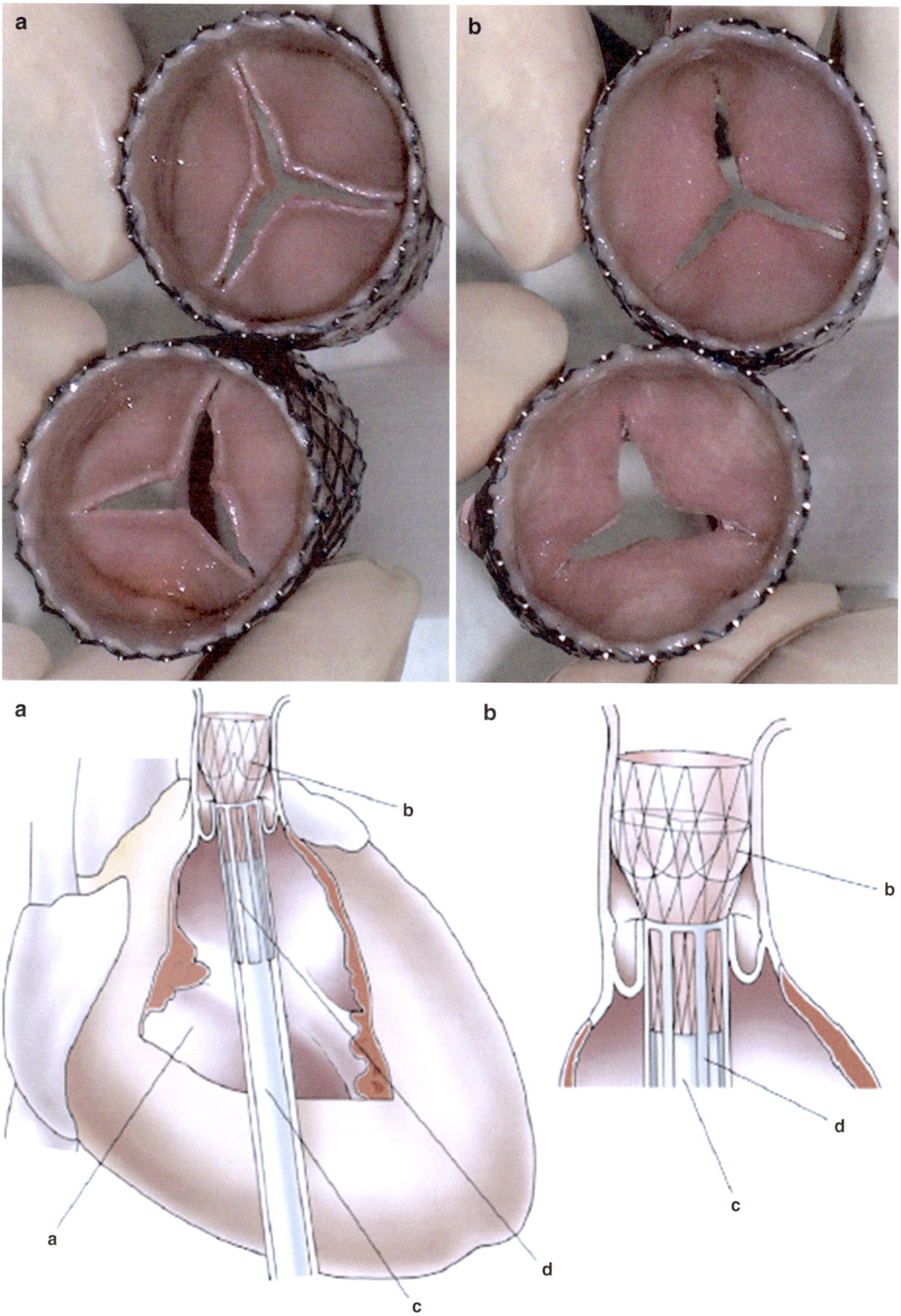

Fig. 11.4 Minimally invasive technique for delivery of Tissue Engineered Heart Valve (TEHV). Macroscopic appearance of TEHV composed of vascular-derived stem cells on a self-expanding nitinol stent prior to implantation, (**a**) Distal view and (**b**) Proximal view. (**c**) Schematic representation of transapical valve delivery. (Reproduced with permission from Schmidt et al. [9])

Similarly, chronic venous insufficiency due to the incompetence of peripheral venous valves can cause significant morbidity associated with venous reflux and distal venous hypertension. A study by Weber et al. showed in vitro study success in combining two evolving technologies, i.e., cardiovascular in vitro tissue engineering and minimally invasive valve replacement techniques. Their data showed that the in vitro fabrication of miniaturized living tissue-engineered venous valves (TEVV) based on autologous (mesenchymal) stem cells on a fully biodegradable (composite) polymer scaffolds integrated into nitinol stent systems is feasible in the ovine model and lays the foundation for an animal in vivo trial in the near future [10]. This encouraging study will need to assess leaflet functionality as well as the in situ remodeling of the TEVV constructs in order to bring this technology closer to a possible future clinical translation. These constructs hold the potential to overcome the limitations of currently used non-autologous replacement materials and may open new therapeutic concepts for the treatment of cardiovascular defects with implantation materials in the future [10].

11.4 Cell Homing Devices and In Vitro Design

11.4.1 Bioscaffolds for Cell Homing

In addition to cell homing, the success of in situ TE/RM is largely dependent on information-rich, biomimetic scaffolds with good mechanical properties that can be adapted to individual organ system without harmful effects. Unlike current filler injections and graft implants, bioscaffolds are cell homing devices with biochemical and biophysical cues that facilitate cell penetration, proliferation, and differentiation [2]. There are myriad biomaterials with potential application in this field that have been reviewed extensively elsewhere [4]. The properties of these biomaterials can be manipulated to regulate the degradation, mechanical strength, and porosity of the scaffolds. By manipulating these properties, the scaffolds can be customized based on the needs of the tissue or organ being regenerated, for example, bone regeneration of large MSK defects requires a bioscaffold that can withstand large mechanical forces. The three-dimensional architecture of scaffolds can be designed with computer-aided design to mimic natural tissue structure and thereby facilitate complex tissue reconstruction. In addition, the design of a composite matrix with various biomaterials may be necessitated for the regeneration of compound tissue defects such as a full thickness avulsion injuring of the mandible involving mucosa, bone, muscle, and skin.

11.4.2 Navigation Cues and Niche Signals

In native tissue, the interaction of soluble factors and the extracellular matrix (ECM) defines the cellular niche and directly impacts stem cell activity. The mechanical and molecular information coded in novel biomaterials must be designed to deliver signals in a precise spatiotemporal and near-physiological fashion to instruct the fate of stem cells homed to the tissue defect. To this end, biomimetic scaffolds should provide structural signals and serve as a reservoir for cell signaling motifs and sequestered growth factors that guide adhesion, amplification, and differentiation [2]. In vascular research, for example, the presence of endothelium-derived macromolecules or their cell interacting domains onto vascular grafts can mimic features of the ECM and thereby assist specific cell adhesion and promote endothelialization [11].

11.4.3 Release Technology

The time-dependent nature of cell signaling and the relatively short half-lives of cell homing factors limit the effectiveness of localized bolus delivery. Release technology is frequently adopted to overcome the short half-life and rabid diffusion of free growth factors in solution (Fig. 11.5). An effective artificial ECM requires a

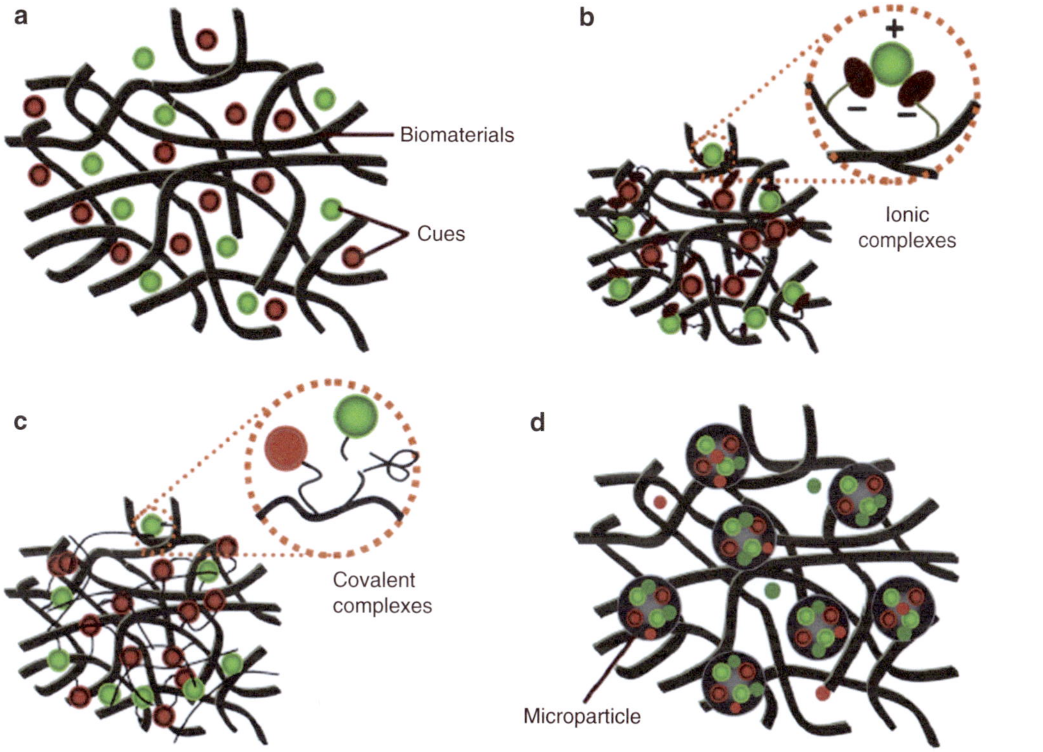

Fig. 11.5 Common methods for controlled delivery of bioactive cues incorporated into biomaterial matrix. Schematic representation of: (**a**) direct loading (**b**) non-covalent immobilization, (**c**) covalent immobilization, and (**d**) encapsulation of cues. Depending on the tissue-specific application, these techniques can be utilized to delivery factors in a tailored spatiotemporal pattern. (Reproduced with permission from Chen et al. [2])

release technology that controls the spatiotemporal delivery of key signaling molecules, prevents unwanted and potentially harmful side effects, and delivers a myriad of protein factors, including homing inducers for tissue regeneration.

The combined use of multiple factors delivered in bioscaffolds may have additive and possibly synergistic effects, offering a strategic advantage over the approach involving the use of a single factor. In addition, the process of regeneration may require several weeks or months for sufficient tissue growth into a defect; therefore, delivery methods must ensure that cues reach the injury site for a prolonged period. Particulate-based protein delivery and gene delivery allow spatiotemporal control of factor release, which may ultimately facilitate the clinical translation of chemotaxis-induced cell homing. For example, microspheres fabricated by a variety of natural and/or synthetic polymers can release proteins from aqueous pockets within the particles and can now be generated to nanoscale dimensions using a single surfactant.

11.5 Novel Biomaterials

11.5.1 Modified Hydrogels

Hydrogels are naturally occurring hydrophilic polymeric networks that can be engineered to have a range of favorable physical and chemical properties for application in TE/RM. Hydrogels can be formulated as injectables and are favorable bioscaffolds for minimally invasive surgery due to their unique characteristics including the ability to fill tissue cavities of any shape and size, quick gelation, and high water content [12]. Monomeric solutions can either be injected devoid of cells to serve exclusively as a cell homing device or they can be pre-seeded with a variety of cells that will be entrapped in the matrix with uniform distribution once they monomers polymerize. Once the polymeric matrix is established, hydrogels are able to maintain their shape and structure in aqueous solution owing to the cross-linking between polymer chains [13]. The hydrogel scaffold can facilitate cellular migration and influence cellular behavior via cell–matrix interactions while also serving as a drug or growth factor reservoir. The following two novel applications of hydrogels highlight their potential and versatility in the field of TE/RM.

Recently, Zeng et al. reported the development and characterization of injectable three-dimensional (3D) microscale cellular niches composed of mesenchymal stromal cells (MSCs), alginate and macroporous poly (ethylene glycol) diacrylate (PEGDA), and PEGDA-derived microcryogels (PMs) for cell delivery [14]. This particular hydrogel formulation was designed to alleviate intervertebral disc degeneration (IVDD). Highly elastic PMs were applied as mechanical skeleton to reinforce alginate encapsulation of MSCs and enable preformed alginate hydrogel to be injectable. This novel method represented a minimally invasive and leak-proof delivery strategy, which prevented cell leakage from the highly pressurized disc. Improved cell retention and survival were achieved with PMs reinforced alginate hydrogel in an ex vivo organ culture model. Injection of such 3D microniches alleviated nucleus pulposus (NP) degeneration in a canine IVDD model. In was concluded that the injectable PMs reinforced alginate hydrogel offered a valuable strategy for MSCs delivery and therapy for restoring intervertebral disc function. This approach should find wide applications to assist other non-injectable hydrogels for cell encapsulation and improved therapy in regenerative medicine [14].

Hydrogels have also been proposed as bioscaffolds for application in cardiac tissue engineering. Williams et al. developed a cardiac extracellular matrix (ECM)–fibrin hybrid scaffold that had tunable composition and elastic moduli to mimic properties of the developing and mature myocardium. ECM of various developmental ages can be used and stiffness controlled by cross-linking via transglutaminase (TG) with minimal effect on cell viability [15]. The ECM–fibrin hybrid solutions were easily injectable through a 25G needle and formed gels in situ. Although the study focused on cardiac ECM, the scaffold has potential to be adapted to a variety of other organs. Injectable ECM-based scaffolds with tunable properties that can direct progenitor cell fate and behavior can enhance future tissue engineering and regenerative medicine strategies.

11.5.2 Shape Memory

The surgical delivery of biomaterials with predefined geometries should be consistent with the principles of minimally invasive surgery to minimize surgical trauma. As such, it is desirable that these materials have shape memory so that they can be compressed into catheters and inserted with small surgical incisions regardless of the scale of the defect. Thornton et al. prepared a number of predefined geometric scaffolds with macroporous alginate hydrogel and introduced them into immunocompromised mice by means of minimally invasive surgical delivery through a small catheter [16]. Scaffolds were rehydrated in situ with a suspension of cells (primary bovine articular chondrocytes) or cell-free medium delivered through the same catheter. Specimens were harvested at 1 h to evaluate the efficacy of cell delivery and the recovery of scaffold geometry at 8 and 24weeks to evaluate neo-tissue formation. A high percentage (88%) of scaffolds that were introduced with a catheter and rehydrated with cells had recovered their original shape and size within 1 h. These delivery procedures resulted in cartilage structures with the geometry of the original scaffold by 2 months and histologically mature appearing tissue at 6 months. The study showed that hydrogels with three-dimensional predefined shapes, formed by covalently cross-linking, can be temporarily collapsed when delivered and regain their shape at a later date illustrating another MI technique.

11.5.3 Extracellular Matrix Derivatives

The extracellular matrix (ECM) is a tissue-specific meshwork of both structural and functional proteins assembled through a process of dynamic reciprocity whereby cells both receive signals from the ECM and contribute to its content and organization. This process is critical to tissue development and homeostasis. Based upon these important functions, ECM-based materials have been used in a wide variety of TE/RM approaches to tissue reconstruction. It has been demonstrated that ECM-based materials, when appropriately prepared, can act as inductive templates for constructive remodeling.

An example of ECM derivatives used for induction of de novo functional, site-appropriate, tissue formation was shown by Badylak and others in the use of a scaffold material composed of porcine-derived ECM configured to mimic the shape and size of the temporomandibular joint (TMJ) [17]. This device was implanted in a canine model of bilateral TMJ discectomy. The results showed that implantation of an initially acellular material supported the formation of site-appropriate, functional host tissue that resembled that of the native TMJ disc. Furthermore, this prevented gross degenerative changes in the temporal fossa and mandibular condyle. The contralateral controls showed no tissue formation and had mild to severe gross pathologic changes of the osseous structures of the joint [17, 18].

11.6 Endoscopic and Arthroscopic Techniques for Cell Delivery in TE/RM

The clinical translation of tissue engineering to minimally invasive therapies is contingent upon the development of novel noninvasive endoscopic and arthroscopic techniques. Bioscaffolds can be delivered on their own as pure cell homing devices, or they can be pre-seeded with cells that can assist in the regenerative process. Cell delivery is particularly important in patient populations where stem cell populations are inactive or relatively depleted such as the elderly or diseased.

The detection, isolation, and sorting of cells hold an important role in cell therapy and regenerative medicine. Custodio et al. developed monoclonal antibodies against cell surface antigens specific to endothelial cells and stem cells that were immobilized on the surface of the microparticles [24]. They demonstrated the ability of biofunctionalized particles to select specific cell types from mixed cell populations and to promote cell expansion, by using human adipose stem cells (hASCs) and human umbilical vein endothelial cells (HUVECs) as examples. The versatility of this method allows the combination of the biotin conjugated microparticles with any biotinylated molecule as antibodies, growth factors, or peptides of interest. They showed that biodegradable and biocompatible particles functionalized with antibodies presented selective affinity to cells, making them potentially suitable for separating subpopulations of cells from complex mixtures. Besides the ability for cell separation, the cultured particles proved to be also suitable for cell expansion. They were able to develop an in vitro versatile, cost-effective, and easy-to-operate system with the capability to simultaneously separate and expand different cells subsets. The aggregation of the functionalized microparticles was shown to successfully form 3D robust structures upon injection into a mold. Thus, the developed microparticles demonstrated they might be potentially useful for further studies accomplishing the formation of a construct in situ upon implantation using minimally invasive procedures.

The minimally invasive delivery of bioscaffolds and cells to a variety of tissue-specific defect poses will need to be addressed prior to clinical translation. An example of such an approach is the study by Subhan et al. where they developed a technique for minimally invasive and accurate delivery of MSCs in a hydrogel to augment the nucleus pulposus (NP) in damaged intervertebral discs (IVD) [19]. Their results demonstrated that the minimally invasive administration of MSCs in hyaluronan hydrogel

(HyStem) can successfully augment the repair of NP in damaged IVD. Ibarra et al. were able to arthroscopically implant autologous matrix-encapsulated chondrocytes in a bioabsorbable scaffold into the knee for cell-based cartilage repair. They demonstrated efficacious and reproducible results with a mean of 36 months of follow-up [20]. Leggett and others were able to utilize gastrointestinal endoscopy to transplant autologous epidermal cell sheets or seeded decellularized biological scaffolds to repair strictures resulting from endoscopic submucosal resection and circumferential endoscopic mucosal resection. This technique can also be used to augment the lower esophageal sphincter with the injection of muscle-derived cells for a novel potential treatment for gastroesophageal reflux disease [21].

11.7 Transplantation of Organ Germs: Salivary Glands

Regenerative tissue engineering techniques have often drawn inspiration from embryology to understand and recapitulate the steps involved in organogenesis. Most organs develop embryologically with reciprocal interactions from at least two distinct cell layers collectively known as organ germs. Therefore, there has been an attempt to bioengineer organ germs for transplantation that will differentiate and form end organ structures in vivo [22]. Although this technique, pioneered by Takashi Tsuji's group in Japan, requires cell harvesting, the transplantation of organ germs would have minimal surgical morbidity and therefore may be considered minimally invasive as compared with whole organ transplantation [22].

One potential application for the bioengineered organ germ method is the formation of salivary glands. Hyposalivation or xerostomia, frequently associated with a history of head and neck radiation or autoimmune dysregulation, can have significant clinical sequela including tooth decay, impaired mastication, swallowing dysfunction, and often decreased quality of life. Current treatment options for xerostomia are often palliative and insufficient; therefore, the development of a engineered salivary gland that responds to gustatory stimulation would have significant clinical impact. Embryologically salivary glands develop with reciprocal epithelial and mesenchymal cell interactions resulting in duct and acina formations, which are the functional unit of salivary glands. Ogawa et al. demonstrated that a bioengineered salivary gland tissue germ fabricated with isolated epithelial and mesenchymal cells from mouse submandibular glands connected with a polygycolic acid monofilament thread guide could be successfully engrafted in a murine model of salivary gland defect [23]. The resultant tissue showed morphologic gland formation and functional amylase positive saliva secretion. This proof of concept study demonstrates the utility of bioengineered organ germ development for important clinical problems including xerostomia.

Conclusions

In situ tissue engineering is a minimally invasive method for the surgical correction of tissue defects or physiologic disease. The examples discussed in this chapter illustrate that the implantation of biomaterials with biologic cues can be used to harness the body's regenerative capacity through a process of cell homing of host stem cells from both vascular and interstitial sources.

References

1. Schurr MO. Minimally invasive therapy and tissue engineering. Minim Invasive Ther Allied Technol. 2002;11(3):83.
2. Chen FM, Wu LA, Zhang M, Zhang R, Sun HH. Homing of endogenous stem/progenitor cells for in situ tissue regeneration: promises, strategies, and translational perspectives. Biomaterials. 2011;32(12):3189–209.
3. Ko IK, Lee SJ, Atala A, Yoo JJ. In situ tissue regeneration through host stem cell recruitment. Exp Mol Med. 2013;45:e57.
4. Rice JJ, Martino MM, De Laporte L, Tortelli F, Briquez PS, Hubbell JA. Engineering the regenerative microenvironment with biomaterials. Adv Healthc Mater. 2013;2:57–71.

5. Chen FM, Zhang J, Zhang M, An Y, Chen F, Wu ZF. A review on endogenous regenerative technology in periodontal regenerative medicine. Biomaterials. 2010;31:7892–927.
6. Marx RE, Carlson ER, Eichstaedt RM, Schimmele SR, Strauss JE, Georgeff KR. Platelet-rich plasma. Growth factor enhancement for bone grafts. Oral Surg Oral Med Oral Pathol Oral Radiol Endod. 1998;85: 638–46.
7. Kjaergard HK, Trumbull HR. Vivostat system autologous fibrin sealant: preliminary study in elective coronary bypass grafting. Ann Thorac Surg. 1998;66:482–6.
8. Adam C. Endogenous musculoskeletal tissue engineering--a focused perspective. Cell Tissue Res. 2012;347:489–99.
9. Schmidt D, Dijkman PE, Driessen-Mo A, et al. Minimally-invasive implantation of living tissue engineered heart valves: a comprehensive approach from autologous vascular cells to stem cells. J Am Coll Cardiol. 2010;56:510–20.
10. Weber B, Robert J, Ksiazek A, et al. Living-engineered valves for transcatheter venous valve repair. Tissue Eng Part C Methods. 2014;20:451–63.
11. Lutolf MP, Hubbell JA. Synthetic biomaterials as instructive extracellular microenvironments for morphogenesis in tissue engineering. Nat Biotechnol. 2005;23:47–55.
12. Qi C, Yan X, Huang C, Melerzanov A, Du Y. Biomaterials as carrier, barrier and reactor for cell-based regenerative medicine. Protein Cell. 2015;6:638–53.
13. Ahmed EM. Hydrogel: preparation, characterization, and applications: a review. J Adv Res. 2015;6(2):105–21.
14. Zeng Y, Chen C, Liu W, et al. Injectable microcryogels reinforced alginate encapsulation of mesenchymal stromal cells for leak-proof delivery and alleviation of canine disc degeneration. Biomaterials. 2015;59:53–65.
15. Williams C, Budina E, Stoppel WL, et al. Cardiac extracellular matrix-fibrin hybrid scaffolds with tunable properties for cardiovascular tissue engineering. Acta Biomater. 2015;14:84–95.
16. Thornton AJ, Alsberg E, Albertelli M, Mooney DJ. Shape-defining scaffolds for minimally invasive tissue engineering. Transplantation. 2004;77: 1798–803.
17. Brown BN, Chung WL, Pavlick M, et al. Extracellular matrix as an inductive template for temporomandibular joint meniscus reconstruction: a pilot study. J Oral Maxillofac Surg. 2011;69:e488–505.
18. Brown BN, Chung WL, Almarza AJ, et al. Inductive, scaffold-based, regenerative medicine approach to reconstruction of the temporomandibular joint disk. J Oral Maxillofac Surg. 2012;70(11):2656–68.
19. Subhan RA, Puvanan K, Murali MR, et al. Fluoroscopy assisted minimally invasive transplantation of allogenic mesenchymal stromal cells embedded in HyStem reduces the progression of nucleus pulposus degeneration in the damaged Interverbal disc: a preliminary study in rabbits. Sci World J. 2014;2014:e818502.
20. Ibarra C, Izaguirre A, Villalobos E, et al. Follow-up of a new arthroscopic technique for implantation of matrix-encapsulated autologous chondrocytes in the knee. Arthrosc J Arthrosc Relat Surg. 2014;30: 715–23.
21. Leggett CL, Gorospe EC, Lutzke L, Anderson M, Wang KK. A new era: endoscopic tissue transplantation. Curr Opin Gastroenterol. 2013;29(5): 495–500.
22. Nakao K, Morita R, Saji Y, Ishida K, Tomita Y, Ogawa M, Saitoh M, Tomooka Y, Tsuji T. The development of a bioengineered organ germ method. Nat Methods. 2007;4(3):227–30.
23. Ogawa M, Oshima M, Imamura A, et al. Functional salivary gland regeneration by transplantation of a bioengineered organ germ. Nat Commun. 2013;4:2498. https://doi.org/10.1038/ncomms3498.
24. Custodio CA, Cerqueira MT, Marques AP, Reis RL, Mano JF. Cell selective chitosan microparticles as injectable cell carriers for tissue regeneration. Biomaterials. 2015;43:23–31

Index

O. Nahlieli (ed.), *Minimally Invasive Oral and Maxillofacial Surgery*,
https://doi.org/10.1007/978-3-662-54592-8

MIX
Papier aus verantwortungsvollen Quellen
Paper from responsible sources
FSC® C105338

If you have any concerns about our products,
you can contact us on
ProductSafety@springernature.com

In case Publisher is established outside the EU,
the EU authorized representative is:
Springer Nature Customer Service Center GmbH
Europaplatz 3, 69115 Heidelberg, Germany

Printed by Libri Plureos GmbH
in Hamburg, Germany